X-RAY IMAGING EQUIPMENT

X-RAY IMAGING EQUIPMENT

AN INTRODUCTION

By

EUCLID SEERAM, R.T., B.Sc.

British Columbia Institute of Technology
Burnaby, British Columbia
Canada

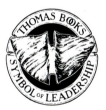

CHARLES C THOMAS • PUBLISHER
Springfield · Illinois · U.S.A.

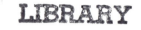
Published and Distributed Throughout the World by

CHARLES C THOMAS • PUBLISHER

2600 South First Street

Springfield, Illinois 62717

With THOMAS BOOKS *careful attention is given to all details of manufacturing and
design. It is the Publisher's desire to present books that are satisfactory as to their physical
qualities and artistic possibilities and appropriate for their particular use.* THOMAS
BOOKS *will be true to those laws of quality that assure a good name and good will.*

Printed in the United States of America
Q-R-3

Library of Congress Cataloging in Publication Data

Seeram, Euclid.
  X-ray imaging equipment.

  Bibliography: p.
  Includes index.
  1. Radiography, Medical--Equipment and supplies.
2. X-ray densitometry in medicine--Equipment and supplies.
3. Imaging systems in medicine. I. Title. [DNLM:
1. Radiography--instrumentation. WN 150 S453x]
RC78.5.S44 1985   616.07'572   84-16163
ISBN 0-398-05078-3

11/26/85   'χ

*This book is dedicated
with love and affection
to my parents, who
taught me the very
essence of life*

PREFACE

AN important challenge in writing a text on x-ray imaging equipment is to meet the varied requirements of the user. Recently, significant changes have occurred in the field of radiology. One such example is the introduction of computers and digital image processing equipment into the domain in imaging. These changes have brought about new directions and activities for all those working in clinical imaging technologies.

The changes in imaging, and particularly x-ray imaging, have placed an increasing demand for textbooks on the fundamental aspects of equipment, which will lay a solid groundwork by introducing simple theoretical considerations and at the same time present a certain level of sophistication.

The purpose of this text therefore is twofold: (1) to present a broad theoretical framework for understanding the principles of x-ray imaging equipment and to lay the basic groundwork necessary for the practical aspects concerning the use of the equipment; and (2) to assist the student in acquiring a further insight into the structure of x-ray imaging equipment through identification and discussion of selected research topics.

Having these goals in mind it is my firm belief that the text is suitable for use in the following ways: (1) as a text for introductory courses in x-ray imaging instrumentation for diploma and undergraduate degree programs in radiography, (2) as a reference text for the professional technologist, and (3) as a supplementary text for courses in applied fields such as biomedical technology.

I have used the brief and comprehensive approach in writing this text in order to maintain the student's interest and attention. Although the later chapters tend to be lengthy, the various subheadings are still described in a concise form.

The text differs from existing ones in several ways. First, it introduces digital image processing and computer concepts — topics that in the past were not within the domain of radiology. Second, it identifies current research topics through reference to several professional journals, a technique which is of vital importance in providing student motivation in the learning process. Thirdly and equally important, it contains summaries of key concepts discussed in the text at the end of each chapter and also includes a small selected bibliography.

The book is divided into four parts. Part A includes ten chapters covering conventional imaging equipment and focusses on topics such as an x-ray imaging scheme, x-ray tables and tube supports, the x-ray machine, exposure timers, scattered radiation reduction methods, geometric tomography, dental and mobile equipment and a chapter on other techniques.

Part B deals with fluoroscopic, x-ray television display and recording principles and equipment. It covers four chapters on the principles of fluoroscopy, image intensification, x-ray television and image monitoring and recording schemes.

Part C lends itself to an introduction of digital imae processing theory and computer concepts which are covered in two chapters.

Part D takes the general principles covered in Part C and relates them to two functional areas of digital imaging technology: computed tomography and digital radiography.

Finally, Part D stands alone and presents a broad overview of quality assurance with respect to what it is and how it is organized.

In selected chapters throughout the text, I have identified and presented the results of current and related research findings. In presenting these, I have used a number of direct quotations so as not to detract from the original meanings. I strongly feel that these research studies will provide a forum for further discussion and perhaps investigation. Students are encouraged to refer to the original works on a particular topic.

The material in this text should be used concurrently with a course in radiologic physics, and, therefore, I have not assumed a previous knowledge of radiologic physics.

It is my firm belief that this text will be up-to-date for several years to come for a number of reasons. First and foremost, the book describes the principles of imaging equipment. Such principles do not change drastically in a short period and a good example to illustrate this point is x-ray production. Today, the principles involved in producing x-rays are essentially the same as those used by Roentgen in 1895, however, they are produced today in a more efficient manner. The second reason is based on the fact that significant changes appear to occur every ten to fifteen years. Recently, radiology has experienced those changes with the introduction of computers and digital image processing technology. These concepts and changes are covered reasonably in this text.

Future trends will always be an issue of current concern in this technology, and those developments when they become firmly established and clinically feasible (out of the research laboratory) will definitely be included in future editions of this text. In the meantime, one must have a firm understanding of the fundamental principles and developments of the current technology, especially as they occurred throughout the years. In other words, this is necessary in order to appreciate new trends and techniques and, more importantly, to understand what makes the new technique better than the old.

These concerns and issues are addressed in this book and they will exist in the domain of x-ray imaging in the years to come.

Good luck in your pursuit of a career in radiography. I trust that you will enjoy the pages that follow.

Euclid Seeram
British Columbia, Canada

INTRODUCTION

THE progress of modern diagnostic imaging and particularly x-ray imaging can be partially attributed to numerous technological developments and innovations that have occurred within recent years.

In the past eighty years, the radiologic community has witnessed several periods in the *technical evolution* of x-ray imaging. These periods commenced with at least *four eras* of *x-ray tubes and generators*. The developments at this time offered a number of advantages including higher x-ray output and the use of shorter exposure times. Today, x-ray tube and generator changes continue to occur at a significant rate.

The *fifth era* in x-ray imaging introduced the *lens and mirror optical system* which are used to view and record x-ray images. This period was shortly followed by the introduction of *image intensifiers, x-ray television* and *automation.*

Refinements in the technology have been so dramatic that the rewards are truly beneficial. Radiologists and technologists alike performed their work with greater speed and accuracy and with less dose to patients.

More recently, a new kind of imaging device has become available for radiological investigation of the head and body. This is the unique and revolutionary *computed tomography* scanner. So remarkable is the technique of computed tomography that, in 1979, Hounsfield of England and Cormack of the United States shared the Nobel prize in medicine for their work in developing a clinically useful machine.

This development marks yet another era in the milestones of diagnostic imaging and that is, the use of the computer as an aid to radiological diagnosis, or more specifically, *digital imaging technology.* Today, applications of the *computer in radiology* have gained widespread attention. These applications range from automation of patient records and radiologic reporting to imaging applications such a computer-aided diagnosis, automated image analysis and computed tomography. To date, computed tomography has had a profound impact on diagnostic imaging such that advances in this technology have generated even newer imaging techniques such as *digital radiography* and *magnetic resonance imaging.*

These modern trends and techniques require an understanding of new concepts, such as, for example, digital image processing theory and computer technology, which until now were not within the domain of diagnostic radiology. These techniques result in three categories of equipment for x-ray imaging. The basis for this categorization depends on the type of image that can be generated. They are as follows:

1. RADIOGRAPHIC EQUIPMENT which is designed to produce *fixed photographic images*.
2. FLUOROSCOPIC EQUIPMENT which permits study of *moving or dynamic images* on a fluorescent screen.
3. COMPUTER-ASSISTED OR DIGITAL IMAGING EQUIPMENT. In imaging, the computer is used to produce a *reconstructed image* from projections.

The impact of these technical developments or diagnostic imaging has been significant. Without a doubt, there will be more and more changes in the future with the ultimate goal of producing optimum image quality with minimal radiation doses. Other goals will include patient and operator *safety, comfort* and *simple and logical operation* of equipment.

The purpose of this brief introduction is to familiarize the student technologist and practitioner alike with the impact of technology on the progress of diagnostic imaging. The main purpose of the text, on the other hand, is to make a general x-ray equipment course a more satisfactory learning experience so that the student will be able to:

(a) acquire a good theoretical framework for understanding the principles of x-ray imaging equipment.
(b) recognize simple malfunction of the apparatus.
(c) gain an exposure to the frontiers of research activities relating to x-ray imaging equipment.
(d) gain an awareness of the increasing use of computers in x-ray imaging.
(e) commence building a vocabularly which would facilitate a better understanding of the literature that uses the language of digital image processing.
(f) lay the basic foundations necessary for the practical aspects of radiography.

The acquisition of these objectives and the ability to accommodate changes in diagnostic imaging technology are important and mandatory characteristics which reflect the future role of the technologist.

E.S.

ACKNOWLEDGMENTS

IT is always a pleasure to acknowledge the assistance of individuals who have supported and contributed to the growth and development of this project, from the point of conception to its completion.

First and foremost, the idea for this book came from my charming wife, Trish, a very special, warm and caring person from whom I continue to learn the meaning of life. Her support and constant encouragement during the years are really what brought this manuscript to completion. To her, I shall like to extend my warmest and most sincere thanks.

The material for this book was conceived at the Ottawa General Hospital School of Radiography through a series of lecture notes given to student radiologic technologists. Their questions and concerns resulted in an expansion of the contents and to these students I am particularly grateful.

I owe special thanks to Sr. M. York, s.c.o., who not only taught me the elements of radiography but provided me with the opportunity to teach x-ray imaging equipment at the Ottawa General Hospital School of Radiography. Her kindness and support will never fade away. Another teacher who has influenced my early years in radiography and to whom I owe my understanding of radiologic physics is Professor C. Hebert, Ph.D., of the University of Ottawa. She has provided me with a good deal of encouragement, and I am indebted to her for her careful and most valuable reviews of the original drafts.

Several other individuals who have assisted me with constructive comments and reviews of selected portions of the original drafts and to whom I extend my appreciation are Dr. G. Copestake, Professor of Radiology, Dr. Liver, Professor of Radiology, and Dr. Bernard, lecturer in Radiology. These three individuals are from the Department of Radiology, Ottawa General Hospital and the University of Ottawa.

I owe special thanks to my friend Pierre Bilodeau, R.T., senior technologist at Sacred Heart Hospital in Hull, Quebec. His fitting disposition and concern to "finish the book man" helped me to maintain the motivation needed to complete this task.

The further growth and development of the manuscript are as a result of my experiences here at the British Columbia Institute of Technology (BCIT). My former department head, Mr. W. Noel, R.T., N.M., a friend and colleague, provided me with the support and help I needed to continue work on this project. Not only do I thank him for his efforts regarding manuscript development but also for his sincere support in teaching radiography both at BCIT and two affiliated clinical facilities. Thanks, Bill.

I must also express my appreciation to Mr. Dave Martin, MSR., B.Sc., (Hons), Department Head, Basic Health Sciences and Acting Department Head, Radiological Technical Services, BCIT. He has given me all the assistance I needed ever since he heard about the project.

To all the students at Vancouver General Hospital and at BCIT who attended the tutorials on x-ray imaging equipment, I am grateful. Not only were they exposed to various portions of the manuscript, but they have provided me with feedback on its form and content. In this regard also, I shall like to express my sincere thanks to Sarah Elizabeth Smith, a very perceptive individual who took the time to read significant portions of the text. Her comments and suggestions from the viewpoint of a student have been invaluable and have shaped the manuscript to its present form.

Another individual to whom I am grateful is Ollie Tomasky, A.C., a colleague and friend in radiography at BCIT, for her support and interest in the project. Her positive comments have always provided me with a drive to complete this work.

Special acknowledgments go to my friend Bill Forrest, clinical engineer at the Vancouver General Hospital, for his hard work in reviewing and commenting on various aspects of the manuscript. I am also thankful to Gary Pickwell, clinical engineering technologist at the Vancouver General Hospital. He took the time to provide answers to my numerous questions on automatic timers and x-ray circuitry.

This book would not have been possible without the efforts of several other individuals. I therefore express my thanks to all the authors, publishers, x-ray manufacturers and their representatives, who not only furnished information but also gave their willing permission to reproduce data and illustrations in the text. I would especially like to acknowledge the help of the Siemens Corporation, Phillips Medical Systems, Picker International, General Electric Company — Medical Systems Division, the Machlett Laboratories Inc., Imatron Inc., American Science and Engineering, Toshiba Medical Systems, ADAC Laboratories, Radiation Measurements, Inc., IBM, and the Technicare Corporation. In addition, I have used material from the following journals: *Electromedica, Medicamundi, Radiology* and the *Proceedings of the Society of Photo-Optical Instrumentation Engineers*. One other individual who provided photographs for use in the text is my friend Roger LeBlanc, R.T., of the Grace General Hospital in Ottawa.

To all the people at Charles C Thomas, Publisher who were involved in the production of this text, I owe my thanks. You have all done a very good job.

I also wish to express my appreciation to all the people in the Word Processing Center at BCIT for their efficient and excellent work.

Finally, my family's encouragement is not to be overlooked. Again, I come back to my wife, Trish. She has influenced and has contributed to my professional and educational development, particularly my university studies. I am very grateful for her help in the proof stages of the publication process.

To my son David, a very special and wise lad, thanks pal for understanding why I dedicated this book to my parents. Remember that my first book was dedicated to you and your mother.

SPECIAL ACKNOWLEDGMENT

I SHALL like to extend my sincere appreciation to Payne Thomas of Charles C Thomas, Publisher for his kind support, encouragement, good counsel and, more importantly, for his patience in awaiting the arrival of the final draft.

SUGGESTIONS FOR THE STUDENT

THE material in this book provides a very broad coverage of x-ray imaging equipment. To assist you in the study of this text, the following guidelines are suggested:

(a) Read through the list of contents and group the chapters according to your course structure.

(b) Read through the appropriate chapters before attending the lectures. This will familiarize you with the language of the course.

(c) Determine the key concepts discussed in the chapter.

(d) Read through the chapter summaries to identify the key concepts. Match these with the ones that you have selected.

(e) Study and understand the diagrams. This is intended to enhance class discussions.

(f) Refer to the original studies when doing an essay on a specific topic. You will find more references in original papers.

(g) The research studies should not be disregarded since they do provide a basis for further discussion.

(h) Try to relate the theory covered in this text to the equipment aspects in the clinical area.

(i) Answer all the questions at the end of the text. This will provide you with a self assessment review and help you to identify areas of weakness.

CONTENTS

Part A

CONVENTIONAL IMAGING TECHNOLOGY

SECTION A: RADIOGRAPHIC EQUIPMENT

SECTION B: FLUOROSCOPIC AND X-RAY TELEVISION EQUIPMENT

Part B

DIGITAL IMAGING TECHNOLOGY

SECTION C: DIGITAL IMAGE PROCESSING AND COMPUTERS

SECTION D: DIGITAL IMAGING APPLICATIONS

Part C

QUALITY ASSURANCE

SECTION E: QUALITY-ASSURANCE OVERVIEW

X-RAY IMAGING
EQUIPMENT

Part A

CONVENTIONAL IMAGING TECHNOLOGY

Section A

RADIOGRAPHIC EQUIPMENT

CHAPTER 1

A DIAGNOSTIC X-RAY IMAGING SCHEME

THE NATURE OF X-RAYS

Discovery and Properties

THE idea of using x-rays to produce visual images of the human body is referred to as *x-ray imaging*.

In 1895, Wilhelm Conrad Roentgen discovered that a highly penetrating radiation is emitted when high-speed electrons strike a target. The *x-rays* (so-called, because their nature was then unknown) produce fluorescence in certain materials, affect photographic film and travel in straight lines. Unlike the particle radiations (α and β-radiation), they are not deflected by electric or magnetic fields. The penetrating ability of the radiation increases with increasing energy of the incident electrons. The intensity of the x-ray beam, on the other hand, is proportional to the number of electrons per second striking the target.

7

After several years of study, it was established that x-radiation exhibits certain phenomena (interference, diffraction and polarization) which are only associated with waves. It was finally possible to determine the wavelengths, and these were found to be much shorter than the wavelengths of ultraviolet light.

An alternative theory of electromagnetic radiation, the *quantum theory*, pictures the radiation as the emission of distinct and separate "packets" of energy, known as *quanta* or *photons*. The energy of the photon is directly proportional to the frequency of the radiation. X-rays are penetrating because they consist of photons carrying a large amount of energy compared to, for example, photons of visible light.

The two most important properties of x-rays, namely, their penetrating ability and their effect on photographic film, led Roentgen to produce the very first image of the human hand (Figure 1:5a). Thus, a new era in the history of medicine had begun; more specifically, it was the birth of *roentgenology*, the science of recording images of the body using x-rays and providing a diagnosis from those images. Later, the term *radiology* emerged to describe the same idea. Today, the term *imaging* is commonly used to indicate any technique which uses some form of energy to produce visual images of an object. Such techniques include ultrasound (high-frequency sound waves), nuclear medicine (gamma rays), thermography (heat energy) and the most recent, magnetic resonance imaging (magnetic fields and radio frequency waves).

COMPONENTS OF THE IMAGING SCHEME

An x-ray imaging scheme consists of a number of components systematically arranged so that each one plays an important role in the production of the image. It is therefore mandatory that the technologist understand how each of these components work and how they fit together in the imaging chain. This is of vital importance, since the technologist is directly responsible for the safe operation of the equipment and the production of optimum image quality.

A typical x-ray imaging scheme (Figure 1:1) consists of the following components:

(a) An x-ray source.
(b) An imaging object.
(c) A detection and recording system.
(d) An image processing system.
(e) A display and viewing system.
(f) A high-voltage generator.
(g) A control unit.

Each of these will now be discussed briefly with a view of describing their general purpose in the total imaging scheme. It is also the intention here to im-

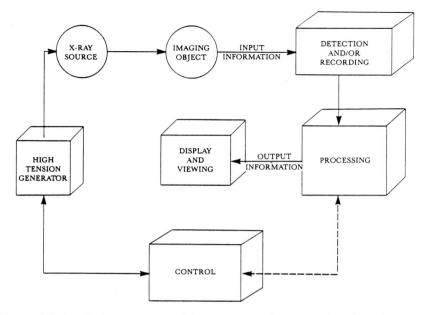

Figure 1:1 A typical arrangement of the components in an x-ray imaging scheme.

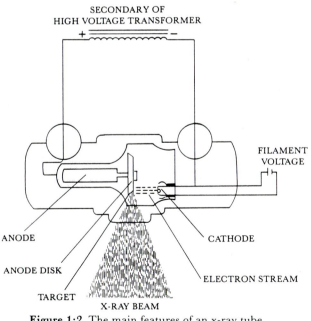

Figure 1:2 The main features of an x-ray tube.

press upon the student that the basic foundations of this text are centered around these components.

The X-ray Source

This is a special kind of glass tube with a highly sophisticated design. In the early days, x-rays were produced in gas-discharge tubes. Today, x-rays are produced in what is popularly referred to as the *x-ray tube,* an evacuated glass envelope consisting of two electrodes — an anode (positive) and a cathode (negative).

In Figure 1:2, the basic features of an x-ray tube are shown. The electron stream is produced by thermionic emission from a heated *filament.* The electrons are then accelerated towards the target by a high potential difference (kilovoltage) applied across the tube. Upon striking the *target,* practically all of the kinetic energy of the electrons is transformed into heat energy. A very small fraction (less than 1%) appears in the form of x-rays. The unavoidable production of heat in the anode poses one of the major problems associated with the generation of x-rays.

The Imaging Object

The object in this context refers to the *patient.* The input information (Figure 1:1) is derived from the patient. *Transmitted x-rays* (x-rays which have passed through the patient) are detected, processed, and later presented in some form for viewing and interpretation.

The fact that different tissues in the patient absorb x-rays in different amounts is the fundamental basis for the formation of the image.

Other kinds of imaging objects are *test phantoms* which are used to provide information on the *performance* of the equipment and to establish a *quality-assurance* program. These test phantoms are becoming more and more commonplace in radiology departments, and already the technologist is responsible for carrying out performance evaluations and quality-control tests on the equipment.

The Detection and Recording System

Transmitted x-rays must be received by some kind of a detection system. In conventional radiography, the detector is a *film or film/screen combination.* In the latter, the screen converts x-rays into light and an image is formed on the film. This method of image formation uses less radiation compared to *non-screen techniques.*

In fluoroscopy, the image receptor (detector) is a *fluorescent screen.* Such a screen fluoresces when struck by x-rays. Today, the fluorescent screen is an essential element of a highly sophisticated image tube called the *image intensifier.* In this case, the image from the intensifier tube (*intensified fluoroscopic image*) can be recorded onto magnetic tape and/or film.

In *computed tomography* (computer-assisted x-ray imaging equipment) the detector system can be either *scintillation crystals* coupled to *photomultiplier tubes* or *gas-ionization detectors*. These are special detectors which convert transmitted x-rays into electrical impulses. These impulses are then converted into *digital* (numerical) data and stored onto magnetic tapes or disks. The digital data are then fed into a digital computer which performs mathematical operations on them to reconstruct an image.

The output image in this case can be recorded photographically so that a permanent record is available or it can be put on magnetic storage devices for reanalysis at some later time.

The Image Processing System

When transmitted x-rays fall upon a detector system, a "latent" image is formed. The image is rendered visible by subjecting it to a processing operation. Today, there are two kinds of processing systems.

The first kind is a *chemical processing* system, analogous to a photographic film processing system. The system is usually a separate unit which houses developer, fixer, wash and drying components. In most radiology departments, automatic film processors are used.

The second kind of processing is done by a *computer* which reconstructs images using special *algorithms* (a specific set of rules for solving problems). This kind of processing demands special computer programs to solve both simple and complex mathematical equations.

The Display and Viewing System

Once the output image is available, there must be some method of displaying and viewing it. For this purpose, single and multiple *viewboxes* are used. The brightness level of these boxes is fixed and the radiologist cannot change it unless he uses a higher intensity lamp. In this viewing and display method, the image cannot be altered in any way.

In computed tomography equipment, the display and viewing system is available as a separate unit featuring an impressive-looking console as shown in Figure 1:3. The image is presented on a television monitor for viewing. The advantage of this method of display is that the operator can now control such factors as image brightness and contrast. The operator can also carry out a number of other operations on the image, such as magnification, measurements, and so on. In the future, such display and viewing consoles may become commonplace in most imaging departments.

The High-Voltage Generator

The high-voltage generator is a separate unit connected in such a way that it provides a high voltage to the x-ray tube. This voltage is mandatory for the production of x-rays.

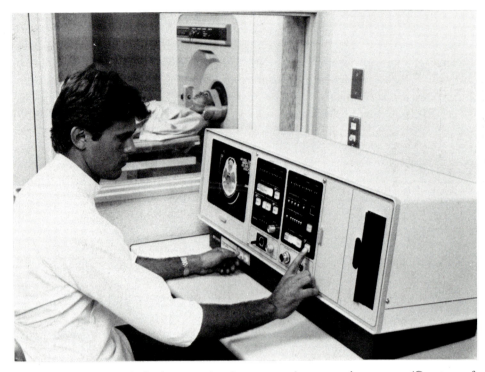

Figure 1:3 Display and viewing console of a computed tomography scanner (Courtesy of Toshiba Medical Systems).

The Control Unit

The control unit is perhaps one of the components in the total imaging scheme with which the technologist is in direct contact. The unit essentially controls several parameters in the imaging scheme. Such parameters include all factors which govern the production of both the quantity and quality of x-rays, as well as the duration of the x-ray exposure. For these reasons, and many more, a *control panel* is characteristic of the control unit.

The control panel consists of a number of knobs, push-button selectors, switches, display meters and so on. By manipulating the appropriate controls and selectors, the technologist sets up all the necessary factors for the examination. He or she may select the kilovoltage (kV), the milliamperage (mA), the duration of the exposure (seconds), which may be controlled by an electronic or automatic timer, and other factors as they relate to the examination. The display meters, on the other hand, indicate to the operator whether the selected factors are utilized when the exposure occurs and whether the system is in proper working condition. Figure 1:4 shows two other control consoles common to x-ray imaging.

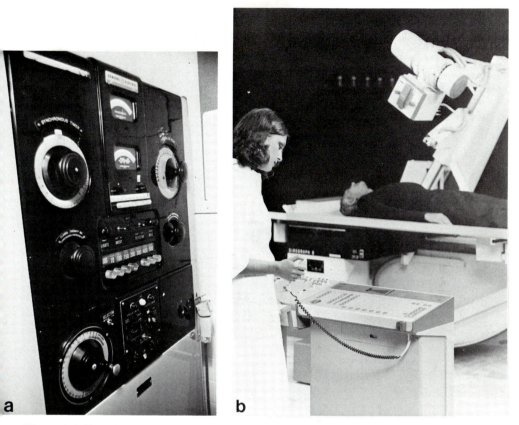

Figure 1:4 Two diagnostic x-ray imaging consoles. (a) Early console and (b) Modern console — (Photograph (b) Courtesy of the Siemens Corporation.)

THE PURPOSE OF AN X-RAY IMAGING SYSTEM

The foregoing discussion emphasizes the importance of each element in the imaging scheme. The primary consideration in such a scheme is related to the acquisition and flow of information.

The information desired by the imaging mechanism is the *image quality* that can be derived as faithfully as possible from the imaging object. Therefore, to be effective and efficient, an imaging system must provide maximum information content (optimum image quality) using the least possible radiation dose. Figure 1:5 shows the improved image quality of today compared to that obtained by Roentgen some decades ago.

Recent innovations and developments in technology have already demonstrated that modern machines do have the capability of operating under conditions which would generate the best possible image. The most important facet, however, in a technologically oriented discipline, such as x-ray imaging, is that

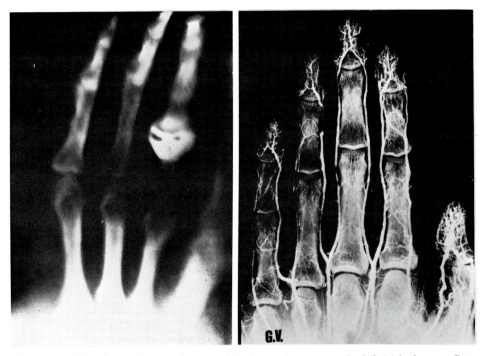

Figure 1:5. Two diagnostic x-ray images of the hand. The one on the left (a) is the very first image produced by Roentgen some eighty years ago. The image on the right (b) was produced recently using a microfocus x-ray tube. The improved image quality is clearly seen in this image. The blood vessels have been made visible by injecting them with contrast material. (Courtesy of the Siemens Corporation.)

the operator must be able to use the machine wisely and within its capability to obtain the maximum potential benefits.

In the remainder of this text, each section in the imaging scheme will be described in some detail, so that the structure and function of the elements involved will become increasingly apparent.

SUMMARY

1. The nature of x-rays is essential to understand x-ray imaging fundamentals. X-rays have several properties; the more important ones, in this context, relate to their penetrating ability and their effect on photographic film.
2. Several major components, of an x-ray imaging scheme including the source of x-rays, the imaging object, the detection and recording system, the viewing and display system, the image processing system, the high-voltage generator and the control unit, are described briefly.

3. X-rays are produced in an x-ray tube, a specially designed glass vacuum tube which has two electrodes — an anode and a cathode.

4. By heating the filament of the cathode and causing them to "boil off" (thermionic emission), electrons can be accelerated across the tube to strike the target on the anode by applying a potential difference (voltage) between anode and cathode. When the electrons collide with the target material, x-rays are produced.

5. The general aim of an x-ray imaging system is identified. Such goal is to produce optimum diagnostic images using minimal radiation doses.

CHAPTER 2

THE X-RAY MACHINE — PART I

THE x-ray tube and its associated circuitry are sometimes referred to as the *x-ray machine*. In Figure 2:1, three basic components of a typical x-ray machine are shown. The electrical power required to energize the machine is derived from the *mains supply*. On the other hand, the high voltage which is needed to produce x-rays is supplied by the *high tension generator* and its associated circuitry.

Once power is supplied to the x-ray tube, there must be some way of controlling and regulating it so that the events in the production of x-rays can occur as smoothly as possible during a radiologic examination. For this purpose, an *x-ray control* is provided. As mentioned in the previous chapter, this is perhaps the part of the system with which the technologist has most contact. For this reason, some common features of the console will be described.

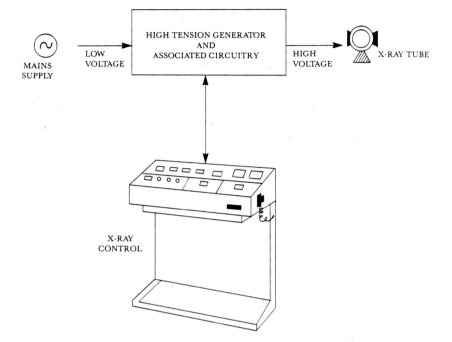

Figure 2:1. Three components of an x-ray imaging system.

ESSENTIAL COMPONENTS

Figure 2:1 can be expanded into Figure 2:2 which shows how the essential components of an x-ray machine are functionally connected. The student should refer to it when reading the rest of this chapter.

Transformers

A transformer is an electrical device which changes the voltage of an alternating current by either increasing or decreasing it. The transformer is usually immersed in oil, which acts as a cooling medium and as an electrical insulator during operation. In the x-ray machine, three types of transformers are present: a step-up transformer, a step-down transformer and an autotransformer.

The *autotransformer* is a special type of transformer. It supplies different amounts of voltage to several circuits in the x-ray machine. For example, the autotransformer supplies both the step-up and step-down transformers with different voltages (V) and ultimately determines the magnitude of the high voltage applied to the x-ray tube.

The *step-up transformer*, or *high tension transformer,* delivers high voltage to the x-ray tube by increasing the voltage tapped from the autotransformer. It is

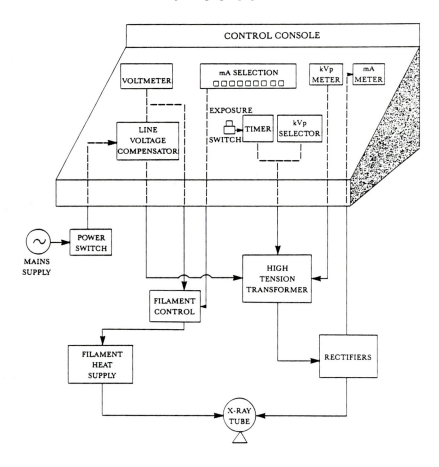

Figure 2:2. Schematic of a basic x-ray machine, showing how the main components are functionally connected. The most common meters and selectors typical of control consoles are also indicated.

designed to increase the AC mains voltage (110V, 120V, 220V, or 440V) to values ranging from about 30 to 150 kilovolts (kV), the range of voltages used in diagnostic radiology.

The *step-down transformer*, on the other hand, is the *filament transformer*. It decreases the AC mains voltage to 10 or 15 volts, necessary to operate the x-ray tube filament since it uses a large current.

Rectifiers

In some x-ray units (dental and low-powered portable sets), the x-ray tube itself acts as a *rectifier*. This is a device which changes AC to DC. High-powered x-ray machines make use of a separate rectifier system, typically referred to as the *rectification circuit*. Since rectification plays an important role in efficient production of x-rays, it will be discussed in some detail in Chapter 8.

High-Voltage Transmission

All the components in the x-ray tube which are subjected to high voltages are located in what is conveniently referred to as the *high-voltage section* of the x-ray circuit. These include: the rectifier system, the step-up transformer, the filament transformer, the x-ray tube, high tension cables, etc.

High tension cables conduct high voltages from the step-up transformer to the x-ray tube. Since there is a high voltage across them, they have a special design. A high tension cable consists of a central core in which there are three conducting wires. Surrounding the core is a special insulator which is, in turn, surrounded by a special sheath of woven copper wire used for grounding purposes. Hence, it is for this reason that high tension cables are sometimes referred to as *shockproof* cables.

High tension cables are quite conspicuous in an x-ray room because they hang from the ceiling and make connections to the x-ray tube via cable receptacles on the tube housing.

THE CONTROL CONSOLE — CHARACTERISTIC FEATURES

The control console is usually located in a cubicle by itself. The cubicle (booth) is lead lined to offer maximum radiation protection. A lead-glass window in the booth allows the technologist to observe the patient at all times.

The control console in an x-ray imaging system houses a number of components such as the peak kilovoltage (kVp) and milliamperage (mA) curcuits; *timing circuits* and other controls, such as voltage level controls.

The control console, therefore, is provided with a panel on which several controls and meters and other function buttons or selectors are located. Throughout the decades, the console has changed its external appearance with more and more features appearing on some units. It is not within the scope of this text to describe each and every feature on a console; only the essential controls and meters which are common to all consoles will be highlighted. These are:

(a) The ON-OFF switch.
(b) A line voltage compensator/indicator.
(c) kVp, mA and time selectors.
(d) Automatic density control.
(e) kVp, mA and time indicators.
(f) The exposure switch.
(g) The Bucky selector.
(h) Room and tube selector.

Figure 2:3 shows some of the controls and meters on a modern console.

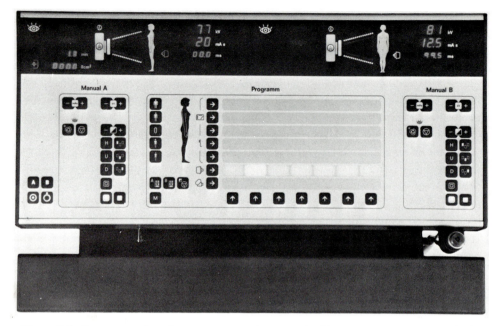

Figure 2:3. Some controls and meters on a modern console. New x-ray generators permit the selection of automatic density control. This photograph shows a smooth-surfaced operating panel which consists of large photoelectronic displays and clearly arranged operating section. The "organ-programmed radiographic technique" permits all "freely" set radiographic parameters to be stored in the simplest way (courtesy of the Siemens Corporation).

The On-Off Switch

There is a main switch on the console which energizes and de-energizes the machine. When the switch is closed (ON-position), power is supplied to the autotransformer and other circuits in the machine.

The Line Voltage Compensator

The AC mains voltage may vary from time to time due to periodic power surges which may be due to the consumption of power by other large electrical equipment operating in the hospital. The purpose of the line voltage compensator is to ensure that a constant voltage is supplied to the autotransformer. Any fluctuation of the mains voltage will affect the x-ray exposure output, which ultimately affects the density of the radiograph.

Older equipment features *manual line voltage compensators* and care must be taken to ensure that the indicator is properly set at all times. Today, machines are provided with *automatic line voltage compensators*. These compensators automatically adjust the voltage in the event of a power surge.

kVp, mA and Time Selectors

These are selectors which the technologist adjusts constantly to obtain exposure techniques for different types of examinations. For example, the technologist may select 80 kVp, 200 mA and 0.4 seconds for an examination of the
average-sized abdomen. These *technical exposure factors* are sometimes established by manufacturers, but in most cases, radiology departments assume
the responsibility of establishing their own technique charts.

The *kVp selector* makes a connection with the autotransformer as illustrated
in Figure 2:4. It allows the technologist to choose the voltage across the x-ray
tube for the duration of the exposure. Some machines are provided with *major
and minor* kVp selectors (Figure 2:4) which change in steps of 10 kVp and 1
kVp, respectively. Other machines may have a *continuous* kVp control selector.
It is interesting to note here that the kilovoltage determines the quality (penetrating ability) of the x-ray beam, amongst other factors.

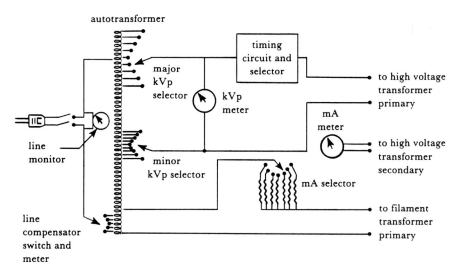

Figure 2:4. The control console circuit. This portion of the total circuit is referred to as the
low voltage section. (From Bushong, Stewart C.; *Radiologic Science for Technologists.* St. Louis, 1982.
The C.V. Mosby Co.)

The quantity of electrons travelling from cathode to anode (tube current) of
the x-ray tube is determined by the *mA selection*. The mA selector makes connections to a variable resistor in the filament circuit. A wide range of mA settings (20 to 1,500 are not uncommon) is available on radiographic equipment,
while values ranging from 0.5 mA to 10 mA can be selected for fluoroscopy.

The *timer* and its associated circuitry determine the duration of the x-ray exposure by controlling the length of time that the high voltage is supplied to the

x-ray tube. Without high voltage, electrons do not flow across the tube and hence no x-rays are produced.

There are several classes of x-ray exposure timers, such as electronic and automatic ones. A detailed description of these timers will be given in a later chapter.

The manual selection of kVp, mA and time by the technologist will ultimately determine the density of the radiograph. In general, by changing any one of these parameters, the technologist has control over the desired radiographic density.

Automatic Density Control

Most x-ray imaging equipment available today incorporate automatic exposure timing. Such automation allows for *automatic density control* (ADC), which means that the desired density (usually chosen by the radiologist) of any anatomical part for small-, medium- and large-sized patients is preprogrammed into the exposure timing circuits. With some automatic timers, the technologist may select only the kilovoltage appropriate to the examination.

Recently, some machines are equipped with a system called *anatomically programmed radiography* (APR). In this system, the technologist can select the examination by choosing the appropriate button or sensor-type touch key (Figure 2:3). This results in the automatic selection of kVp, mA and time factors for that examination. When using the APR system, patient positioning is critical for accurate results.

Presently, some x-ray generators, particularly those used in special vascular procedures, automatically provide very fast selection of optimum exposure factors for an object. In this concept, very low doses are delivered to the patient (before the examination), the absorption by the patient is measured and a comparison is then made with the generator and x-ray tube output, so that optimum values of mA and kVp are automatically computed to give the best possible contrast.

The use of automatic exposure timing devices has proved to be of benefit to both the patient and operator. It must be realized that automation in this context does not produce "push-button" technologists but, rather, demands a good knowledge of their (automatic timers) working principles. Good skills are necessary for proper use of these timing devices.

kVp, mA and Time Meters

The tube voltage, tube current and the exposure time are displayed on kVp, mA and time meters, respectively. The meters display and indicate that the preset exposure factors are obtained when the exposure occurs.

There are other meters and selectors on the control console, but these will not be discussed here since they differ from machine to machine.

The Exposure Switch

The exposure switch on x-ray machines must be of a *dead-man type*. This means that it is "so constructed that a circuit-closing contact can be maintained only by continuous pressure on the switch" (N.C.R.P. 1973). Such a switch is considered a safety device.

In the past mechanical switches were used, but recently electronic switches have become available because of the drawbacks (one of which is related to exposure timing) imposed by mechanical switches.

On fixed radiographic equipment the switches are located on the control panel. In some cases, however, the switch is a separate unit connected to an exposure cord. In this situation the technologist should remain in the control booth when making the exposure.

The operation of most x-ray exposure switches is based on the following two actions:

(a) Activation of one position (usually indicated on the switch or machine) starts the anode (in rotating anode x-ray tubes) rotation. This action also heats the filament of the tube.

(b) Activation of the other position on the switch (expose position) commences the x-ray exposure and allows it to continue only for the preset duration.

The Bucky Selector

The *Bucky selector* is one that is used only when the part to be x-rayed is of a certain thickness. It is so called after its inventor *Gustave Bucky,* who developed a special device called a grid to improve image contrast.

When x-raying thick parts, increased scattered radiation is produced (in the part) which reaches the film. These scattered rays degrade the quality of the image. By introducing the grid between the patient and film, the scattered rays are removed and image quality improves.

The Bucky is located just beneath the x-ray table and consists of a tray (to hold the film cassette), the grid and its associated circuitry.

Tube Selector

In some departments, two x-ray rooms may share the same control console. In this respect, the technologist must select the correct tube for the appropriate room. This is important, since a patient may be irradiated unnecessarily if the incorrect tube is selected.

SAFETY CONSIDERATIONS

Safety considerations for x-ray imaging equipment is a subject by itself.

Since the machine is one huge electrical circuit designed to produce ionizing radiation, safety is usually discussed in terms of:

(a) Electrical safety.

(b) Radiation safety.

Electrical Safety

The x-ray machine consists of a number of safety devices apart from the dead-man-type exposure switch. These devices are intended to prevent the possibility of electrical hazards to the operator, patient and the machine itself. Examples of these devices are *fuses* and *circuit breakers,* which protect the machine from electrical overloads by preventing the passage of greater load than is necessary for normal operation.

The entire x-ray machine is *grounded* to reduce the possibility of electric shock to the patient and operator. In any circumstance, when the technologist discovers a potential electrical hazard during operation of the machine, the mains supply switch must be turned off immediately. This switch is always within the reach of the technologist and is usually located in the control booth.

Radiation Safety

It is becoming increasingly apparent that even small doses of radiation can cause biological damage. One of the fundamental goals of the radiology department is to prevent unnecessary radiation exposures during an examination.

There are several methods to reduce and prevent unnecessary radiation exposure. The elements of radiation protection involve a number of topics, each of which is important to a good radiation protection program. Such elements relate to:

(a) The fundamental principles of radiation protection.

(b) Equipment design.

(c) Good operational practices.

The principles of protection require an understanding of *time, shielding* and *distance* concepts. For example, since the radiation dose is directly proportional to the time of the exposure, it would be best to use the shortest possible exposure time for an examination in order to keep doses to minimal levels.

Shielding of the gonads with lead aprons, for example, will significantly reduce the gonadal dose, thus minimizing the probability of genetic effects.

Radiation dose is inversely proportional to the square of the distance (inverse square law). This means that the greater the distance between the source of radiation and the exposed person, the smaller the radiation dose.

The design of x-ray imaging equipment must meet certain requirements established by national and, in some cases, international agencies on radiation protection, such as the International Commission on Radiological Protection (I.C.R.P.).

In other words, the equipment incorporates radiation protection mechanisms to minimize radiation hazards to both patient and operator. For example, *collimation* of the primary beam (restriction of the beam only to the region of interest) by a collimator significantly reduces the radiation dose to the patient.

Filtration is another means of protecting the patient. Filters (usually aluminum for most diagnostic work) are positioned between the x-ray tube and patient to absorb low-energy x-rays (do not play a role in the formation of the image) before they get to the patient. Hence, a reduction in dose.

X-ray tubes and generators are designed to produce radiation more efficiently, with the ultimate goal of delivering small doses to patients.

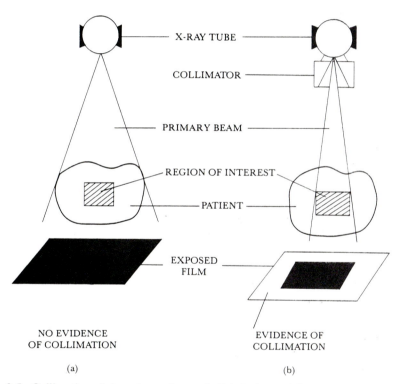

Figure 2:5. Collimation of the primary beam. In (a) the beam falls on an area greater than the region of interest. In (b) the beam is restricted only to the region of interest.

Finally, it is how well the technologist practices the rules of radiation protection which determines the effectiveness of a radiation protection program. At all times, particular attention must be given to guidelines and recommendations established by radiation protection agencies. For example, the technologist must collimate the radiation beam and always strive to show some evidence of collimation on the film (Figure 2:5).

Through an understanding of the principles of operation of the components just identified and their role in the imaging scheme, the technologist will be able to use the machine wisely and within its full capabilities. This knowledge, coupled with good operational practices, ensures maximum benefits for the patient, technologist and the imaging department.

SUMMARY

1. The production and control of x-rays require the use of a special machine called the x-ray machine.
2. The machine is a complex electronic circuit consisting of a number of devices such as transformers, rectifiers, voltmeters, milliammeters, timing apparatus and so on.
3. A transformer is a device used to either increase or decrease the voltage of an alternating current. Three types of transformers are identified: the autotransformer, the high tension transformer and the filament transformer.
4. A rectifier changes alternating current to direct current. A rectification circuit is necessary for the efficient production of x-rays.
5. High tension cables conduct high voltages from the step-up transformer to the x-ray tube. A high voltage is needed to produce x-rays.
6. Several elements characteristic of a typical control console are highlighted. These include the mA, kVp and time selectors and meters, the on-off switch, the Bucky selector, the line voltage compensator, the exposure switch, automatic density control and the tube selector.
7. The line voltage compensator ensures that a constant voltage is supplied to the autotransformer, since any fluctuation will affect the x-ray exposure output.
8. The kVp determines the penetrating power of x-rays produced by the tube, while the mA determines the quantity of x-rays. The timer, on the other hand, determines the duration of the exposure.
9. Automatic exposure timing is discussed briefly through identification of automatic density control and anatomically programmed radiography. In automatic exposure timing, a desired density for a specific part of the anatomy is preset in the timing circuits.
10. Meters and selectors provide visual display of all exposure factors used for an examination.
11. The exposure switch on an x-ray machine must be of a dead-man type.
12. Safety considerations are discussed in terms of electrical and radiation safety. Electrical safety involves the use of devices which prevent the

possibility of electrical hazards to the operator, patient and the equipment itself.

13. A brief description of radiation protection principles is given to provide an awareness of the importance of radiation protection in diagnostic x-ray imaging.

CHAPTER 3

X-RAY TABLES AND TUBE SUPPORTS

THE x-ray table and tube support are important elements in the x-ray imaging scheme, since they play a role in the production of the image and influence the efficiency with which the examination can be carried out. Figure 3:1 identifies the general layout of two x-ray tables and a tube support system in a radiographic room. These units have undergone significant developments throughout the years and the changes have brought about a number of advantages, such as improved patient comfort, improved image quality and examination of the patient in a number of planes (horizontal, vertical), a practice which is essential in present-day imaging trends.

X-RAY TABLES

The x-ray table is usually considered as a special unit on which the patient is positioned for the examination. In view of the developments in table design and function, a simple categorization of x-ray tables has evolved. Such categorization is based on the type of examination that can be performed on the table. These two categories (Figure 3:1) are:

(a) Radiographic tables.
(b) Radiographic-fluoroscopic tables.

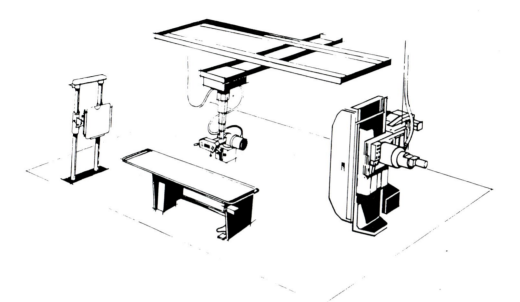

Figure 3:1. A diagramatic representation of two x-ray tables and an x-ray tube support system. The x-ray tube is suspended over the radiographic table while the fluoroscopic table is shown as a separate unit on the right (courtsey of the Siemens Corporation).

Radiographic Tables — General Features

A *radiographic table* is one on which examinations are done with or without a Bucky diaphragm (to be discussed later) and in conjunction with an x-ray tube positioned over the table.

Examinations of the extremities, chest, abdomen, pelvis, vertebral column and skull are just a few examples of studies that can be done on a radiographic table.

There are two types of radiographic tables.:

(a) Fixed radiographic tables.
(b) Tilting radiographic tables.

Type (a) implies that the table is stationary and fixed in the horizontal plane. The examinations carried out on this type of table are therefore restricted only to those in the horizontal plane. Figure 3:2 shows a fixed radiographic table. Type (b) is a more versatile table on which examinations are carried out, with

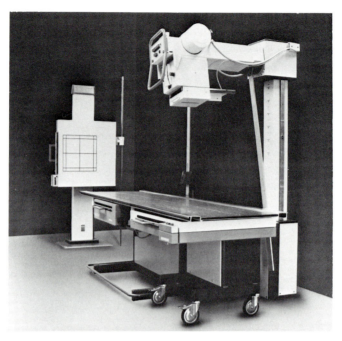

Figure 3:2. A fixed radiographic table (courtesy of the Siemens Corporation).

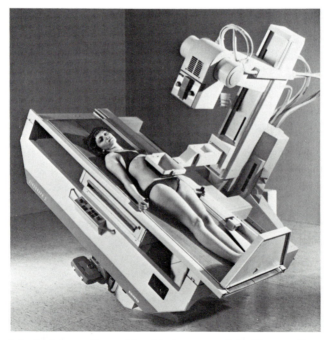

Figure 3:3. A tilting radiographic table (courtesy of the Siemens Corporation).

various degrees of angulation ranging from the horizontal plane (180°) to the vertical plane (90°). The mechanism of table tilting has given rise to several types of tilting tables. Two of the most popular types of tilting tables include the *90°- 90° tilting table* and the *90°- 15° Trendelenberg* (patient's head tilting down). In Figure 3:3, a tilting radiographic table is shown.

In the 90°- 90° type, the patient can be tilted 90° to the upright position ("head-up") or 90° to the "head-down" position.

Tilting the table is usually accomplished by a *motor drive and gear mechanism* which are located (in general) at the base of the table. This mechanism consists of a flywheel and brake which provide fast and smooth stops during tilting.

The framework of the table is rigid and is made of steel or any other equivalent material in order to support the weight of the patient.

The base of the table is made of similar material and is fixed securely to the floor. This is necessary to ensure that the table is free of vibrations during a procedure. As an added radiation protection feature, the framework of some radiographic tables are encased by sheets of metal which act as barriers against scattered radiation (Figure 3:4).

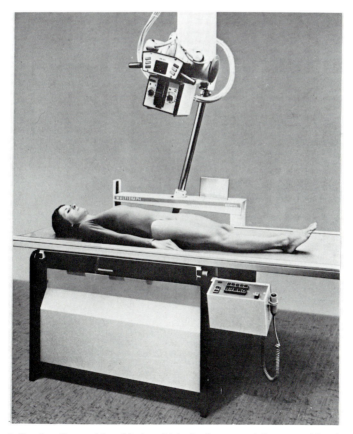

Figure 3:4. A fixed radiographic table in which the framework is encased by sheets of metal which act as barriers against scattered rays (courtesy of the Siemens Corporation).

The tabletop is made of a radiolucent material such as *Bakelite*. Bakelite is a synthetic resin which was developed in the United States by L.H. Baekland in 1909. It is prepared chemically by reacting phenolic compounds (e.g. phenol or cresol) and aldehydes (e.g. formaldehyde). Recently, *Arborite*® and plastic are used in the construction of tabletops. Usually, these are bonded onto some other material to give supporting strength. Tabletops are generally smooth and free of crevices so that they do not trap barium and other radio-opaque materials, which may appear on the image as artifacts.

There are three types of tabletops:

    (a) Fixed.
    (b) Moving.
    (c) Floating.

In the *fixed* type, the tabletop is stationary and in some cases the patient has to be moved along the length of the table to facilitate positioning. In the *moving* type, the top is designed to travel along the length (longitudinal) of the table. In this case, certain aspects of patient positioning (for example, centering) can be accomplished by moving the tabletop with the patient.

A *floating* table top implies that the top can travel along the length and across the width of the table. It can also travel obliquely or transversely, as illustrated in Figure 3:5. The tabletop can be locked in any position by using hand- or foot-operated electromagnetic locks.

When a floating tabletop is used, even though patient centering is affected

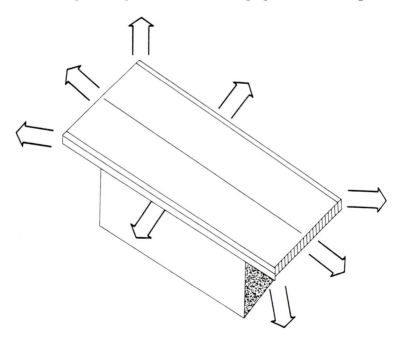

Figure 3:5. The direction of movement of a floating tabletop. This feature facilitates patient positioning.

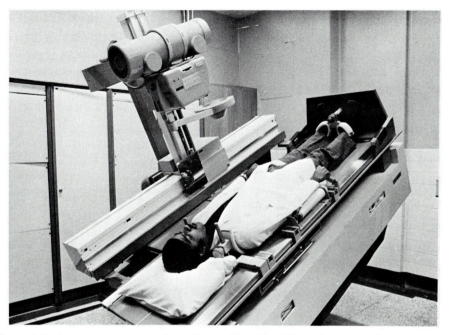

Figure 3:6. Accessory equipment for radiographic tables. Shown here are a foot support and straps, shoulder pads, hand grips and a compression band.

by moving the tabletop, the central ray must remain continuously centered to the Bucky diaphragm. In some units, this centering is always maintained.

The *Bucky diaphragm* is a special unit which is positioned just beneath the tabletop. It consists of a framework to support a *grid* (absorbs scattered radiation produced by the patient, since these rays only degrade image quality), a *cassette tray* and a separate *electronic circuit* to move the grid during the exposure. In some cases, the entire assembly is mounted on bearings that rest on a pair of rails to provide free movement along the length of the table. This allows the technologist to position the cassette under the part of the patient that is examined. For floating tabletops, the Bucky assembly is generally fixed so that the patient is now positioned over the cassette by moving the tabletop.

All radiographic tables should include the following added accessories, as demonstrated in Figure 3:6:

(a) A strong lightweight *foot support* for the patient to stand on during tilting of the table from the horizontal to the vertical position. In a 90°-90° tilting type, the table is made to accommodate the foot support at either end.

(b) *Shoulder pads, handgrips, head clamps,* and so on. These are especially useful in procedures which require careful immobilization of the patient.

(c) A *compression band* or belt to assist in immobilization and compression of fatty tissue.

Radiographic-Fluoroscopic Tables — General Features

As the name implies, a radiographic-fluoroscopic table (R-F table) is designed to provide both radiographic and fluoroscopic images using tilting and non-tilting techniques. R-F tables are sometimes referred to as combination tables, universal tables or mulitpurpose tables.

Older R-F tables incorporate two x-ray tubes: an *overtable tube* for conventional radiography and an *undertable* tube for *under-table fluoroscopy* (or undercouch fluoroscopy). R-F tables have all the general features of radiographic tables, however, there are certain added features which deserve mention here. These are:

(a) The tabletop is always a moving type, since it is important to move the patient during a fluoroscopic examination for positioning and other purposes.

(b) The undercouch tube is always encased by sheets of metal which line the sides of the table. The thickness of the sheeting is used to limit the amount of radiation due to scattering and leakage from the patient and x-ray tube, respectively.

(c) A spotfilm device, or serial changer as it is sometimes referred to.

The Spotfilm Device

The spotfilm device is a unique piece of apparatus which enables the radiologist to make instantaneous recordings of the fluoroscopic image. The features which make the spotfilm device unique are:

(a) A fluorescent screen. The characteristics of the screen are discussed in the chapter on fluoroscopy.

(b) A scattered radiation grid (stationary or moving), which can be moved in or out of the exposure field during fluoroscopy and radiography, to improve the contrast of the image.

(c) A cassette receptacle to accommodate various sizes of cassettes.

(d) Lead masks which divide or "split" the film so that a number of views can be obtained on a single film. Dividing the film in this manner is referred to as *cassette programming.* Various formats of programming are usually indicated on the spotfilm device or at the control panel if the unit is a remote-controlled one. Cassette programming is such that no further exposures occur when the program is completed, a feature which protects the patient from unnecessary radiation.

(e) A compression cone fitted to the undersurface of the spotfilm device. This allows the radiologist to palpate the patient during the examination without having to place his hand directly into the radiation field.

(f) An associated complex electronic circuit which has a twofold purpose:

(1) It controls all movements of the spotfilm device.

(2) It allows for switch-over from fluoroscopy to radiography.

(g) Lead-lined drapes which hang from the unit to protect the operator from scattered radiation arising from the patient.

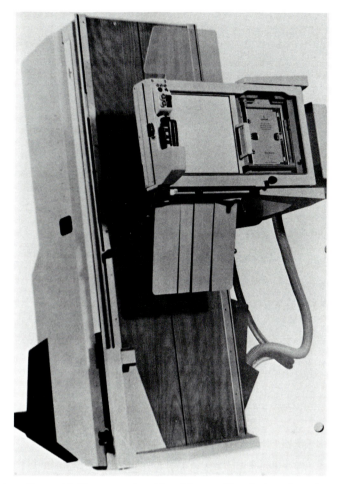

Figure 3:7. A radiographic/fluoroscopic table with spot film device, featuring a fluorescent screen for direct viewing (courtesy of the Siemens Corporation).

When the radiologist makes an exposure for radiographic recording, several events occur automatically:

(a) The cassette (which is out of the exposure field during fluoroscopy) is introduced into the exposure field.

(b) Fluoroscopy is terminated.

(c) Recording is done by conventional radiographic methods. This means that the anode of the undertable tube is brought up to fullspeed of rotation, the filament current (undertable tube) is increased for radiography, and the focal spot size changes because of the high exposure values used in radiography. All these changes occur in about 0.8 seconds.

Figure 3:7 shows a radiographic table with spotfilm device and fluorescent screen for direct viewing of the fluoroscopic image.

Movements of the Spotfilm Device

The spotfilm device is coupled to the undertable x-ray tube. The distance between the tabletop and the spotfilm device is variable (18 cm-53.5 cm) to accommodate various patient sizes and to allow the radiologist to apply compression during certain fluoroscopic procedures. The distance between the undertable tube and the tabletop is fixed and usually ranges from 38 cm to 51 cm. This distance is significant from the point of view of patient dose. In this regard, various radiation protection agencies have made recommendations with respect to minimum target-skin distances during fluoroscopy.

The spotfilm device can also move along the length and across the width of the table. These movements are all motorized and contribute to the ease with which the patient can be examined during fluoroscopy.

Collimation

An interesting feature of R-F tables is collimation of the primary beam during fluoroscopy. Limiting the beam to the region of interest is achieved by an arrangement of diaphragms which are positioned either close to the undertable tube port or close to the underside of the table. Both manual and automatic adjustment of the diaphragms are possible. Figure 3:8 illustrates the technique of collimation during fluoroscopy.

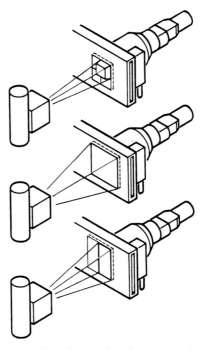

Figure 3:8. The technique of collimation during fluoroscopy for different spot exposures (courtesy of the Siemens Corporation).

Spotfilm Device with Image Intensifier Tube

The introduction of x-ray image intensification techniques (brightening of the fluoroscopic image) has eliminated the method of direct observation of the fluorescent screen. An image intensifier tube is positioned in place of the original fluorescent screen on the spotfilm device as seen in Figure 3:9. The intensified image is picked up by a television camera tube and the signal is transmitted to a television monitor for viewing.

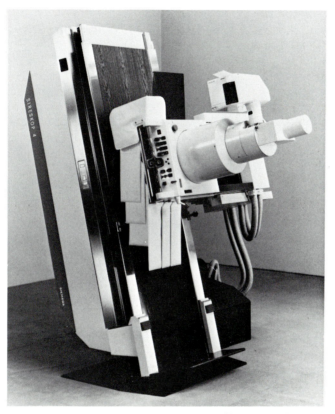

Figure 3:9. A radiographic/fluoroscopic table with spot film device, featuring an image intensifier tube (courtesy of the Siemens Corporation).

Overhead Fluoroscopy

Another method of fluoroscopy, *overhead fluoroscopy*, is available in some radiology departments. This method has eliminated the need for an undertable x-ray tube and the spotfilm device.

The technique makes use of the overhead x-ray tube and the Bucky diaphragm. The x-ray image intensifier tube is now positioned under the table. During fluoroscopy, the film is out of the exposure field. For radiographic recording the film is brought over the image intensifier (exposure field) and the

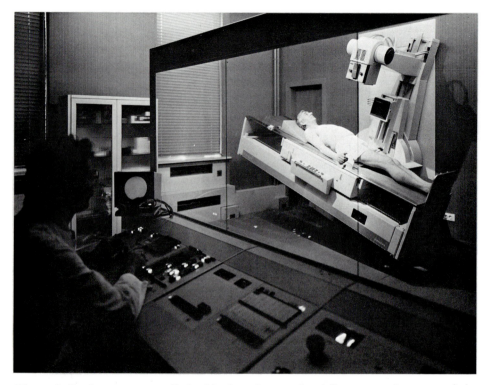

Figure 3:10. A remote-controlled table featuring overhead-fluoroscopy (courtesy of the Siemens Corporation).

exposure is then made. A remote-controlled overhead fluoroscopic x-ray table is seen in Figure 3:10.

A disadvantage of overhead fluoroscopy is that of increased scattered radiation doses compared to undercouch fluoroscopy. In this regard, personnel must remain in the control booth during fluoroscopy.

SPECIAL TABLES

There are several specialized x-ray tables available today. These include tomographic tables, urologic tables, tables used in the operating room and those used in computed tomography and angiography. Tables for computed tomography and angiography will be identified in subsequent chapters. Figure 3:11 identifies a tomographic table, two urologic tables and a table for use in computed tomography.

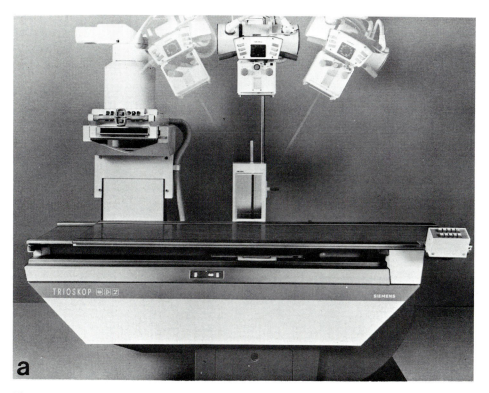

Figure 3:11. Three other types of radiographic tables (a) a tomographic table with radiographic/fluoroscopic capabilities, (b) a urologic table, and (c) a table for computed tomography. (courtesy of the Siemens Corporation).

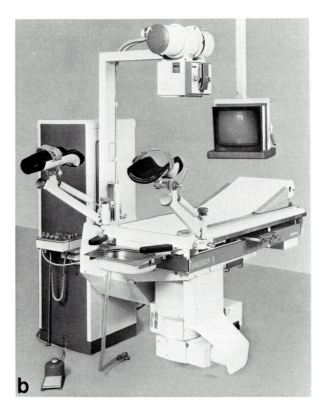

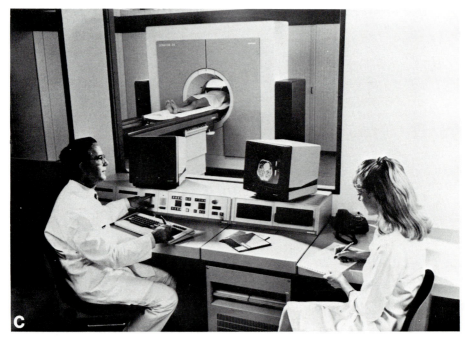

X-RAY TUBE SUPPORTS

The purpose of a tube support system is twofold:

(a) to support the weight of the x-ray tubehead.
(b) to facilitate easy maneuverability of the tubehead during radiography and fluoroscopy.

An x-ray tube support system is designed so that it is free of vibrations, safe with respect to electrical and mechanical hazards, and provides all possible movements of the tubehead. The movements must be smooth and controlled by locking mechanisms.

A typical tube support (Figure 3:12) consists of the following:

(a) A *central column* which is the main weight-supporting structure.
(b) A *crossarm*. This is attached to the central column. The x-ray tube is mounted on the crossarm.
(c) A *counterbalanced* system which ensures that the x-ray tube remains suspended (fixed) when locking or braking devices are not in use.
(d) Mechanical or electromagnetic locks.

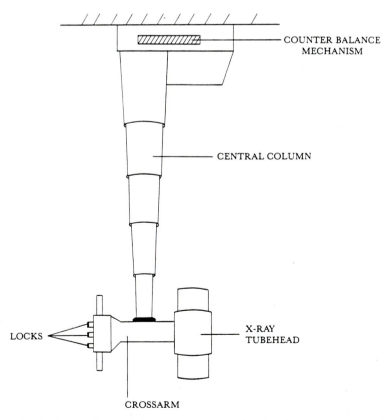

Figure 3:12. A typical x-ray tube support system, showing the main components.

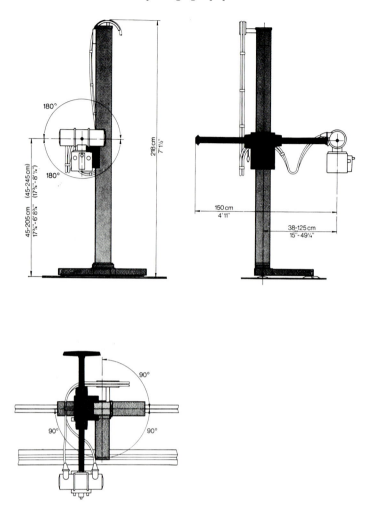

Figure 3:13. The floor tube support system. (courtesy of the Siemens Corporation).

Types of Tube Supports

There are several types of tube supports, but only the more common ones will be described here. These include the floor support, floor-to-ceiling support, and the ceiling-suspended support.

The characteristic features of the *floor support* or stand are a main supporting central column mounted on a T-support base, which is affixed onto a rail system on the floor, and a telescoping crossarm which supports the x-ray tube. The column is pivot-bearing, and this allows the whole unit to rotate through 270° with stop locations at every 90°. This support is illustrated in Figure 3:13.

The *floor-to-ceiling* support system shown in Figure 3:14 involves a slight modification of the floor stand, in that the main supporting column extends to

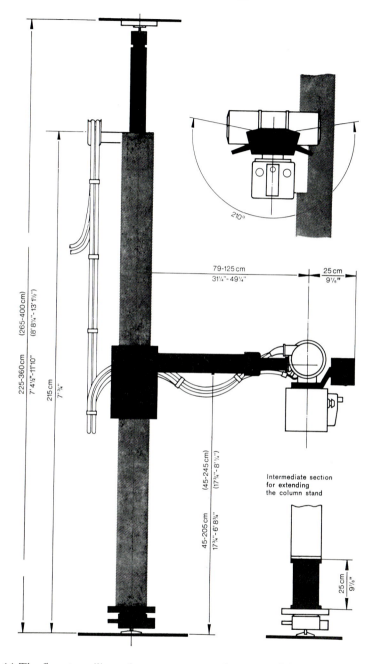

Figure 3:14. The floor-to-ceiling tube support system (courtesy of the Siemens Corporation).

fit onto rails mounted on the ceiling and the floor. The column is pivot-bearing to permit rotation of the tube and crossarm through 270° with stop locations at every 90°. The crossarm is also a telescoping column like the floor-support crossarm.

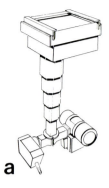

a

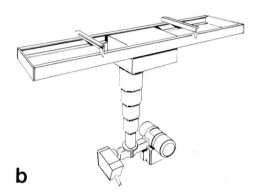

b

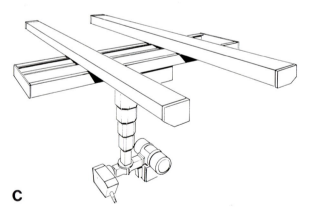

c

Figure 3:15. The basic design of the ceiling-suspended tube support system allows tube movement in almost any direction (courtesy of the Siemens Corporation).

The *ceiling-suspended* tube support is perhaps the most versatile system, in that it permits tube movements in almost any direction in the x-ray room (Figure 3:15). Sturdy rails are attached to the ceiling with transverse bridges affixed to these rails. The telescoping central column alters the source-to-image distance and the crossarm allows the tube to rotate through 360° (Figure 3:16).

The cross-arm of the tube shield can be swivelled about the vertical axis of the telescopic column by +180 / −170° = 350° in a horizontal plane. Moreover, the tube shield can be rotated about a horizontal axis up to ± 130° = 260°.

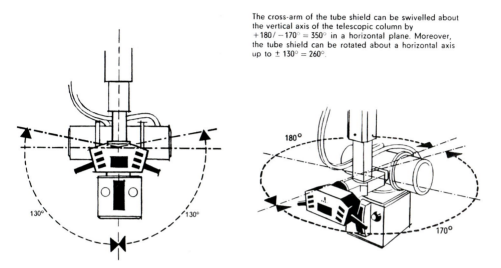

Figure 3:16. Various movements afforded by the cross-arm of the ceiling-suspended tube support (courtesy of the Siemens Corporation).

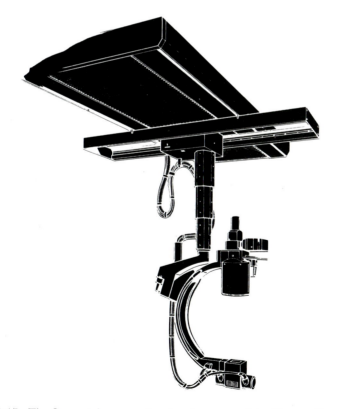

Figure 3:17. The C-arm tube support system (courtesy of the Siemens Corporation).

Another tube support system is one used in mobile x-ray image intensifier fluoroscopy units for use in the operating room. The *C-arm* support, as it is referred to, usually supports the x-ray tube and image intensifier tube (for mobile C-arm units). The C-arm support system shown in Figure 3:17 features a

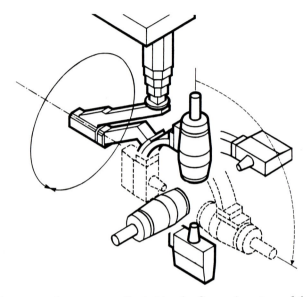

Figure 3:18. The range of movement afforded by the C-arm (courtesy of the Siemens Corporation).

ceiling-mounted telescoping column with a C-arm. A combination of mechanical and electromagnetic locks secures the unit in its appropriate position. The range of movement afforded by the support system is shown in Figure 3:18.

Tube Movements

The efficiency and versatility of a tube support are related to several factors, including the different kinds of movement afforded by the system. Essentially, there are four tube movements that are of importance to the technologist.

LONGITUDINAL. This indicates that the tube travels in the horizontal plane along the length and across the width of the tube.

VERTICAL. This movement describes the x-ray tube travel in the vertical plane, thus varying the source-to-image distance for overhead radiography and for adjusting the centering point for upright views of a patient.

TRANSVERSAL. This motion implies that the tube moves diagonally across the table or across the x-ray room.

ROTATIONAL. Rotation of the tube is possible in both horizontal and vertical planes. In the horizontal plane, both crossarm and tube can rotate through

360°. In the vertical plane, however, only the tube rotates through various degrees. Precise rotation of the tube is extremely important for *angled beam techniques*.

Locking Mechanisms

All movements of the x-ray tube and support systems are controlled by locking mechanisms which can be either *mechanical* or *electromagnetic* in design. Mechanical locks are simple in operation and are found on some x-ray equipment. Electromagnetic locks include the use of a special electrical circuit and are based on the principle of electromagnetic induction. These locks are operated by push-button or throw-type switches usually found on the control arm of the tubehead.

SAFETY MECHANISMS

If an x-ray tube were to fall on a patient during an examination, the consequences can be very severe. Safety mechanisms are always incorporated into a tube support system to eliminate this hazard. In Figure 3:19, one type of "fail-safe" mechanism is shown. The normal suspension cable pulls against the pressure created by the spring, and this in turn causes the collar to remain parallel to the crossarm. If the cable breaks, the downward force of the crossarm (caused by the weight of the x-ray tube) and the upward force (created by the spring) result in a breaking action. The counterweight imparts stability to the whole system.

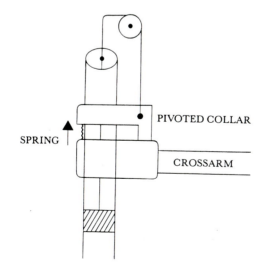

Figure 3:19. A fail-safe mechanism characteristic of a tube support system (from *X-ray Equipment for Student Radiographers*. Chesney, D.N. and Chesney, M.O. Blackwell Scientific Publications Oxford 1971).

Ceiling-suspended tube support systems have fail-safe mechanisms which incorporate safety cables in their telescoping central columns. When the electromagnetic lock is not activated, the weight of the x-ray tube is counterbalanced by the tension on the spring.

The x-ray table and tube support are two pieces of the equipment which are constantly used by the technologist during an examination. Careful and wise use of the equipment will therefore ensure speed, accuracy and safety for both the patient and the technologist.

SUMMARY

1. The chapter presents essential features of x-ray tables and tube supports that are of importance to the technologist.
2. Two types of tables are described: the radiographic and the radiographic-fluoroscopic tables.
3. The radiographic table is a standard table on which examinations can be done with or without a Bucky diaphram, in conjunction with an x-ray tube position over the tabletop.
4. Two types of radiographic tables include those which are fixed in the horizontal plane and those which can tilt from the horizontal plane to the vertical plane.
5. X-ray tabletops are made of a radiolucent material such as plastic and Bakelite. Tabletops can be classified as fixed, moving and floating.
6. The floating tabletop implies that the top can be moved in any direction, thus making it easier to position the patient compared to fixed and moving tops.
7. A characteristic feature of tables is the Bucky diaphragm or assembly. The assembly consists of a tray to hold the cassette, a grid, and a circuit to move the grid. The Bucky is used when thick parts are x-rayed. Its purpose is to improve the contrast of the image by absorbing scattered rays from the patient.
8. Added accessories for radiographic tables include a foot support, shoulder pads, head support, handgrips and a compression band.
9. A radiographic-fluoroscopic table implies that both radiography and fluoroscopy can be carried out on the table. It has all the features of a radiographic table but consists of two x-ray tubes: one for radiography and the other (usually mounted under the table) for fluoroscopy.
10. A characteristic feature of a radiographic-fluoroscopic table is the spotfilm device. This device allows the radiologist to make instantaneous recordings of the images displayed on a television screen. Several elements of the spotfilm are also discussed.

11. Most spotfilm devices today feature an image intensifier tube in place of the convential fluoroscopic screen. This method reduces the radiation dose in fluoroscopy.

12. The technique of overhead fluoroscopy makes use of the overhead tube and the Bucky diaphragm (radiography) and therefore eliminates the need for a spotfilm device and undertable x-ray tube.

13. The x-ray tube support or stand holds the x-ray tubehead and provides for easy movement of the tubehead during a procedure.

14. The main features of a tube support are its central column, crossarm, counterbalanced mechanism and locks.

15. Tube supports are of several types and only the main features of the floor support, floor-to-ceiling and ceiling-suspended supports are described.

16. Movements afforded by tube supports include longitudinal, vertical, transversal and rotational.

17. Tube supports incorporate "fail-safe" mechanisms to ensure that x-ray tubes do not fall on patients in the event of failure of the counterbalanced mechanism.

CHAPTER 4

X-RAY EXPOSURE TIMERS

ONE of the parameters which influences radiographic density in clinical x-ray imaging is the exposure time. All x-ray machines are provided with exposure timers, and, therefore, it is mandatory that the technologist have a firm understanding of the principles of the timer. Such principles will not only allow the technologist to use the timer to its full potential but will also provide him/her with a further understanding of the limitations imposed by each type of timer.

The position of the timer and its associated circuit is shown in Figure 4:1. Two points should be noted in this regard:

(a) Since the timer is located on the control panel, it is maintained at a low voltage to reduce the danger of electrical shock.

(b) The circuit of the timer is such that it makes a connection or forms a "bridge" with the kVp control and the primary of the high-voltage transformer which provides the kVp for the x-ray tube.

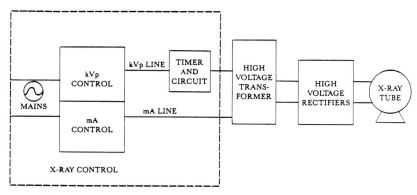

Figure 4:1. Simplified block diagram of an x-ray machine indicating the position of the x-ray exposure timer. The timer is located on the x-ray control panel and it forms a bridge with the kVp control and the high voltage transformer. The autotransformer is not shown in the figure.

PURPOSE OF THE TIMER

The primary purpose of the timer is to determine the duration of the x-ray exposure (or "beam-on" time) by terminating the high voltage supplied to the x-ray tube. In terminating the exposure, *relays* and *contacts* are used to function essentially as switches.

TYPES OF TIMERS

X-ray exposure timers range from simple and inexpensive devices to complex, expensive electronic circuitry. They include the clockwork timer, the electromagnetic synchronous timer, the electronic timer, the mAs timer and the automatic timer. Since electronic and automatic timers are more popular in imaging departments, they will be described in some detail in this chapter.

Clockwork Timers

Clockwork timers were used in the past on low-powered x-ray units. The timing is based on the principle of a clockwork mechanism. The mechanism is such that a dial (calibrated in seconds) is used to apply tension on a spring. When the exposure occurs, the tension is released and the dial unwinds to its original starting point: the zero position. The time taken for this action is the exposure time.

Clockwork timers can provide exposure times as short as 0.25 seconds, and, therefore, their use in clinical imaging is restricted only to certain examinations. Today, these timers are obsolete.

Electromagnetic Synchronous Timers

Electromagnetic synchronous timers were also used in the past and they have become obsolete in modern imaging.

The timer consists of an electric motor which works in synchronization with the frequency of the mains supply (60 Hz). The synchronous motor, as it is often called, is always running when the x-ray unit is turned on. A pointer (which rotates between two points corresponding to various time intervals) is engaged to the motor during the exposure through an electromagnetic clutch. This action causes the pointer to rotate back to its starting position which represents zero time.

The minimum exposure time offered by this type of timer is one sixtieth sec.

Electronic Timers

The *electronic timer* used in x-ray imaging is a more complex timer than the previous two timers just described. It is primarily designed to give very short exposure times for use in a variety of examinations, particularly those in which functional dynamics are important.

The three most essential components of an electronic timer are : a capacitor, a variable resistor and a suitable device to terminate the x-ray exposure. This is illustrated in Figure 4:2.

Principles of Operation

The operation of an electronic timer requires that the capacitor be charged to a certain critical value through the variable resistor. The time (*t*) taken for the capacitor to charge up (to the critical value) is proportional to the product of the resistance (*R*) of the resistor and the capacitance (*C*) of the capacitor. The smaller the value of R, the shorter is the exposure time.

When the capacitor is being charged or discharged, it follows an exponential curve. The product RC is called the *time constant* of the circuit. In fact, it is

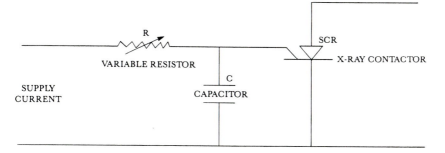

Figure 4:2. Typical arrangement of the essential components of an electronic timer. Shown here are a variable resistor (rheostat), a capacitor and a silicon-controlled rectifier (switching device). The silicon-controlled rectifier functions to terminate the x-ray exposure. Only a basic representation is shown here and therefore the diagram is not totally accurate.

the time taken for the capacitor to become about two-thirds charged. In cases where the proportionality constant is not known, problems must be solved by taking ratios, where

$$\frac{t_2}{t_1} = \frac{R_2 C}{R_1 C} = \frac{R_2}{R_1} \text{ (for a particular capacitor).}$$

Hence, one must know one value of t corresponding to one value of R.

When a capacitor has been charged up to a critical voltage (say 200 volts), an electromagnetic relay opens a contact to terminate the exposure.

In the past the relay was triggered by a thyratron (a gas-filled three-electrode valve tube). Today, solid-state devices such as a *silicon-controlled rectifier* (SCR-DC device) or a *Triax* (an AC-SCR) are used.

When a technologist makes an exposure using the electronic timer, the following events occur:

(a) The capacitor begins to charge up.
(b) At the same time (during activation of the exposure switch), the SCR is turned on and the exposure commences.
(c) When the capacitor acquires a certain critical voltage, the SCR device is turned off, hence terminating the exposure.

The circuitry for the electronic timer is complex and is not within the scope of this text. Electronic timers are very accurate and provide very short exposure times (as short as one millisecond).

Because of the time required for the high-voltage cables to lose their charge and the hysteresis current in the high-voltage transformer, the primary contactor is limited in time to 0.002 second. Therefore, *grid-controlled switching* must be used if very short exposure times are required.

Electronic timers are suitable for use in angiography and other special procedures, as well as in examinations where patient motion (voluntary and involuntary) poses a problem.

The mAs Timer

The *mAs timer* is a special electronic timer. The mA (x-ray tube current) is integrated into a capacitor such that it (capacitor) acquires a certain charge. Once the capacitor reaches this charge, the exposure terminates. The time taken for the capacitor to charge up is the exposure time.

The mAs for an examination is selected by the technologist at the control panel. However, since the mA is used in the process of charging the capacitor, the timing mechanism is positioned in the high-voltage section of the x-ray machine.

The mAs timer can provide very short exposure times using the highest mA (within the safe limits of the tube) for any value of mAs selected by the technologist.

These timers are still being used on some x-ray machines.

AUTOMATIC TIMERS

The idea of *automatic timing* in x-ray imaging was proposed as early as 1929 by Franke, but it was not developed until recently because of technical limitations.

The automatic timer consists of several components which act to convert the x-ray beam into electrical signals. These signals in turn act on a timer circuit in the x-ray generator to terminate the exposure at the appropriate time, when sufficient radiation has reached the film to produce the proper film density.

Types of Automatic Timers

There are two types of automatic exposure timers available in x-ray imaging:

(a) Those which use a photocell or a photomultiplier tube and are based on the principle of fluorescence. These are referred to as *phototimers*.

(b) Those which use an ionization chamber and are based on the principle of ionization. These are referred to as *ionization timers*.

Phototimers

A phototimer consists of a fluorescent screen which converts x-rays to light (Figure 4:3). The light is appropriately directed to a phototube (photocell) or a photomultiplier (PM) tube. Since the PM tube is a more recent development, it will be described here. The use of this tube (PM tube) eliminates the need for amplifier circuits which are necessary when the phototube in used.

The PM tube consists of a photocathode which converts the light from the

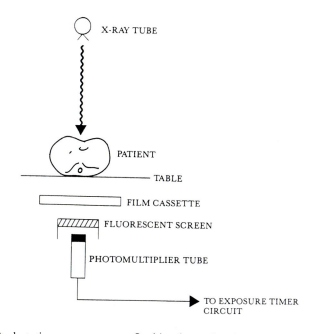

Figure 4:3. A phototimer arrangement. In this scheme the photomultiplier tube is positioned behind the cassette (*exit detector*) although in some units, the tube is positioned in front of the cassette (*entrance detector*). The current from the photomultiplier tube is used to charge a capacitor through a variable resistor. This scheme has been kept simple on purpose to maintain clarity.

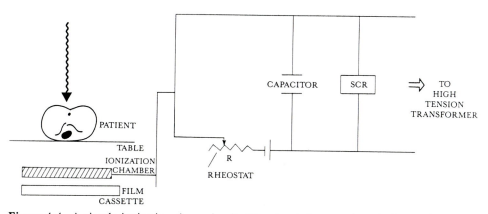

Figure 4:4. A simple ionization timer circuit. The circuit is somewhat similar to the electronic timer in that the current from the ionization chamber is used to charge the capacitor through the rheostat. See text for further explanation.

fluorescent screen (which may be positioned in front of the cassette or behind it) into electrons. These electrons are multiplied in the tube itself by a series of dynodes. The important point here is that the number of electrons is directly proportional to the incident light on the photocathode.

The current resulting from the PM tube is used to operate a timing circuit (Figure 4:3) in the x-ray generator. The circuit is similar to the electronic timer circuit, in that it contains a capacitor, a variable resistor (rheostat), and SCR device and an electromagnetic switch.

The current from the PM tube is used to charge the capacitor through the variable resistor. When the capacitor reaches a certain preselected value, the SCR device conducts and opens the x-ray exposure contacts, thus terminating the exposure. The SCR device will always conduct when the same accumulated quantity of light has reached the photocathode, that is, when the proper amount of radiation has reached the film.

The charge on the capacitor determines the film density which is normally selected by the radiologist during installation of the timer. The density is not fixed but can be altered by varying the resistance in the circuit. This can be done by the technologist at the control panel.

In high-powered x-ray generators (three-phase generators), the phototimer is generally used in conjunction with a technique referred to as *forced extinction* or *millisecond termination* (to open the switch). This allows the timer to stop the exposure much more accurately and to provide exposures as short as two to four milliseconds. This capability permits the technologist to select high mA and/or kVp for examinations in which motion unsharpness is a problem.

Timers which operate without forced extinction can provide consistent film densities only if the mA and kVp factors are set to require exposure times longer than twenty to thirty milliseconds, for three-phase equipment.

In imaging departments where faster screen speeds (rare-earth screens) are used, accurate phototiming (even with forced extinction) will occur only if the exposure times are longer than two to four milliseconds.

Ionization Timers

The basis of an *ionization timer* is an ionization chamber which contains a volume of air between two metal electrodes. The volume of air is referred to as *measuring fields* or *detector fields*.

The chamber is usually a flat parallel-plate ionization chamber which is radiolucent and therefore it is positioned in front of the image receptor (film cassette) and behind the scattered radiation grid.

Principles of Operation

The principle of the ionization timer is illustrated in Figure 4:4. When transmitted x-rays pass through the chamber, an ionization current is produced which is proportional to the intensity of radiation incident on the film. This current is used to charge a capacitor (*C*) in the timing circuit through a variable resistor (*R*) to a preselected value. Once this value is reached, the SCR device conducts and opens the exposure contacts, thus terminating the exposure.

Measuring Fields and the Dominant

Automatic exposure timers may have one or more measuring fields arranged in a variety of ways.

In general, there are three types of fields which allow the technologist the freedom to choose fields suitable to the particular examination. These fields include a single, double or triple area of sensitivity. Of these three, the three-field automatic timer is the most popular.

The Single-Field Automatic Timer

The *single-field* automatic timer has one area of sensitivity positioned in the center of the unit. It is designed primarily for use in fluoroscopy with the spot-film device, since small film sizes (24 × 34 cm or 18 × 24 cm) are generally used.

The Two-Field Automatic Timer

The two-field automatic timer consists of a large and small area of sensitivity. The use of these fields is dependent on the primary structure of interest rather than the size of the film.

The primary structure of interest in the context of automatic exposure timing is called the *dominant*. For example, in a routine chest examination the dominant represents the lung fields.

In using the two-field automatic timer the small field is usually selected for a small dominant such as the cervical spine. On the other hand, the large field is chosen for a large dominant such as the stomach in an upper gastrointestinal examination or the colon in a barium enema examination. In the latter two examinations, it is advisable to use the large field even if smaller film sizes (24 × 30 cm) are used. With smaller film sizes (18 × 24 cm), the small field should always be used.

The Three-field Automatic Timer

This is the most widely used automatic timer. The position of the three fields is shown in Figure 4:5. Depending on the examination and the dominant, a single field or all three fields may be used. For example, the two outer fields are selected for routine chest examinations and the middle field is selected for examinations of the spinal column.

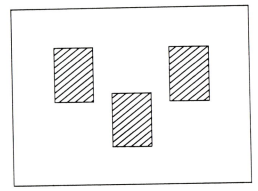

Figure 4:5. Typical arrangement of a three-field selector of an automatic exposure timer. See text for further explanation.

Density Selection

At the time of installation of the automatic exposure timer, adjustments are made to the timing circuit to produce a film density (normal setting) chosen by the radiologist.

In certain cases (such as patient pathology, a change in film/screen combination, and so on), the technologist may have to alter the density to produce films of density comparable to the normal density. This change in density can be made through the *density selector* located on the control panel.

In general, the density selector is set at the normal (usually denoted by N on most machines) indicator. The density may be selected as +1 or +2 and –1 or –2 by moving the selector to these settings. The settings will provide a 50 percent (+1) and a 100 percent (+2) increase in mAs and a 25 percent (–1) and a 50 percent (–2) decrease in mAs. Other machines may be programmed to provide different values of mAs.

In altering the density setting through the density selector, the technologist changes the reference voltage for a special circuit called a comparator circuit. Each position on the density selector (that is, normal, +1, +2, –1, –2) has a certain voltage value, referred to as a fixed voltage reference, in the comparator circuit.

The Concept of Back-Up Time

Automatic exposure timers incorporate a mechanism in the circuit which acts as a safety factor. This is the *back-up time* or *back-up mAs*. It is the time or mAs limit that cannot be exceeded for any exposure setting.

The kVp and mA selected by the technologist will influence the exposure time. If safe times are not observed, the maximum tube loading may be exceeded and will damage the x-ray tube.

The automatic timer can only operate within certain time limits. Whenever the timer is used, a pre-adjusted maximum time is selected for the examination, and if the actual exposure time (once the radiation has passed through the object) is too short, then the film density will be lighter (than the normal density). The film will be underexposed. In this case the timer has reached the *upper time limit* (back-up time), and usually an audible tone is sounded and the exposure is terminated (due to x-ray tube limit). The film still requires more radiation to meet the desired density and therefore it appears underexposed.

Minimum Response Time

On the other hand, if high technical factors (kVp and/or mA) are selected for a thin body part (which attenuates very little radiation), for example, the exposure time may be shorter than the *lower time limit* of the automatic timer. This lower time limit is the *minimum response time* which is defined as the shortest time permissible by the timer. For some units the minimum response time is about 1 millisecond or less. If the minimum response time is reached for a particular exposure, the film is darker than the normal density since the timer will not terminate the exposure fast enough. The actual exposure time is shorter than the minimum response time.

Practical Considerations in Using Automatic Timers

It is important to realize that a number of factors must be carefully considered for successful use of the automatic timer. If programming the kVp, mA, focal spot size, collimation and so on is required by the technologist, then the following must be observed:

(a) *Proper selection of kVp, mA and focal spot size.* In general, high mA values (short exposure times) are appropriate when motion is a problem. In the absence of motion problems, lower mA values with small focal spot are preferable. High kVp techniques are selected for barium examinations and in cases where high grid ratios (16:1) are used.

(b) *Source-to-image distance (SID).* If the distance is altered during the examination, the density will not be affected. The technologist must, however, pay attention to the exposure time, magnification and definition factors.

(c) *Contrast Considerations.* The contrast scale may be changed by the technologist. If the original kVp is lowered, the exposure time will be twice as long as the original technique. For example, if the kVp is lowered from 80 to 70, from 70 to 60 and from 60 to 55, the exposure time will be about two times as long than the original technique. On the other hand, if the kVp is increased (say from 80 to 95, 90 to 105 and from 100 to 120), the exposure time will be about one-half that obtained with the original technique.

(d) *Collimation (field size).* The small field (two-field timer) or the center field (three-field timer) is always selected for a field size of 18 × 24 cm or smaller.

(e) *Anatomical region and field selection.* The anatomical region (dominant) must be properly positioned and aligned over the appropriate field of the timer for optimum results. In general, with a three-field automatic timer, the center field is used for the spinal column, skull, shoulder, hip, knee and so on. For larger areas requiring larger film sizes such as a 35 × 43 cm, a combination of two or all three fields may be selected for regions such as the abdomen, pelvis, chest, stomach and small and large bowel.

It is important to note that on some units employing automatic exposure timing, the mA selection is not required by the technologist; only the kVp and focal spot size are usually selected. In other units which are based on the *anatomically programmed radiography* (APR) concept, all factors including mA, kVp, focal spot size and the measuring field are selected automatically when the region is selected by the technologist at the control panel. This allows the technologist more time to position the patient accurately over the appropriate measuring field.

Advantages of Automatic Timing

Automatic exposure timing is gaining widespread use in present-day imaging trends, especially in general radiography and fluoroscopy. Automatic exposure timing ensures:

(a) Radiographs of consistent density, regardless of patient size and thickness.

(b) Reduced patient dosage since exposures are correct most of the time.

(c) An increase in workload since there is no need for unnecessary repeats due to incorrect exposures.

(d) Automatic compensation for exposure values if the source-to-image receptor distance changes.

(e) Applications in other radiographic techniques such as in mammography, tomography, mobile radiography and so on.

TESTING EXPOSURE TIMERS

In some instances exposure timers may function inaccurately and it is therefore mandatory to perform certain tests to check the accuracy of these timers. A number of tests are available and they range from simple procedures that may be carried out by the technologist, to more complex tests usually performed by the clinical engineering department or the x-ray service engineer.

The type of test procedure for a specific timer will depend on the power requirements of the x-ray unit (single- or three-phase power), type of rectification circuit and so on.

Single-Phase X-ray Machines

The Spinning Top Test

For timers which operate on single-phase power, the *spinning top test* is ideal to check the accuracy of the timer, since the radiation is produced in pulses. For half-wave and full-wave rectified units, the voltage waveform is essentially similar except for their *pulsation frequency* (number of pulses per second).

In half-wave rectification, the pulsation frequency is 60 cycles per second, whereas the number of pulses produced per second is 120 for full-wave rectification.

The device used to check these timers is the *spinning top*. This is shown in Figure 4:6. It consists of a metal disk (usually brass) which can be made to spin manually since it rests on a brass base by a spindle at its center. Located at the periphery of the disk is a single hole.

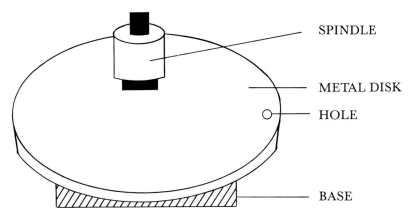

SPINDLE

METAL DISK

HOLE

BASE

Figure 4:6. Schematic representation of a spinning top used to test the accuracy of x-ray exposure timers for single-phase machines.

In performing the test procedure, the top is placed on an unexposed film, exposure factors are selected with a short exposure time (say one tenth sec), the top is set spinning and the exposure is made. When the film is processed, a series of dots appear on the film. Each dot represents a pulse. If the exposure timer is functioning correctly, the number of dots is given by the following relationship:

Number of dots (pulses) = pulsation frequency × exposure time

The spinning top test is not suitable for exposure times shorter than 0.25 second since the dots are too close together, which makes it difficult to count.

The following examples will clarify this situation.

Example 1

An x-ray technologist uses the spinning top test on a half-wave rectified unit (single-phase power) to check the accuracy of the exposure timer. The exposure factors are set at 100 mA, one fifteenth sec, and 75 kVp. If the timer is accurate, how many dots will appear on the film?

Solution

The pulsation frequency is 60 pulses per sec for a half-wave rectified x-ray machine

$$\text{Number of dots} = \text{pulsation frequency} \times \text{exposure time}$$

$$= 60 \text{ pulses/sec} \times \frac{1}{15} \text{ Sec}$$

$$= 4$$

Therefore, 4 dots are seen on the film and this indicates that the timer is accurate.

Example 2

Exposure factors of 100 mA, 80 kVp and 0.1 sec are selected on a single-phase full-wave rectified x-ray machine. If the timer is functioning correctly, how many dots should appear on the film?

Solution

The pulsation frequency is 120 pulses/sec.

$$\text{Number of dots} = \text{pulsation frequency} \times \text{exposure time}$$

$$= 120 \times \frac{1}{10}$$

$$= 12 \text{ dots}$$

If more or less than 12 dots appear on the film, this would indicate that the timer is inaccurate.

The spinning top may also indicate whether the high tension rectifiers are malfunctioning. The technologist may conduct this test if he/she observes that there is a decrease in the mA or mAs readings after the machine has been used for a period of time for examinations of the same body part.

When rectifiers fail, the voltage waveform of the x-ray tube (hence the pulsation density) changes. The procedural setup for this test is similar to that of checking the timer. A variation in density of the dots is a good indication of rectifier failure. In this case, the technologist should consult the x-ray service engineer.

Three-Phase X-ray Machines

Other Tests

The spinning top test cannot be used successfully to check the accuracy of the timer for three-phase x-ray units since these machines do not produce x-rays in pulses. A number of tests are available for three-phase equipment.

One such test involves the use of a solid-state detector (photoconductor) which is coupled to an integrated circuit. When the photoconductor is exposed to radiation, a current results. The current is subsequently displayed on an oscilloscope and the time is obtained by measuring the length of the display.

In some x-ray machines a *testpoint* is usually available in the control panel. The testpoint is designed to show the *actual length of exposure* (ALE). In this method, the oscilloscope is connected to the testpoint. The time is read off the scope during the exposure.

A third method of testing timers (also mA, kVp, and filament current) is the *high tension bleeder technique*. In this method, a special resistor divider network (Dynalizer®) is used, which is connected to the x-ray tube, the high tension transformer and an oscilloscope as shown in Figure 4:7. When the exposure is made, a waveform is displayed on the oscilloscope and the time is measured (between the amplitude of the waveform), usually at the 80 percent level. Some test units provide a digital display of the time.

On some x-ray machines a high-voltage divider is built into the machine (this eliminates the need for the Dynalizer®) and all that is necessary is to connect the oscilloscope to it.

These tests are generally conducted by the clinical engineer in the department, since the technologist is usually not trained for this type of testing.

A Simple Test to Check the Accuracy of the Automatic Timer

This test may be carried out by the technologist in conjunction with the clinical engineer.

A plastic pail full with about 18 cm of water (large enough to simulate an average-sized abdomen) is used. It is positioned over the appropriate field of the automatic timer and an exposure is made. The film is then processed and the density is checked using a densitometer. A film density of approximately

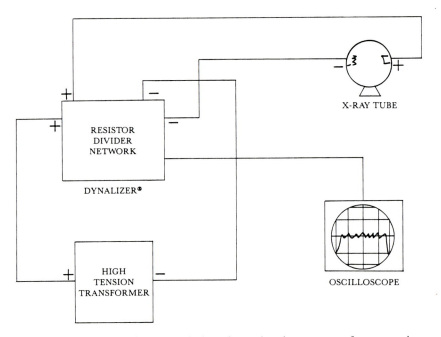

Figure 4:7. The high tension bleeder technique for testing the accuracy of exposure timers on three-phase machines. The voltage waveform is displayed on an oscilloscope and the time is measured between the amplitude of the waveform usually at the 80 percent level.

one above base fog is usually acceptable and indicates that the automatic timer is accurate. Any deviation from this reading indicating that the film is too light or too dark reflects an inaccurate timer. Therefore, it is necessary to recalibrate the timer.

SUMMARY

1. The purpose of the exposure timer in an x-ray unit is to determine the duration of the exposure by terminating the high voltage supplied to the x-ray tube.
2. The timer is maintained at a low voltage to reduce the danger of electrical shock, since it is located on the control panel.
3. There are at least five classes of x-ray exposure times. These include clockwork timers, electromagnetic synchronous timers, electronic timers, mAs timers and automatic timers.
4. Clockwork timers are based on the clockwork mechanism principle and were used in the past on low-powered x-ray machines.
5. Electromagnetic synchronous timers were also used in the past. They are obsolete in present-day imaging. They consist of an electric motor synchronized with the frequency of the AC mains supply.
6. Electronic timers are common to modern imaging. They consist of es-

sentially a capacitor, a variable resistor and a suitable device to terminate the exposure.

7. The timer works on the principle of charging the capacitor to some critical value through the variable resistor (R). The time (t) taken for the capacitor to charge up to the critical value is proportional to the capacitance (C) of the capacitor. The smaller the value of R, the shorter the exposure time.

8. The product RC is called the time constant of the circuit.

9. Electronic timers provide accurate and very short exposure times and, therefore, grid-controlled switching is used.

10. The mAs timer is a special electronic timer in which the mA is integrated into a capacitor such that it acquires a certain charge. Once this charge is reached, the exposure terminates.

11. Automatic x-ray timers convert x-ray photons into electrical signals which act on a timer circuit to terminate the exposure when sufficient radiation has reached the film to produce the proper film density.

12. Automatic timers may be phototimers or ionization timers.

13. The phototimer is made of a fluorescent screen coupled to a photomultiplier tube. The screen converts the radiation into light which is then directed into the photomultiplier tube. The tube then converts the light into electrical signals which are used to charge a capacitor through a variable resistor. When the capacitor reaches a certain preselected value, the exposure terminates, thus providing the desired film density.

14. Ionization timers make use of a chamber which contains a volume of air referred to as measuring fields or detector fields.

15. When radiation falls on the chamber, an ionization current is produced and it is used to charge a capacitor in the timing circuit to some preselected value. Once this value is reached, the exposure is terminated to give the desired film density.

16. Ionization timers may consist of one, two or three fields.

17. The film density may be controlled by a density selector which allows appropriate increase or decrease in mAs.

18. The back-up time or back-up mAs is the time or mAs limit that cannot be exceeded for any exposure setting.

19. An automatic timer may operate only with certain time limits, an upper and lower time limit. The lower time limit is the minimal response time and it is the shortest time permissible by the timer.

20. Several practical points in using automatic timers were identified. These include the proper selection of kVp, mA and focal spot size, the influence of source-to-image distance on density, contrast considerations, the effect of collimation, anatomical region and field selection.

21. The advantages of automatic timing are listed.

22. The exposure timer may be checked for accuracy through a number of tests, such as the spinning top test and the high tension bleeder technique. Each of these tests were described.

CHAPTER 5

X-RAY TUBES FOR DIAGNOSTIC IMAGING

Part One

THE x-ray tube is one of the main components in an imaging scheme, since it provides the radiation necessary to image objects. It is mandatory that technologists have a firm understanding of the design and function of the tube for two reasons. First, there are several factors which influence the safe operation of the tube, and, second, the proper use of these factors will contribute favourably to the overall life expectancy of the tube.

The x-ray tube has undergone significant changes throughout the years, with each change effecting a more efficient performance. One of the major concerns in x-ray tube design is dealing with the problem of heat production and dissipation. This chapter will trace the development of the x-ray tube and will describe the more important features of the tube rather than deal with the physics of x-ray production

BRIEF HISTORICAL NOTES

The growth and development of x-ray tubes can be traced back to 1895 when Roentgen discovered x-rays. At that time he used a *Crookes tube* (a partially evacuated glass tube) containing a small amount of gas (for conducting a

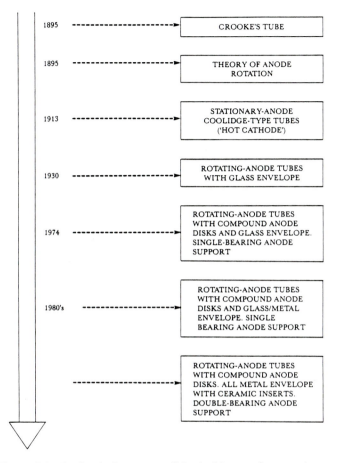

Figure 5:1. An "evolutionary trend" in the history of x-ray tubes.

current) and two electrodes, an anode (positive) and a cathode (negative).

The Crookes tube did not perform efficiently due to the absorption of gas as the temperature of the electrodes was increased and also to the penetration of ions into the glass wall. As the tube lost its volume of gas, higher voltages were required for its operation. Moreover, the tube current and voltage could not be varied independently, since the only way of increasing the current was to increase the voltage.

In 1913, Dr. Coolidge introduced the *"hot-cathode"* or *Coolidge tube* as it is sometimes called. This tube is a high-vacuum tube consisting of an electrically heated cathode from which electrons are "boiled off" and which are accelerated to a positively charged fixed anode.

Later, other tubes meeting the same design criteria as the Coolidge tube appeared on the scene and, collectively, they were referred to as *stationary-anode x-ray tubes.*

In 1897, Professor E. Thomson proposed a theory of rotating the anode as a means of increasing the amount of heat that the anode can withstand, since this was the major limitation of the stationary-anode x-ray tube. This theory led to the introduction and development of the *rotating-anode x-ray tube*. Since then, the rotating-anode x-ray tube has been the focus of attention in the further development of x-ray tube technology, primarily with respect to the anode disk and the envelope which houses the electrodes. Figure 5:1 presents a brief "evolutionary trend" in the development of x-ray tubes.

Today, the rotating-anode tube is most widely used in almost all examinations. However, the stationary-anode tube is still being used in low-powered (low output) mobile and dental x-ray units.

X-RAY TUBE REQUIREMENTS FOR IMAGING

To meet the increasing demand for optimum image quality in imaging with the least possible radiation dose to the patient, there are a nubmer of requirements with respect to the design of the x-ray tube. The tube must therefore be designed to provide:

(a) very sharp images (high definition).
(b) very short exposure times so that moving structures can be imaged without unsharpness (due to motion).
(c) specific radiation output for optimum imaging of certain structures (for example, low kVp technique to image soft tissues).
(d) repeated exposures which are necessary for rapid serial imaging.
(e) the capability of withstanding high electrical loads.
(f) rapid heat dissipation.

The remainder of this chapter will present a description of the features of the x-ray tube which play a role in meeting the above requirements.

X-ray tubes for imaging fall into two classes, the basis of which depends on the type of anode characteristic of each. They are:

(a) stationary-anode x-ray tubes.
(b) rotating-anode x-ray tubes.

Both of these tubes will now be described with emphasis on the rotating-anode x-ray tube.

THE STATIONARY-ANODE X-RAY TUBE

A stationary-anode x-ray is shown in Figure 5:2. The tube consists of two electrodes — an anode and a cathode — which are enclosed in an evacuated glass envelope.

The *cathode* is the negative electrode which consists of a *filament* from which

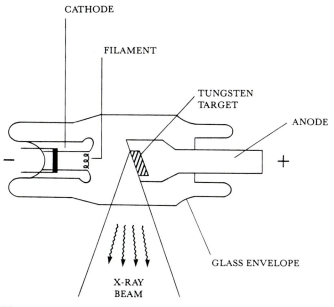

Figure 5:2. Principal features of a stationary-anode x-ray tube.

electrons are "boiled off" by the process of thermionic emission.

The *anode* is the positive electrode located at the opposite end of the tube and faces the cathode. By applying a potential difference (kV) between the anode and cathode, the electrons which are "boiled off" the filament (to be discussed under the section on rotating-anode tubes) are accelerated at high speeds across the vacuum to strike the anode. This voltage influences the intensity and spectral distribution of x-rays emerging from the tube. The voltage range used in diagnostic imaging varies from 30 to 150 kilovolts.

If this voltage is not applied to the tube, then the electrons which are emitted form a "cloud" around the filament. This cloud of electrons, called the *space-charge*, prevents the further emission of electrons.

When the voltage increases, more electrons from the cloud are directed towards the anode and this increases the tube current (mA). When the mA does not increase even although the voltage across the tube increases, a certain value is reached. This value is called the *saturation current*. However, as the tube voltage is varied, changes do occur in the mA and hence a space-charge compensator is included in the x-ray circuit to reduce the influence of tube voltage upon tube current.

A *vacuum* is necessary in the design of x-ray tubes because the presence of air in the tube will result in oxidation of the hot filament wire and a short tube life. Moreover, collisions of electrons with air molecules reduce their speed, thus affecting the quality of the x-ray beam produced. This is an important consideration, in that all x-ray tubes, during manufacture, are subject to a process referred to as *degassing*.

In the degassing process, the component parts of the tube are exposed to very high temperatures to expel any trapped air molecules. However, prolonged use may result in a *gassy* tube and this has an ultimate effect on x-ray exposure.

The Anode Structure

The first stationary-anodes were made of a solid copper block. Embedded in the face of the copper anode is a rectangular piece of metal (such as tungsten), referrred to as the *target*. The small area of the target onto which electrons are focussed is called the *focus* or *focal spot* and it is the source of the emission of x-rays.

The anode face is inclined at a small angle (the *target angle*) to the central ray of the beam as is illustrated in Figure 5:3. An effective focal area which is square and smaller than the actual focal spot is projected onto the film. The principle of inclining the anode, or using a bevelled edge, is called the *line focus principle* and it was developed by Goetze.

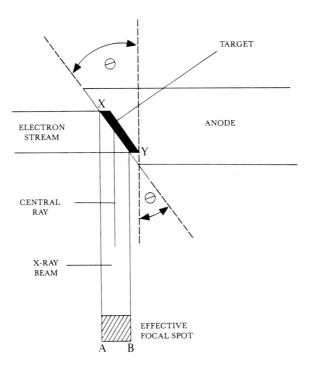

AB = XY   SINE θ

Figure 5:3. The line focus principle. The anode face is inclined at some angle θ, to the central ray of the x-ray beam.

In Figure 5:3, the relationship between the side *AB* of the effective focal spot and the length *XY* of the rectangular area on the target is given by the following:

$$AB = XY \sin\theta$$

Hence, the smaller the angle θ, the smaller the effective focal spot size.

The effective focal spot size influences the detail that can be imaged. In general, the smaller the effective focal spot size, the sharper are the images seen on the film.

In producing x-rays, about 99 percent of the electrical energy applied to the tube is transformed into heat and about less than 1 percent is converted into x-rays. The problem of heat production in the tube is of paramount importance and is one of the influencing factors in the design of the tube and, more specifically, the anode.

The materials used for anode construction must not only meet the requirements for x-ray production but must also serve as good conductors of heat. It is for these reasons (as well as others) that tungsten and copper are used in stationary-anode tubes.

Tungsten is used as a target material because it has the following properties:

(a) a high melting point (3370°C) and, therefore, it can withstand very high temperatures.

(b) a high atomic number (74). The *efficiency of x-ray production* is directly proportional to atomic number and, therefore, increases with increasing atomic number. Efficiency is given by the following relationship:

$$\text{Efficiency of x-ray production} = \frac{\text{x-ray power output}}{\text{power input}} \times 100\%$$

$$= \frac{KZIV^2}{VI} \times 100\%$$

$$= KZV \times 100\%$$

where *K* is a constant.
V is the tube potential.
I is the tube current.

(c) low vapor pressure at high temperatures. This property maintains the vacuum.

(d) high thermal conductivity. It conducts heat very rapidly.

(e) it can easily be shaped into any desired form (such as a rectangle, circle or a square).

The tungsten target is embedded in the copper block as stated earlier and the heat developed in the tungsten spreads to the copper by conduction and, therefore, it becomes very hot. Copper is used for the anode because it is one of the best conductors of heat and, therefore, it can remove heat very rapidly from the target.

Limitations of the Stationary-anode Tube

The limitations imposed by stationary-anode x-ray tubes are several and include the following:

(a) with continuous tube operation (repeated exposures), the temperature of the tungsten and copper becomes high enough to decrease the rate at which copper conducts heat. As a result, heat dissipation becomes a problem.

(b) the area of the target bombarded by electrons is limited to a small size.

(c) the *loading capacity* of the tube is limited. Loading capacity refers to the electrical load (kVp, mA and time) that the tube can withstand.

Stationary-anode Tubes for Computed Tomography

Although stationary-anode tubes are limited to low-powered mobile and dental units (low output machines), they have found application in the early generation computed tomography (CT) machines. This aspect of stationary-anode tubes is discussed further in Chapter 17 on Computed Tomography.

In essence, stationary-anode tubes can provide higher x-ray intensity for long exposure times typical of first-generation CT machines (translate-rotate scheme), compared to rotating-anode tubes. The scan times characteristic of these machines generally range from 10 seconds to several minutes.

In modern CT machines this scan time is significantly shorter and therefore precludes the use of stationary-anode tubes. For these scanners, the rotating-anode tube is used since it provides higher power (higher intensity) for short exposure times compared to stationary-anode tubes.

THE ROTATING-ANODE X-RAY TUBE

The rotating-anode x-ray tube is shown in Figure 5:4. Shown in Figure 5:4a are a cathode assembly, a rotating-anode and associated units (rotor, stator and ball bearings) which are (excluding the stator) encased in an evacuated glass envelope. The glass envelope and stator coils are both encased in what is commonly referred to as the tube housing. Also shown are the high tension cable receptacles, an exit window, oil filling and an expansion chamber. Each of these elements will now be described.

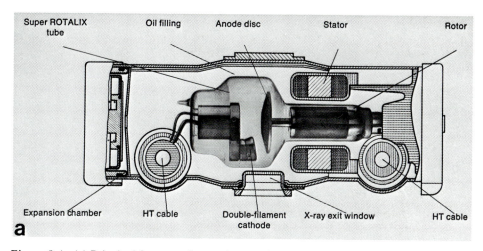

Figure 5:4. (a) Principal features of a rotating-anode x-ray tube (courtesy of Philips Medical Systems); (b) External appearance of a rotating-anode x-ray tube (courtesy of the Siemens Corporation).

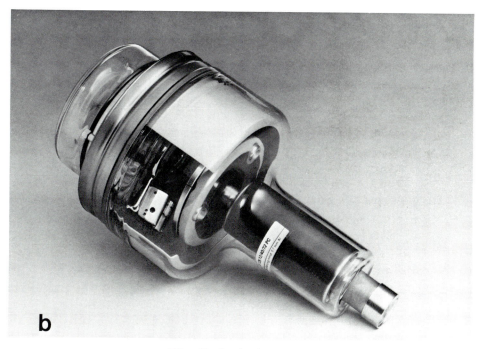

The Cathode Assembly

The *cathode assembly* consists of a filament and focussing device (cup). The filament is the source of electrons in the tube. It is made of a very thin piece of tungsten wire arranged so that it forms a helical or spiral winding to increase the surface area of the wire.

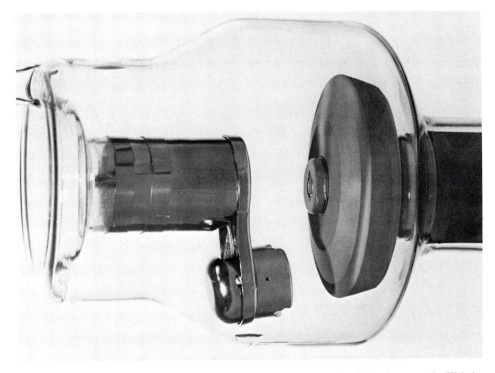

Figure 5:5. An "electronic lens" or focussing cup shown on the left of the photograph. This is sometimes referred to as a Wehnelt cylinder and it directs the electron stream to the target of the rotating anode. (courtesy of Machlett Laboratories, Inc.)

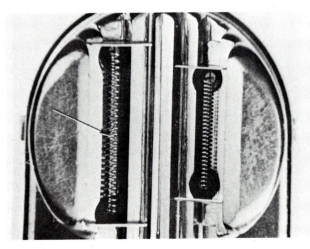

Figure 5:6. Dual filaments of an x-ray tube, positioned side-by-side. The arrow indicates a break (gap) in the large filament. Note the helical winding. (courtesy of Machlett Laboratories, Inc.)

Electrons are "boiled off" the filament when it is subjected to very high temperatures (about 2000°C). The rate at which electrons are emitted depends on the temperature and surface area of the filament. The greater the surface area and the higher the temperature applied to the filament, the greater the rate of electron emission. When electrons leave the filament, they must be directed to the target of the anode. This is accomplished by the focussing cup or *Wehnelt cylinder* which acts as an "electronic lens" (Figure 5:5).

X-ray tubes may have one filament, in which case they are referred to as *single focus tubes,* or they may have two filaments (large and small) and are, therefore, referred to as *dual focus tubes.*

The dual filaments are usually mounted side by side as shown in Figure 5:6. When dual focus tubes are used, the filament heating circuit only allows one filament to be heated. Dual focus tubes provide: (a) a choice of focal spot size, (b) higher mAs and shorter exposure times are possible with the larger filament (larger focal spot), and (c) the smaller filament (small focal spot) permits fine details to be imaged more clearly than the larger focal spot.

Prolonged use of the tube (especially with heavy exposures) may result in evaporation of the tungsten filament. Evaporation causes a metal coating to develop on the walls of the glass envelope of the tube and this results in arcing within the tube. Arcing may render the tube useless. Evaporation will reduce the diameter of the filament, which may break when there is about 10 percent decrease in diameter, thus creating a gap in the winding.

The life of pure tungsten filaments is considered adequate for tube currents below 300 mA or even 500 mA. If tube currents are increased above these values, filament life becomes an important factor in the premature failure of the tube. With an ever-increasing trend towards the use of higher mA generators, there is a need for a more efficient electron emitter. In this regard, *thoriated tungsten filaments* have become available for higher mA techniques, having been used successfully in high-vacuum, high-voltage rectifier valve tubes for several decades.

Thoriated tungsten filaments provide greater efficiency than pure tungsten filaments. This means that filament life is increased with the use of high mA values. Laboratory studies have shown that the operation of thoriated tungsten tubes at 2000 mA values is quite stable. With further research it is expected that thoriated tungsten filaments will allow operation from 3000 mA to 5000 mA levels.

The Rotating-anode Disk

The rotating anode of earlier x-ray tubes was made of a pure tungsten disk supported by a short molybdenum stem affixed to the center of the disk. The other end of the stem is usually mounted to the *rotor* (copper cylinder) of a small induction motor. Since the disk is an extremely important feature in the performance of the tube, it will be discussed in some detail under a separate section.

The Vacuum

If the x-ray tube is not completely evacuated, then electrons from the filament collide with gas molecules thereby losing some or all of their kinetic energy. The filament also deteriorates due to oxidation. The loss in energy ultimatley affects the quality of the x-ray beam emerging from the tube. To prevent these collisions, tubes are evacuated to pressures less than 10^{-5} mm Hg.

The vacuum seal is not perfect and, therefore, the tube may become "gassy" with time.

The Glass Envelope

The purpose of the glass envelope is to support the anode and cathode structures and to maintain the vacuum. The envelope is made of hard, heat-resistant glass capable of withstanding mechanical stresses and high voltages. The portion of the glass envelope where the useful x-ray beam emerges from the tube is called the *tube exit window*. The window is made much thinner than the rest of the envelope. This is necessary, since a thicker portion of glass will change the quality of the beam by attenuation.

The Tube Housing

The glass envelope (tube insert) is encased in the x-ray *tube housing* or *tube shield*. The housing has a threefold purpose:

(a) It provides mechanical support for the tube insert.
(b) It provides radiation shielding (ray-proofing).
(c) It provides electrical insulation from the high voltage applied to the tube.

The tube housing is cylindrical in shape and is made either of aluminum, an alloy of aluminum or steel. It is fitted with insulated receptacles (two) for the high tension cables which originate from the high tension transformer.

The housing also features a *tube port* to allow the passage of useful x-rays. The port is radiotransparent and is, therefore, made of glass or aluminum (in some tubes).

The housing is lined with thin sheets of lead, since the x-rays produced in the tube are scattered isotropically (in all directions).

THE ROTATING-ANODE DISK

A very brief description of the rotating-anode disk was given earlier in the chapter. In this section, a detailed account of the disk is given, since it (the disk) has undergone significant changes throughout the years.

Source-image distance, cm

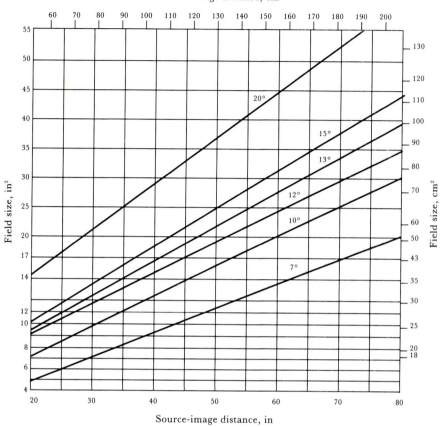

Source-image distance, in

Figure 5:7. Field coverage and source-to-image receptor distances for six different target angles. (courtesy of Machlett Laboratories, Inc.)

Diameter of the Disk

The diameter of the disk ranges from about 50 mm to 125 mm. The diameter is one of the factors which determine to maximum permissible load that the tube can withstand. The larger the disk, the greater the electrical load that can be applied to the tube.

The disks of earlier rotating anodes were made entirely of pure tungsten, since its favourable properties such as its high atomic number and good thermal and mechanical characteristics allow it to serve as an ideal target.

The Target Angle

The *target angle* is defined as the angle between the bevelled track (at the circumference of the disk) on the anode and the central ray of the x-ray beam.

This slope functions in the same manner as that of the stationary-anode tube. Target angles for rotating-anode tubes range from about 7° to 20°.

The target angle influences a number of factors which have practical implications, such as field coverage (film size or image intensifier) at specific source-to-image receptor distances and loading on the focal spot (to be discussed subsequently). The field coverage and source-to-image receptor distances for several target angles are shown in Figure 5:7.

For a given effective focal spot size, the total area of electron bombardment varies with the target angle (Figure 5:8); the smaller the angle the greater the loading. For example, the relative loading on a 15° tube is about 100 percent, compared to about 200 percent for a 7° tube. The trade-off for a given focal spot size is between coverage on the one hand and loading on the other.

Target Angle vs Loading

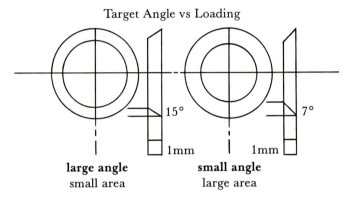

large angle
small area

small angle
large area

Figure 5:8. The effect of target angles on field coverage and tube loading. The smaller the target angle, the smaller the coverage, but the greater the loading. The trade-off for a given focal spot size is between coverage and loading. (courtesy of Machlett Laboratories, Inc.)

In general, for radiographic work at 100 cm source-to-image receptor distance using a 35 cm × 43 film, the most widely used target angle is 12°. For angiographic work with 35 cm × 35 cm film at 100 cm source-to-image receptor distance, the best angle is 10° which gives a 20 percent increase in the permissible loading with a corresponding reduction in exposure time (Machlett Laboratories Inc., 1983).

Anode Heel Effect

The target angle results in a beam distribution across the film which varies in intensity — that is, not all points on the film receive the same beam intensity. This variation in intensity of the beam is such that it (intensity) is greater at the cathode end of the tube compared to the anode end. This effect is known as the *anode heel effect*.

The Focal Spot

The *focal spot* of a rotating-anode disk is the area on the disk subject to electron bombardment in the production of x-rays.

Tubes with two focal spots are usually referred to as dual focus tubes. These tubes consist of small and large focal spots. The heat capacity is limited for small focal spots and greater for large focal spots. In addition, the smaller the focal spot, the less the geometric unsharpness and the better the detail of the image.

During use of the tube when mA and kV are being changed, the size of the focal spot may change. This effect is called *blooming* and it has implications when measuring the size of the focal spot. Higher mA values have a more pronounced effect on the size of the focal spot than kVp and, in general, the size of the focal spot is measured with low mA values.

Rotation of the Anode Disk

The energy necessary to rotate the anode disk is supplied by the stator of an induction motor (Figure 5:4). The stator is mounted outside the glass envelope of the tube. When three-phase AC is supplied to the stator, a rotating magnetic field results and eddy currents are induced in the copper cylinder (rotor) which is pulled around in the direction of the magnetic field.

The speed of anode rotation depends on the frequency of the mains supply. A frequency of 60 Hertz (60 cycles per second) results in a rotation speed of 3600 rpm (revolutions per minute). In older tubes, average speeds of rotation range from about 3000 to 3600 rpm. If the stator is supplied with 150 cycles per second, then the speed of rotation increases to 9000 rpm. In recent rotating-anode tubes, speeds up to 10,000 rpm (180 Hertz) are possible (high-speed rotation).

The purpose of increasing the rotation speed is to increase the specific load values (maximum permissible electrical load in watts or kilowatts) of the tube. For example, a speed of 9000 rpm increases the specific load by about 70 percent compared to a speed of 3000 rpm, since the heat is spread over a larger area of track.

Free and smooth rotation of the disk are facilitated through the use of steel ball bearings which are lubricated with metallic barium, silver or lead, since ordinary lubricants reduce friction in the rotor assembly. High-speed rotation is much harder on the bearings compared to lower speeds.

Before making an exposure, it is necessary for the anode to acquire its maximum speed of rotation. It is for this reason that the induction motor is energized about one second before x-rays are produced. Should both the rotor switch and the exposure switch be activated simultaneously, there is a delay of about one second before the exposure commences.

NEW ANODE DISK TECHNOLOGY

The Compound Anode

As stated earlier, the disks of older rotating-anode tubes were made entirely of pure tungsten. In recent years, a new kind of anode disk has become available for rotating-anode tubes. This is the *compound anode disk* shown in Figure 5:9. A compound anode is constructed of two or more materials in combination. The disk consists of a *base body* onto which a *coating layer* is applied. The coating layer is the active layer from which x-rays are produced, while the base body serves to absorb and store heat produced in the coating layer.

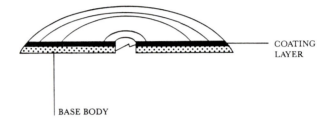

Figure 5:9. Construction of a compound anode disk. The coating layer or substrate is applied to the base body which absorbs and stores heat produced in the coating layer.

Disk Materials

The materials used in the construction of compound anode disks are several and include *rhenium, tungsten, molybdenum, graphite, zirconium* and *titanium.* A typical combination is shown in Figure 5:10 and consists of rhenium-tungsten-molybdenum (RTM). The base body is molybdenum, while the coating layer is made of an alloy of rhenium (about 10%) and tungsten (about 90%).

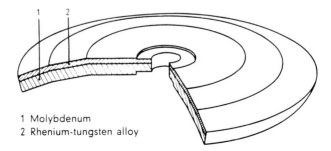

Figure 5:10. Construction of the Rhenium-Tungsten-Molybdenum (RTM) compound anode disk. (courtesy of the Siemens Corporation.)

The elements used for the coating layer must have a higher atomic number than molybdenum and also a higher melting point. Molybdenum has too low an atomic number to be used as the target (efficiency of x-ray production is proportional to atomic number).

RTM compound anode disks have several advantages over pure tungsten disks and these include:

(a) Lesser rotational problems because of its lighter weight.
(b) Extreme resistance to the aging process.
(c) Greater heat-storage capacity.
(d) Less roughening of the target area.
(e) A high and uniform dose for the entire life of the tube.

In certain radiographic procedures which require an exposure series such as in tomography, the RTM compound anode disk presents a few problems. The heat developed around the focal path causes mechanical stress which ultimately leads to distortion and fracture of the disk. Distortion reduces the target angle, the field size and the quantity of useful x-rays produced.

In dealing with these problems, several methods have been developed by x-ray tube manufacturers (for example, the Philips Metallurical Laboratory in Eindhoven). These methods include the use of slits and grooves in the disk (stress-relieved disks), blackening the disk and the use of other elements such as titanium, graphite and zirconium in the construction of the disk.

Disks with Slits

These disks are provided with equally distributed slits which are angled about 20° to the axis of rotation as shown in Figure 5:11. This angulation ensures that electrons cannot pass through the slit to strike the glass envelope. This technique prevents cracking and is three times less liable to distort when compared with disks having no slits.

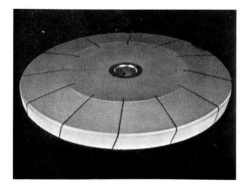

Figure 5:11. A compound anode disk with slits (from Schreiber, P.: New anode disk technology in super rotalix tubes. *Medicamundi* Vol. 20, No. 2, 1975).

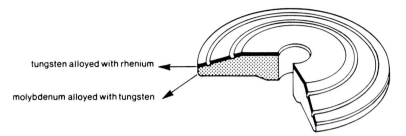

tungsten alloyed with rhenium

molybdenum alloyed with tungsten

Figure 5:12. Construction of a compound anode disk with grooves (from Schreiber, P.: New anode disk technology in super rotalix tubes. *Medicamundi* Vol. 20, No. 2, 1975).

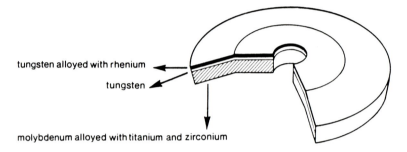

tungsten alloyed with rhenium

tungsten

molybdenum alloyed with titanium and zirconium

Figure 5:13. Construction of a Tungsten-Zirconium-Molybdenum (TZM) compound anode disk (from Schreiber, P.; New anode disk technology in super rotalix tubes. *Medicamundi,* Vol. 20, No. 2, 1975).

Disks with Grooves

These disks are constructed with concentric grooves on both sides of the focal path and extend into the molybdenum base body as shown in Figure 5:12. A major advantage of this technique is that fluoroscopy can be done with the disk stationary without significant problems.

Blackening the Anode Disk

The blackening of the rear surface of the disk can be applied to disks with slits or grooves. A blackened anode disk alone reduces anode temperatures and distortion by threefold, whereas a blackened disk with slits reduces distortion by a factor of nine.

In general a blackened disk increases the fluoroscopic output of the tube and permits a quicker sequence of load series, since the anode temperature is reduced. This is so because of the increased rate of heat loss by radiation (a black body is the best radiatior of heat).

Use of Elements Titanium and Zirconium as Disk Materials

More recently, a new disk has become available for the rotating-anode tube. This is the *titanium-zirconium-molybdenum* (TZM) disk shown in Figure 5:13. It consists of three layers instead of two, characteristic of the RTM disk. The base body or substrate is made of molybdenum alloyed with titanium and zirconium, while the coating layer is made of a tungsten-rhenium alloy about 0.7 mm thick. Between the coating layer and the base body is a separate layer made entirely of tungsten of about 0.7 mm thickness.

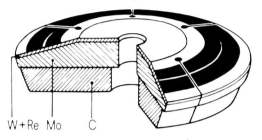

W+Re Mo   C

Figure 5:14. Construction of a *stress-relieved* compound anode disk using graphite (C) as the base body. (courtesy of the Siemens Corporation.)

Because of its special properties (grain structure and porosity), the base material of the TZM disk resists cracks and distortion without the need for slits or grooves. Another advantage of the TZM disk is that distortion is less than one tenth of that of the RTM disk of comparable geometry.

Use of Graphite as Base Body

Another material which has been used in the construction of the compound anode is *graphite* (Figure 5:14). In Table 5:1, a comparison of some properties of tungsten, molybdenum and graphite is given.

Graphite is used because of its high specific thermal capacity (approximately ten times that of tungsten), an emission coefficient of almost one, and a *heat permeation number* very close to tungsten and molybdenum. (The heat permeation number refers to the density, specific heat and thermal conductivity of a material.) The efficiency of the base of body depends on the heat permeation number such that the higher the heat permeation number, the faster heat is transferred from the focal path of the coating layer to the base body.

The graphite compound anode has a lower momentum (mass × velocity) when moving at the same speed (as the RTM disk) and, therefore, it can be made to start and stop more quickly. However, there are still problems associated with this disk. Because of the poorer conductivity of graphite compared with molybdenum, the focal path becomes hotter than the focal path of a standard RTM disk under the same conditions. In addition, there are problems in binding the coating layer to the base body in the graphite compound anodes and, therefore, it has not gained widespread use. Table 5:2 compares the graphite and RTM compound anode disks.

Table 5-1

COMPARISON OF SOME PROPERTIES OF
TUNGSTEN, MOLYBDENUM AND GRAPHITE

From Friedel and Haberrecker: Increased output of rotating-anode
x-ray tubes. *Electromedica* 4-5/1973.

	TUNGSTEN	MOLYBDENUM	GRAPHITE
Thermal conductivity at 1000°C.	*96	90	15-55
Density	*19.3	10.2	1.6-1.8
Thermal capacity at 1000°C.	* 4.1	7.4	48
Heat permeation number at 1000°C.	* 8.7	8.5	3.5-7.0
Emission coefficient at 1000°C.	0.15	0.15	0-85
Atomic Number	74	42	6
Reaction with Tungsten	—	—	at 1400°C and up, tungsten carbide is formed

*relatve units

Table 5-2

COMPARISON OF THE GRAPHITE COMPOUND
ANODE AND THE RTM DISK

From Friedel and Haberrecker: Increased output of rotating-anode
x-ray tubes. *Electromedica* 4-5/1973.

	GRAPHITE COMPOUND ANODE	RTM ANODE DISK
Total weight	800 g	800 g
Thermal capacity	350,000 joules	200,000 joules
Output at 1.0 s load	50 kW	50 kW
Output at 2.0 s load	17.5 kW	10 kW
Cooling period after load series of 72000 joules	2 min.	4 min.

INSULATION AND COOLING

During operation of the x-ray tube, almost all the electrical energy applied to it is converted into heat energy. If this heat is not dissipated, than a number of problems may arise. To deal with heat dissipation, the housing of the tube is filled with a non-conducting type of oil placed between the glass envelope and the inner walls of the housing. The purpose of the oil is twofold:

(a) It acts as an electrical insulator and protects the housing from the high voltage applied to the tube.
(b) It plays a role in the dissipation of heat by absorbing the heat developed at the anode and distributing it all around the housing. It therefore acts as a cooling medium.

During continuous operation of the tube, the temperature of the oil increase, thus causing it to expand. This expansion, if unattended, may break the housing and the oil may leak to the outside of the casing. Provision is thus made to deal with the expansion of oil by including metallic or rubber *bellows* in the tube housing (see Figure 5:4), which provide a little more room for the oil to expand when the bellows are compressed. If, however, the heat storage capacity of the housing is exceeded and there is no more room for expansion, a microswitch connected to the bellows is activated to prevent further exposures until the tube cools down.

Heat-Dissipation Processes

Heat dissipation in the x-ray tube is accomplished by three processes, namely, conduction, convection and radiation (see any radiology physics text for an explanation). These processes are illustrated in Figure 5:15.

Cooling Methods

The original methods of cooling the x-ray tube include the circulation of oil by convection currents and the use of electric fans (air circulators) positioned outside the tube on the housing.

Another method of cooling which has recently become available in x-ray imaging involves the use of a *heat exchanger*, which forces the oil through the housing to the outside of the housing and back to the inside.

The heat exchanger consists of an oil pump, a flexible tubing and a radiator and fan. The oil pump, radiator and fan are housed in a compact enclosure which is connected to the tube by means of the flexible tubing. This arrangement is seen in Figure 5:15. The oil in the housing is circulated by means of the pump through the radiator (where the heat is removed by the fan) and then it is returned to the housing. This method is sometimes referred to as *forced circula-*

tion of oil and it offers the following advantages:

    (a) increased cooling rate of the housing.

    (b) increased radiographic and fluoroscopic heat loading.

    (c) more frequent rotor starts.

    (d) reduction in the generation of *"hot spots."* (During extensive use of the tube with heavy exposures, hot spots are formed in the region of the stator windings and the anode. These spots will lower the dielectric constant of the oil in these regions and, hence, the performance of the tube is limited with a possibility of breakdown of the insulation at high voltage.)

    (e) helps to extend the life of the tube.

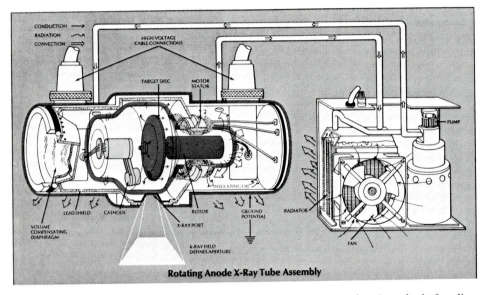

Rotating Anode X-Ray Tube Assembly

Figure 5:15. Heat dissipation processes in a rotating anode x-ray tube. A method of cooling using a heat exchanger (oil pump, flexible tubing, radiator and fan) is also illustrated. (courtesy of Machlett Laboratories, Inc.)

Measurement of the Anode Disk Temperature

In 1938, a method of controlling the anode temperature using a photoelectric cell was described. Today, more and more x-ray tubes incorporate this added feature and different methods are available to monitor the anode disk temperature.

One such method uses color indicators (green, yellow, and red) to provide a simple warning system to prevent thermal overloading of the tube. The green indicates commencement of an exposure or exposure series, while the yellow light indicates that the series or single exposure should be terminated and that no other exposure should be made. The red light means that all exposures should be terminated immediately.

Another method shown in Figure 5:16 makes use of an infrared sensor which "looks" at the anode through an optical window in the housing. An electronic readout indicates to the x-ray generator how hot the anode is, how much more work can be done, and when to terminate all exposures.

SPECIALIZED TUBES FOR IMAGING

A number of specialized x-ray tubes have been designed and built for use in certain radiographic procedures. Only three will be considered here very briefly.

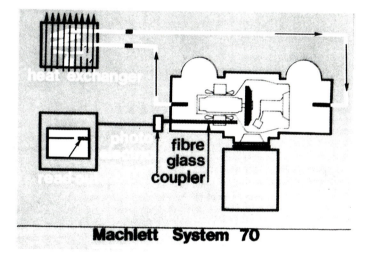

Figure 5:16. A method of controlling anode temperature, using a photoelectric cell. The cell "looks" at the anode through the fibre glass coupler and provides an indication of the temperature on the read-out device. (courtesy of Machlett Laboratories, Inc.)

X-Ray Tubes for Stereoradiography

Stereoradiography involves the production of an image which can be observed (using a stereoscopic viewer) with the illusion of depth. Such an image is formed by exposing two films with the tube in a different position for each exposure.

The same result can be obtained through the use of a *stereoradiographic x-ray tube*. This tube consists of a rotating anode which is bombarded at the same time by two streams of electrons originating from two separate cathode assemblies.

X-Ray Tubes for Field Emission Radiography

The field emission x-ray tube differs from the conventional x-ray tube in the way in which the electrons are obtained. The cathode of the tube is a metal needle from which electrons are extracted by a high electric field and not by thermionic emission. Field emission x-ray tubes allow the use of high kVp and high mA (greater than 1000 mA); hence, very short exposure times are possible. Field emission imaging has been applied to a number of diagnostic procedures and, therefore, it will be described in greater detail in a later chapter.

The Grid-Controlled X-Ray Tube

The *grid-controlled x-ray tube* consists of three electrodes: an anode, a cathode and a *control grid*. The function of the grid is to permit the tube itself to control the x-ray exposure. This is accomplished by applying a voltage (2-3 kV) between the filament and the grid such that when the voltage on the grid is negative with respect to the filament, electrons cannot move towards the target and hence x-rays cannot be produced. X-rays are only produced when the voltage on the grid is equal to that of the filament. The grid controlled x-ray tube offers the following advantages:

   (a) very short exposures during angiogrpahy.
   (b) commencement and termination of these exposures almost instantaneously.
   (c) pulse cine-fluorography (see Chap. 13).

RECENT DEVELOPMENTS IN X-RAY TUBE TECHNOLOGY

Tube with Glass/Metal Envelope

The glass envelope of conventional tubes poses an inherent limitation on loadability (results in limited heat storage capacity and less efficient heat dissipation), since the physical properties of glass are seriously affected by tungsten deposits. This subjects the glass to electron bombardment and ultimately premature breakdown. Another limitation imposed by glass envelopes is that they require relatively large and ultimately heavy tube housing. This in turn results in poor cooling conditions (less effective cooling).

Recently, a new kind of tube has been introduced to diagnostic x-ray imaging. The tube is a rotating-anode tube with the same features described previously except for the following differences:

   (a) The tube envelope consists of glass end-pieces which are bonded very securely to a metal envelope as shown in Figure 5:17.

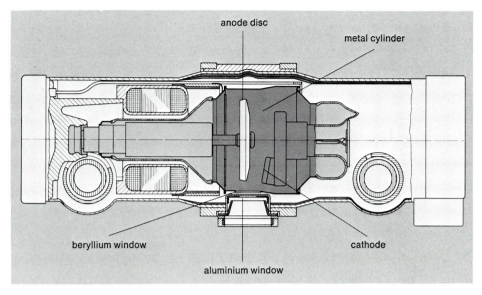

Figure 5:17. Rotating-anode x-ray tube with glass end-pieces bonded to a metal envelope. Two other features are the "large-volume" anode disk and the two exit windows. (courtesy of Philips Medical Systems.)

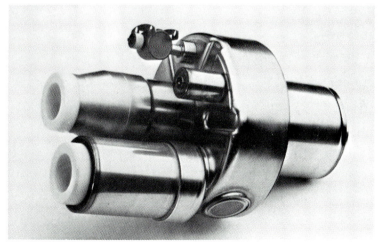

Figure 5:18. The metal-ceramic x-ray tube with double bearings. (courtesy of Philips Medical Systems.)

(b) The metal envelope encases the electron optical field between the anode and cathode. This results in a higher cathode emission and, hence, high tube currents with corresponding short exposure times. The metal portion of the envelope is unaffected by metal deposits, such as tungsten, during the life of the tube.

(c) Two windows are provided. The first is a beryllium window and the second is an aluminum window as shown in Figure 5:17. Compared with conventional tubes, these two windows provide optimum pre-filtration of the radiation beam, minimal extrafocal radiation and decreased scattered rays.

(d) A "large-volume anode disk" ensures higher heat storage capacity and more efficient heat dissipation.

This new tube is suitable for use in angiography, Bucky techniques and cinefluorography where short exposure times and sustained operation are necessary.

Metal/Ceramic Tube with Double Bearings

Another type of x-ray tube which has appeared even more recently is the *metal/ceramic tube with double bearings*. This tube, shown in Figure 5:18, represents the latest development in x-ray tube technology.

A schematic of the tube is shown in Figure 5:19. The most characteristic

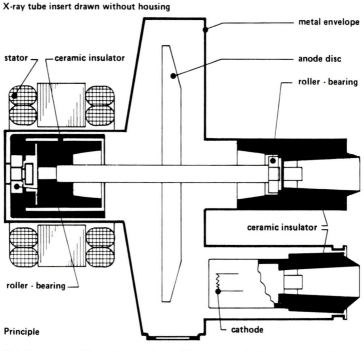

Rotating anode with bearings on both sides of the axle, inside an all-metal envelope with ceramic inserts for electrical insulation.

Figure 5:19. Schematic of the metal/ceramic x-ray tube with double bearings. (courtesy of Philips Medical Systems.)

features are the metal envelope, ceramic insulation double-bearing axle and the large disk. The metal envelope features high loadability and is earthed to facilitate the capture of stray electrons and, as a result, reduces the production of extra-focal radiation. The metal envelope has better mechanical stability and thermal and electrical properties than glass. At high temperatures, the metal envelope has a high heat conductivity and cools rapidly compared with glass. This makes it very useful in angiography which requires high thermal cooling.

The metal envelope is not susceptible to metal deposits due to evaporation. The exit window on the envelope is made of beryllium, which provides very low radiation absorption. An interchangeable aluminum filter is also provided. This inherent filtration can be changed to suit the needs of particular examinations. The thickness of the oil (inherent filter) is reduced and this, in turn, reduces the amount of scattered rays produced by the oil.

Ceramic Insulation

The ceramic portion of the tube is highlighted in Figure 5:19. The Al_2O_3 ceramic acts as insulating material. It is bonded to the housing to ensure a vacuum-tight seal. The ceramic insulation portion of the tube also contains the cathode and double-bearing anode.

The ceramic insulators are also provided with receptacles for the high tension cables and ensures insulation for voltages up to 150 kV without the need for extra insulation. Apart from this, an extra portion of ceramic insulation is built into the rotor end of the anode and rotates with it. This arrangement ensures insulation of the disk and axle at high voltages.

Double-Bearing Axle

In conventional rotating-anode tubes, disks are provided with a single-bearing construction. In the metal/ceramic tube, the disk is mounted onto a double-bearing axle. This design ensures that the bearing load is more uniform (compared with conventional tubes) and therefore extends the life of the tube.

The Disk

The new tube design features larger disks (120 mm diameter) compared with the 90 mm-100 mm diameter disks of conventional rotating-anode tubes. The larger disks provide improved cooling and, despite the greater inertia (of the larger disk), the specially designed anode drive and stator supply allow exposure commencement times as short as one second.

Advantages

The new concept in x-ray tube design and construction provides several advantages. In summary, these include:

   (a) A twofold increase in heat storage capacity.

(b) Improved image quality, since there is greater loadability of the 120 mm disk and absorption of secondary electrons by the metal envelope. This means that there is an improvement in the signal-to-noise ratio, since the amount of scattered radiation is reduced.

(c) Longer tube life, since the double-bearing axle provides greater stability and the metal envelope is unaffected by metal deposits.

(d) The new tube housing acts as a mechanical carrier and provides radiation protection, as well as cooling.

(e) Provides a greater number of exposures per series and, therefore, reduces waiting time between exposures. This makes the tube particularly suitable for serial radiography (angiography), tomographic exposure series, cine-work and remote-controlled radiography and fluoroscopy.

Part Two

X-RAY TUBE RATINGS

To achieve optimum performance of the x-ray tube, it is necessary to understand the factors which govern the safe operation of the tube. The data generated from these factors are generally referred to as *x-ray tube ratings*. The data can be available in table or in graphical form, in which case they are referred to as *rating charts*. Three factors which are of concern when discussing x-ray tube ratings are:

(a) the maximum tube voltage (kVp).
(b) the maximum tube current (mA).
(c) the maximum energy dissipation in the form of heat.

The Maximum Tube Voltage

The *maximum tube voltage* is the maximum permissible instantaneous kilovoltage that can be applied to the tube without causing damage. The maximum kVp depends upon a number of factors, such as:

(a) the distance between the anode and cathode.
(b) the shape of the anode and cathode structures and the shape of the glass envelope.
(c) the type of circuit which supplies the high voltage to the x-ray tube. These circuits include self-rectified, single-phase half-wave rectified and three-phase full-wave rectified. The voltage rating increases when a full-wave rectified circuit is used rather than a self-rectified tube. For three-phase full-wave rectification at short exposures, the voltage

rating is higher than when single-phase full-wave rectification is used. For longer exposures, however, the ratings are higher with single-phase rectification than with three-phase rectification. (For a more complete discussion, see any standard radiologic physics text.)

(d) occasional transient surges in voltage. The x-ray tube can tolerate these surges only if they are below 10 percent of the miximum voltage rating.

The Maximum Tube Current

The maximum average mA is dependent on the limitations placed on the current and voltage applied to the filaments (large and small) of the tube. Filaments are assigned maximum ratings for two modes of operation:

(a) *Continous mode*, where the filament is maintained at exposure levels of a long duration, such as in fluoroscopy.

(b) *Intermittent mode,* where the filament is boosted to operating voltage for exposure levels of a short duration (less than 30 seconds), such as in radiography.

Typical voltage and current values range from 3-7.5 volts and 3.5 amperes to 4-12 volts and 3-5.5 amperes for small and large filaments, respectively. For radiographic exposures, the filament current should not exceed 5.5 amperes. In fluoroscopy, the filament current is much lower than in radiography, since a continuous application of current to the filament causes a steady rise in the temperature of the filament.

The Maximum Energy

The *maximum energy* is the maximum heat energy which can be produced by the tube (within safe limits) in a given period of time.

The ratings for maximum energy are related to the focal spot, the anode, and the tube housing.

The Heat Unit

The unit of measurement for maximum energy ratings is the *heat unit* (HU), which is defined as the energy produced by one kilovoltage and one milliampere in one second. For different x-ray circuits, the HU is given as follows:

(a) *For single-phase equipment:*
$$HU = kVp \times mA \times seconds$$

(b) *For three-phase equipment:*
$$HU = kVp \times mA \times seconds \times \underline{1.35}$$

(c) *For constant potential generators:*
$$HU = kVp \times mA \times seconds \times \underline{1.41}$$

The maximum energy ratings for the anode and housing of the tube are given in terms of *heat-storage capacities*. The heat storage capacity is the number of heat units that the anode and tube housing can absorb without causing damage due to overheating.

Maximum Energy Ratings for the Focal Spot

Rating charts are provided by manufacturers for all x-ray tubes installed in a department. To find out whether the focal spot of the tube can withstand a particular exposure (kVp, mA and time), the rating chart should be consulted. Figure 5:20 shows a radiographic rating chart for an x-ray tube. The following examples will explain how to use this chart.

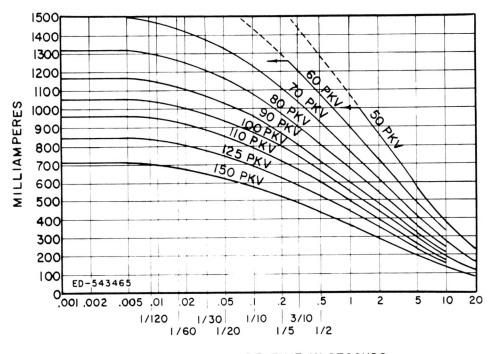

MAXIMUM EXPOSURE TIME IN SECONDS

Figure 5:20. A radiographic rating chart. See text for further explanation. (courtesy of Machlett Laboratories, Inc.)

Example 1:

Is an exposure of 1100 mA, 80 kVp, one sixtieth sec permissible?

Solution

1. Locate 1100 mA on the ordinate (vertical axis) and the 80 kVp curve. Where these two lines intersect, the maximum exposure time is found to be in excess of 0.05 (1/20) second.

2. Since 1/60 second is less than 1/20, the exposure factors can safely be applied to the tube.

Example 2.

If a technologist sets an exposure time of 0.2 seconds and a tube voltage of 100 kVp, what is the maximum mA that can safely be applied to the tube?

Solution

1. Locate 0.2 seconds on the horizontal axis and the 100 kVp curve.
2. Where they intersect, trace a line towards the vertical axis.
3. The point where that line reaches the vertical axis indicates the mA that can be used.
4. The answer is 800 mA.

Example 3:

What is the maximum kilovoltage that can safely be applied to the tube if an exposure, using 1 second at 600 mA, is required?

Solution

1. Locate the 600 mA value on the vertical axis and then the 1 second time on the horizontal axis.
2. Trace these two lines to the point where they intersect.
3. The point of intersection falls on the 90 kVp curve.
4. The answer is 90 kVp.

The points which fall under each voltage curve indicate that combinations of mA and time (secs) do not exceed the loading capacity of the focal spot when that voltage is used. On the other hand, those points which fall above each voltage curve express mA and time (secs) combinations which will overload the tube and cause damage.

Maximum Energy Ratings for the Anode

The heat developed at the focal spot is transferred to the anode structure and, hence, the heat-storage capacity of the anode becomes an important factor. The heat-storage capacity refers to the thermal characteristics of the anode. An anode theremal characteristics chart is used when the time for a single exposure or exposure series is greater than the time covered by the radio-graphic rating chart. Figure 5:21 shows a typical anode thermal characteristics chart. Such a chart shows two types of curves:

(a) *The "Input" Curve:* These curves show the amount of heat stored in the anode after a specified long, single exposure or a number of rapid, successive exposures. The cooling during operation of the tube is taken into consideration here. (For example, the delivery of 1200 HU/sec input energy to the anode is equal to the anode heat-storage capacity after 15 mins; the delivery of 1000 HU/sec input energy could be continued for a long time.)

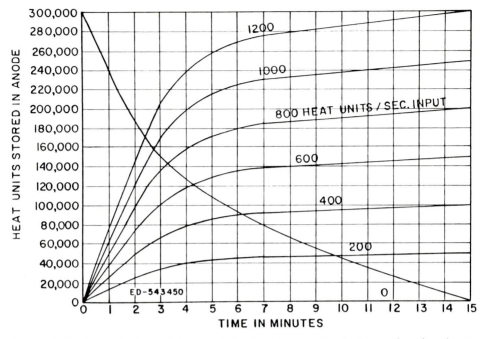

Figure 5:21. An anode thermal characteristics chart. See text for further explanation. (courtesy of Machlett Laboratories, Inc.)

(b) *The Cooling Curve:* This curve shows the amount of heat stored in the anode after a specified period of cooling.

Two other characteristics which must also be considered in this chart are:

(a) The maximum anode heat-storage capacity. For this chart (Figure 5:21), it is 300,000 HU.

(b) The maximum anode cooling rate. This is the rate of heat dissipation of the anode when its temperature is at its maximum. (The cooling rate for this chart is given to be 60,000 HU/min.)

In Figure 5:21 it is clear that a single exposure of 300,000 HU or a rapid exposure series which will produce a total of more than 300,000 HU should not be used. The Figure also shows that for the maximum 300,000 HU, it will take the anode 15 minutes to cool to zero heat units. The use of the chart may be explained through the following example:

Example 4:

In a radiographic series consisting of 16 exposures, the technique 100 kVp, 400 mA and one half second is used for each exposure.

(a) Is this technique permissible according to Figure 5:21?

(b) If an exposure series is made for 15 exposures using the technique 100 kVp, 400 mA and ½ sec for each exposure, how long does it take the anode to cool down to 100,000 heat units?

Solution

(a) The number of heat units for each exposure

$$= 100 \text{ kVp} \times 400 \text{ mA} \times \tfrac{1}{2} \text{ sec}$$
$$= 20,000 \text{ HU}$$

Therefore, the number of HU for 16 exposures

$$= 20,000 \times 16$$
$$= 320,000 \text{ HU}.$$

This amount of heat exceeds the anode heat-storage capacity of 300,000 HU.

Hence, the technique is not permissible.

(b) The number of heat units for 15 exposures

$$= 20,000 \times 15$$
$$= 300,000 \text{ HU}.$$

This is the maximum heat-storage capacity of the anode.

Therefore, it will take approximately 5.5 minutes for the anode to cool down to 100,000 HU. (In order to arrive at this answer, trace down the vertical axis until 100,000 HU point is reached, then trace along the horizontal axis to the point of intersection with the cooling curve. From this point, trace down to the horizontal time axis. That point reads about 5.5 mins.)

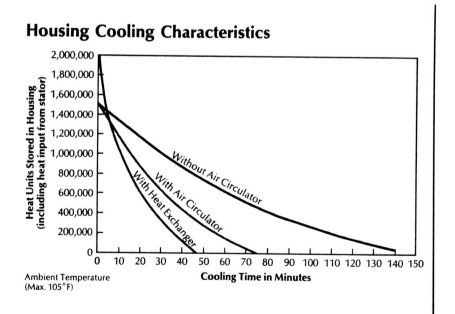

Figure 5:22. An x-ray tube housing cooling chart. See text for further explanation. (courtesy of Machlett Laboratories, Inc.)

Maximum Energy Ratings for the Housing

In the process of heat dissipation, heat developed at the focal spot is transferred to the anode and hence to the oil in the housing. The tube housing then heats up and, therefore, the heat-storage capacity (of the entire housing) must be considered when determining the maximum energy rating of the tube. The housing cooling chart is referred to only when the time for an exposure series is greater than the time covered by the anode thermal characteristics chart. Figure 5:22 shows a housing cooling chart. This curve shows the amount of heat stored in the tube housing after some specified period of cooling. Two concepts are illustrated in this chart:

(a) The maximum heat-storage capacity of the housing. In Figure 5:22, the maximum heat-storage capacity is 2,000,000 HU, with the heat exchanger.

(b) The maximum cooling rate of the housing. For this chart, the cooling rate is given by the manufacturer as 96,000 HU/min with the heat exchanger.

Ratings for Rapid Sequence Imaging

The ratings for rapid serial radiography can be expressed as follows:

Too many exposures within a limited period of time may dangerously overheat the tube. This can occur in three different ways:

(1) The surface of the target can be overheated by repeating exposures before the surface heat has had time to dissipate into the body of the anode.

(2) The entire anode can be overheated by repeating exposures before the heat in the anode has had time to radiate into the surrounding oil and the tube housing.

(3) The tube housing can be overheated by making too many exposures before the housing has had time to lose its heat to the surrounding air.

Reference to the anode thermal characteristics chart and housing cooling charts can ensure that overheating during a series of exposures does not occur as indicated in items 2 and 3 (above). However, a second reference must be made to the radiographic rating chart to ensure that a series of exposures does not result in overheating as described in item 1. The following condition must be met in all cases of exposures made in rapid sequence:

THE TOTAL HEAT UNITS OF A SERIES OF EXPOSURES MADE IN RAPID SEQUENCE MUST NOT EXCEED THE HEAT UNITS PERMISSIBLE AS INDICATED BY THE RADIOGRAPHIC RATING CHART, FOR A SINGLE EXPOSURE OF A DURATION EQUAL TO THE ELAPSED TIME REQUIRED TO COMPLETE THE SERIES OF EXPOSURES.

The above rule presumes that each individual exposure is safe and that the series is performed at a constant exposure rate, ie, all individual exposures in the series are of the same number of heat units and separated by the same time interval. THE ABOVE RULE IS NOT APPLICABLE TO CINERADIOGRAPHY.

Where the time interval between individual exposures exceeds the time range of the radiographic rating chart, it can be presumed that no danger of focal track overheating exists and that the only precautions to be taken are those against exceeding anode or housing heat storage capacity. (Machlett Laboratories, 1981.)

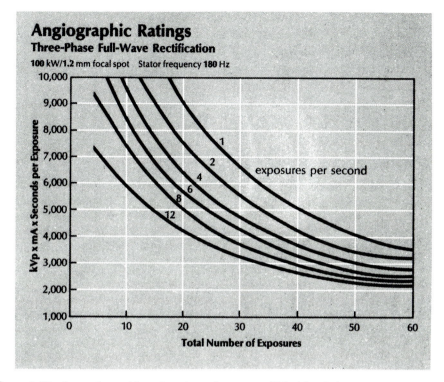

Figure 5:23. An angiographic rating chart. (courtesy of Machlett Laboratories, Inc.)

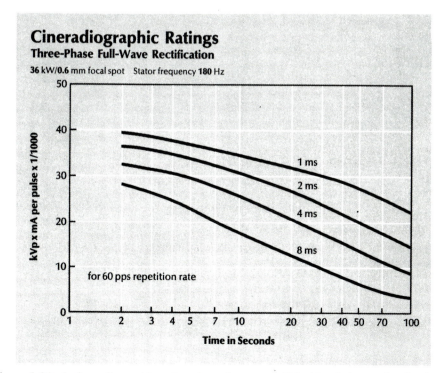

Figure 5:24. A cineradiographic rating chart. (courtesy of Machlett Laboratories, Inc.)

Table 5-3

X-RAY TUBE FAULTS, THEIR CAUSES AND EFFECTS

COMPONENT	FAULT	CAUSE OF FAULT	EFFECTS OF FAULT
Filament	failure to heat	fault in filament circuit	no x-rays produced
	break	vaporization causes thinner filament — high mA values	no passage of tube current and hence no x-rays are produced
Vacuum	"gassy"	prolonged use — vacuum seal is not perfect	milliamperage increases to high values
Glass envelope	formation of reflecting surface on glass	heavy exposures cause vaporization of metal parts of the tube. The vaporized tungsten forms the reflecting surface	reduction of insulating properties of the glass envelope
	hole	insulating properties reduced	vacuum ruined
	cracking	careless handling — stress from anode's weight. Overexpansion of oil.	general performance of tube can be affected
Ball bearings	deformation	prolonged use — extreme high temperatures.	termination of the useful life of tube — reduced rotation speed
Stator	failure to turn the rotor	no power supply to stator circuit	cracking of the anode disk
Anode (the target area)	pitting or erosion of the target track	heavy exposure factors which raise the temperature of the target to very high values	causes unsharpness in the radiographic image — reduces the intensity of useful beam of radiation — increase in exposure values as time progresses
Disk	distortion of the disc	very high temperature rise	wobbling of disc production of unsatisfactory radiographic images.
	localized melting — cracking of the surface	excessive rise in temperature	reduction in the radiation output

Special charts for angiography (Figure 5:23) and cineradiography (Figure 5:24) are supplied by the manufacturer and should be made available to the imaging department for use by the technologist.

In summary, the use of these charts is essential to safeguard the x-ray tube and its housing from damage which may be caused by overheating due to an exposure series made in rapid succession.

COMMON FAULTS IN THE X-RAY TUBE

Continuous operation of the x-ray tube may bring about, in time, deterioration of its various parts. The faults which develop affect the efficiency of x-ray production and in some cases may terminate the life of the tube. Table 5:3 lists some commonfaults which may develop in the x-ray tube, their causes and effects. Most of the faults that develop in the anode disc may be due to frequently repeated overloading of the tube.

EXTENDING THE LIFE OF THE X-RAY TUBE

The introduction of new radiographic techniques require the use of higher power levels (greater electrical loads), and, therefore, it is important for the technologist to consider certain factors in order to extend the life of the x-ray tube. These factors appear in a booklet entitled *How to Get Maximum Life from your Rotating-anode X-ray Tubes* (Machlett Laboratories, 1981) and are as follows:

(a) *Anode Temperature Rise* —
The values shown on the Radiographic Rating Chart must not be exceeded. Where techniques permit, use less than the indicated maximum rating for extended life. It is not a good practice, particularly with three-phase generators, to use the full rating on a cold (room-temperature) anode. Lower rated exposures should always precede a full maximum value exposure to reduce the "thermal shock" to the cool anode.

(b) *Anode Storage Capacity* —
For multiple exposures, the Cine radiographic, Angiographic and Anode Cooling Charts must be considered and rigidly adhered to. Again the best practice is to use less than indicated maximum values for extended life.

(c) *Anode Rotation* —
Frequent restarts of the anode adds housing heat that detracts from the ability to accept heat from the anode. Indiscriminate use of high speeds tends to excessively wear the bearings and sudden movements of the tube should be avoided while at high speeds.

(d) *Housing Storage Capacity* —
The indicated maximum capacity must be carefully observed to avoid overheating the housing. An even more serious consideration is to ensure that the capacity isn't exceeded so much that ruptures of the oil seals occur.

Air circulators can aid in cooling the housing and should be used in under-table applications where conditions warrant. Periodic cleaning of the blower is necessary and extended "on" time must be used to continue cooling after the last exposure series has ended.

(e) *Filament Life Extension* —
Excessive boost times must be avoided in all cases and the charts followed closely to avoid shortening the useful life. Reduction of suggested mA values for most radiographic techniques with the required increase in (within limits) can greatly extend the filament life.

These five factors should perhaps be posted in all x-ray rooms to remind the technologist that the life of the tube may be extended if these factors are observed.

In summary, to extend the life of the x-ray tube:

(a) Reduce the filament preparation time.
(b) Avoid excessive heat.
(c) Observe and consult rating charts, input and cooling curves.
(d) Use lower tube currents when possible.
(e) Wait for the tube to cool between exposures.
(f) Use high-speed anode rotation only when needed.

SUMMARY

1. X-ray tubes are of two types: the stationary anode and the rotating anode.

2. An x-ray tube designed for imaging must provide very sharp images, short exposure times, specific radiation output, repeated exposures, rapid heat dissipation and the capability of withstanding high electrical loads.

3. The stationary-anode tube is described with reference to anode structure, since the filament (cathode structure) design is almost the same as in the rotating-anode tube.

4. A vacuum is necessary in an x-ray tube, because the presence of air molecules will result in oxidation of the filament and short tube life. The quality of the beam is also affected, since electrons may collide with the air molecules, resulting in a loss of their kinetic energy.

5. The stationary anode consists of a copper block in which a rectangular piece of metal (tungsten) is embedded. This piece of metal is the target. The face of the anode is inclined at an angle (target angle) to the central ray of the beam.

6. Tungsten is used as a target material because of its high melting point, high atomic number, low vapor pressure and its high thermal conductivity.

7. The stationary-anode tube is limited with respect to its loading capac-

ity, heat dissipation and small size of its target area.

8. The rotating-anode tube is different from the stationary-anode tube with respect to its anode construction.

9. The cathode assembly of x-ray tubes (stationary or rotating) consists of a filament and focussing cup. The filament is made of a thin piece of tungsten arranged in a helical winding to increase its surface area. The focussing cup acts as an electronic lens to direct the electrons to the target area.

10. The rotating anode is made of pure tungsten shaped into a disk (earlier tubes) which is supported by a molybdenum stem. The force of rotation of the disk is brought about by the stator of an induction motor.

11. The diameter of the disk influences the maximum permissible load which the tube can withstand. The disk has an angle of bevel which may range from 7°-20°.

12. The focal spot is the area on the disk subject to electron bombardment.

13. The rotation speed depends on the mains frequency. Typical speeds are in the order of 3600 rpm, but higher speeds are possible through an increase in the frequency to the stator. Increasing the rotation speed increases the specific load on the tube. Free and smooth rotation are facilitated by steel ball bearings lubricated with metallic barium, silver or lead.

14. The compound anode disk is one which is made of two or more metals. It consists of a base body onto which a coating layer is applied. The new disk materials include rhenium, zirconium and titanium used in conjunction with tungsten, molybdenum and graphite. A typical compound anode disk is the RTM disk, which consists of molybdenum (base) and 10 percent rhenium and about 90 percent tungsten (coating layer). The advantages of compound anode disks are listed.

15. The RTM compound anode disk presents a few problems with respect to mechanical stresses which lead to distortion and fracture of the disk. Several methods have been developed to deal with this problem. These include making disks with slits, grooves, blackening the disk and using titanium and zirconium as disk materials. These are described.

16. Oil is used as an electrical insulator and protects the tube housing from the high voltage applied to the tube. It also plays a role in the dissipation of heat. Heat dissipation is accomplished by conduction, convection and radiation.

17. Apart from cooling of the tube which is facilitated by convection currents and small electrical fans positioned outside the tube housing,

another method of cooling using a heat exchanger is discussed and the advantages are listed.

18. Specialized x-ray tubes for imaging are discussed with respect to stereoradiography, field emission imaging and the grid-controlled x-ray tube for use in angiography and pulsed cine fluorography.

19. Recent developments in x-ray tube technology are described with respect to tubes with glass/metal envelope and the metal/ceramic tube with double bearings.

20. The main features of the glass/metal envelope tube are the glass endpieces bonded to the metal envelope. The metal envelope results in a higher cathode emission and is unaffected by metal deposits. Other features include two windows, a beryllium and an aluminum window and a large-volume anode disk.

21. The most characteristic features of the metal/ceramic tube are the metal envelope, ceramic insulation double-bearing axle and the large disk. The double bearings ensure that the bearing load of the disk is more uniform compared with the conventional design.

22. The advantages of this new technology are listed.

23. X-ray tube ratings are discussed with respect to maximum tube voltage, maximum tube current and maximum energy dissipation in the form of heat.

24. The maximum kVp depends on several factors such as the spacing between the anode and cathode, the shape of the anode and cathode structures, the shape of the glass envelope, the type of circuit which provides the high voltage to the tube and occasional transient surges in voltage.

25. The maximum average mA depends on the limitations placed on the current and voltage applied to the filament.

26. The maximum energy are related to focal spot, the anode and tube housing. Maximum energy ratings are expressed in heat units. A heat unit is the energy produced by one kV and one mA in one second. The heat unit expressions are given for single-phase, three-phase and constant potential generators.

27. The heat-storage capacity refers to the thermal characteristics of the anode. A typical anode thermal characteristics chart shows two curves: an input curve (amount of heat stored in the anode after a specified long single exposure or a number of rapid, successive exposures) and a cooling curve (amount of heat stored in the anode after a specified period of cooling).

28. Two other points to be noted on this chart are the maximum heat-storage capacity and the maximum anode cooling rate.

29. The maximum energy ratings for the tube housing are also described with respect to the maximum heat-storage capacity and the maximum cooling rate.

30. The ratings for rapid serial radiography are described.
31. Common faults in the x-ray tube are given in table form.
32. Finally, the life of the x-ray tube may be extended by paying careful attention to factors such as the anode temperature rise, anode storage capacity, anode rotation, the housing storage capacity and the filament life.

CHAPTER 6

SCATTERED RADIATION REDUCTION METHODS

SCATTERED RADIATION

THE beam of x-rays emanating from the x-ray tube is called the *primary beam*. Upon interaction with the imaging object (patient), a fraction of the beam is absorbed. Another fraction is transmitted through the patient (*primary transmission*), while the remainder is *scattered* at various angles. Most of these scattered rays are also transmitted through the patient (*scatter transmission*). The total radiation reaching the film is the sum of the primary and scatter transmission. The process is illustrated in Figure 6:1.

Effects of Scatter on Image Quality

Scattered radiation is detrimental to image quality, because it reduces contrast and increases image background noise. These rays also decrease image resolution due to penumbral effects which are attributed to the geometry of the beam.

Factors Influencing Scattered Radiation

Through an understanding of the factors influencing the amount of scattered radiation produced in an object, the reduction methods become more apparent. The main concern of *anti-scatter techniques* (reduction methods) has been focussed on improving contrast by studying a number of parameters such as the *contrast reduction factor* which is equivalent to the primary radiation fraction and the scatter fraction.

The *primary radiation fraction,* P, is defined as the ratio of primary radiation to that of primary radiation plus scattered radiation reaching the film (Burgess and Pate, 1981). The *scatter fraction,* F, is defined as the ratio of intensity of scattered radiation to that of the scattered and primary rays reaching the film

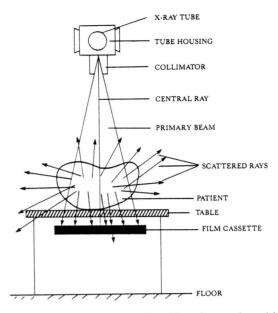

Figure 6:1. The production of scattered radiation. Upon interacting with the patient, a fraction of the primary beam is absorbed. Another fraction is transmitted through the patient while the remainder is scattered at various angles. Sources of scatter include the x-ray tube housing, the collimator, the x-ray table, the film cassette and the floor.

(Niklason, Sorenson and Nelson, 1981).

It has been demonstrated experimentally that as *patient thickness* increases and as the x-ray *field size* (area irradiated) gets larger, P decreases while F increases. This results in reduced contrast, since more scattered rays are produced with increasing field size and thicker body parts such as the abdomen.

Apart from patient thickness and field size, another factor which influences scatter production is *kilovoltage*. From practical experience, when low kVp techniques are used, contrast is much better than with higher kVp techniques. As the kVp is increased, there is more scatter production and therefore more of these rays get to the film, thereby degrading image contrast. The student must realize, however, that there are definite advantages and disadvantages associated with the use of high and low kVp techniques.

Sources of Scatter

Any object with which the primary beam interacts is a potential source of scatter. In diagnostic x-ray imaging, the patient is the main source of scatter. The other sources are shown in Figure 6:1 and include the x-ray tube housing, the collimator, the x-ray table, the film cassette and the floor. The remainder of this chapter will deal with methods of reducing the production of scatter in the patient.

ANTI-SCATTER TECHNIQUES

The purpose of anti-scatter techniques is to improve image contrast by decreasing the amount of scattered radiation reaching the film. Several anti-scatter techniques are available and have been used quite extensively in diagnostic x-ray imaging. These include:

   √ (a) Reduction of kVp to practical limits.
      (b) The compression technique.
   √ (c) The air gap technique.
   √ (d) Limitation (restriction) of the x-ray field size.
      (e) The scattered radiation grid technique. Since this is the most widely used anti-scatter technique, it will be treated in detail under a separate section.
      (f) The scanning slit technique.

kVp Reduction Technique

In clinical radiogrpahy, the kVp and mAs are responsible for film density, although other factors are involved (for example, distance). Essentially, the kVp is used to control penetration and contrast. Reducing the kVp improves the contrast of the image, however, the kVp must be high enough so that the primary beam will penetrate the part.

By lowering the kVp to acceptable limits, there is less Compton interaction and more photoelectric absorption (x-ray interactions with matter). This simply means that at lower kVp values more of the primary beam is absorbed by higher atomic number elements (for example, bone). Most of the scattered rays produced at the surface of the patient closest to the x-ray tube will not pass through the body (low scatter transmission) to reach the film.

There is a definite relationship between kVp and mAs in maintaining film density. It follows that if the kVp is lowered, then there must be a corresponding increase in mAs. This technique conversion is not within the context of this text and, therefore, it will not be treated here.

The Compression Technique

The *compression technique* is often used in clinical radiography to decrease patient thickness. It is more commonly associated with the intravenous pyelogram (a contrast examination of the urinary tract) and mammography (Chapter 10). Although its use in pyelography is mainly to compress the ureters so that the contrast may fill the renal pelvis and calyces, it can also be used to decrease the thickness of the part by applying compression to the appropriate region.

Effective compression may be accomplished through the use of a *compression device* such as the compression band (Figure 6:2a). The band is about 25 cm (10 inches) wide and is usually made of radiolucent vinyl. It is anchored at one end to a universal clamp and the opposite end is attached to a quick-release wind-up ratchet which is usually affixed to the operator's side of the tabletop. The band is adjustable and can be tightened by the ratchet mechanism. The use of the band is illustrated in Figure 6:2b.

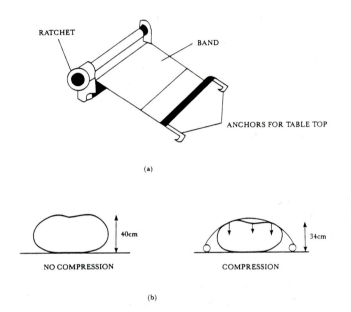

Figure 6:2. (a) The compression band. (b) Schematic representation of the use of the band.

Although the compression technique is useful in immobilizing the patient and decreasing patient thickness, it provides two other advantages. First, by providing a uniform thickness, the exposure at the image plane is more uniform, and, second, image sharpness is improved since the object is now closer to the film (Bushong, 1980).

When the compression band is used as an anti-scatter technique to improve contrast, there is a reduction in the amount of scattered radiation reaching the film because of the decreased thickness.

The Air Gap Technique

The *air gap technique* is based on the fact that scattered rays are more divergent than primary rays. If a space or gap (about 15 cm) is left between the object and the film, most of the scattered rays will fall out of the gap and will not reach the image receptor (film), thus improving contrast. This principle is illustrated in Figure 6:3.

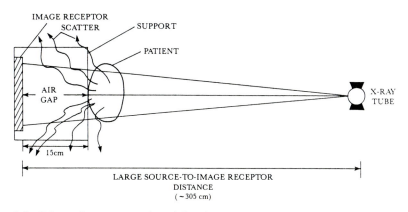

Figure 6:3. Schematic representation of the air-gap technique. The gap is the space between the patient and the image receptor and it is usually about 15 cm. Since scattered rays are more oblique than the primary beam, they fall out of the gap before striking the image receptor. A large source-to-image receptor distance is also characteristic of the air-gap technique in order to reduce magnification.

In clinical practice, the following points must be considered when using the air gap technique:

(a) Since the object-to-image receptor distance is increased, there is *magnification.*

(b) However, magnification is minimized through the use of a *larger source-to-image receptor distance.* In this regard, the primary rays are almost parallel in the vicinity of the object. From the beam geometry, penumbra is reduced; therefore magnification is reduced. The source-to-image receptor distance in chest examinations (based on the air gap technique), for example, is about 305 cm (10 feet).

(c) The long source-to-image receptor distance introduces the problem of patient exposure. There is an *increase in exposure* which is attributed to the inverse square law (radiation increases inversely as the square of the distance).

(d) Because of the increased source-to-image receptor distance, a *higher tube output* is needed to maintain proper film densities.

Limitation of Field Size

The amount of scattered radiation produced in the patient can be reduced by limiting or restricting the primary beam only to the area of interest. This is accomplished through the use of *beam limiting devices* or *beam restrictors,* which are introduced into the path of the primary beam in such a way that they are as close as possible to the exit window of the x-ray tube.

The technique of restricting and shaping the beam is referred to as *collimtion,* although the term *coning* is often used synonymously.

X-ray Imaging Equipment

Table 6-1

ESSENTIAL FEATURES OF CONES, CYLINDERS AND DIAPHRAGMS

BEAM RESTRICTOR	DESCRIPTION	DIAGRAM
CONE	Structure felt to resemble a geometric cone. It describes a solid, bounded by a circular base where every point on the base is joined (by line segments) to a common vertex. (Significant penumbral effects.)	 VERTEX HEIGHT BASE RIGHT CIRCULAR CONE
CYLINDER	The word cylinder is derived from the Greek "kylindros" meaning roller. This is a more efficient beam restrictor than the cone. Reduces penumbral effects compared to the cone.	 HEIGHT RIGHT CIRCULAR CYLINDER
DIAPHRAGM	Metal plates with different sizes and shapes of apertures. They are commonly used in radiography of the skull.	 CROSS SECTION APERTURES CIRCULAR SQUARE RECTANGULAR
EXTENSION CYLINDER	Cylinder which can extend by means of the telescoping effect. This is a very efficient beam restrictor. Useful in spot films of L_5 -S_1 junction and coned views of the orbits.	

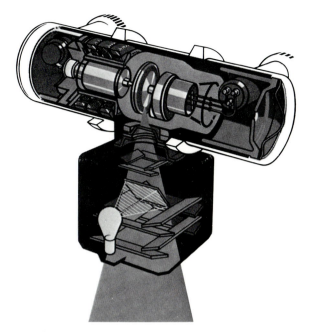

Figure 6:4. A multileaf collimator affixed to the x-ray tube. (courtesy of the Siemens Corporation.)

The Collimator

A simple *collimator* is one which shapes and limits the primary beam by moving two pairs of lead leaves (about 0.32 cm thick) to produce either square or rectangular apertures, much the same way as a camera shutter works. Therefore, the leaves have become to be known as *collimator shutters*.

Today, all diagnostic x-ray tubes are fitted with multileaf collimators. Although the technical details in the design of multileaf collimators are not within the scope of this text, there are certain features which are important. Figure 6:4 shows a multileaf collimator affixed to the x-ray tube. The characteristic features are:

    (a) a set of lead shutters
    (b) a light-beam indicator
    (c) a housing for the shutters and light-beam indicator
    (d) a timer (not seen in the figure)
    (e) a transparent plastic beam definer (not seen in the figure) located at the base (side closer to the patient) of the housing
    (f) a field coverage table

The collimation scheme is further outlined in Figure 6:5. The near shutters are positioned in close proximity to the x-ray tube focus. This arrangement

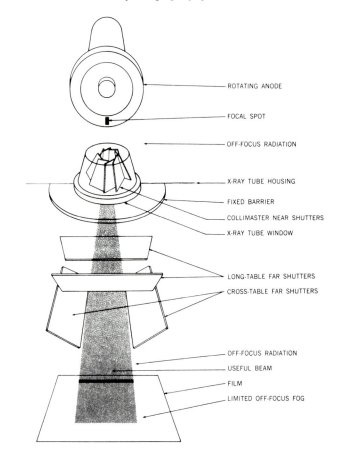

ROTATING ANODE

FOCAL SPOT

OFF-FOCUS RADIATION

X-RAY TUBE HOUSING

FIXED BARRIER

COLLIMASTER NEAR SHUTTERS

X-RAY TUBE WINDOW

LONG-TABLE FAR SHUTTERS

CROSS-TABLE FAR SHUTTERS

OFF-FOCUS RADIATION

USEFUL BEAM

FILM

LIMITED OFF-FOCUS FOG

COLLIMASTER BEAM SHAPING SYSTEM

Figure 6:5. Schematic representation of one type of collimation scheme. See text for further explanation. (courtesy of Machlett Laboratories, Inc.)

partially serves to "cut off" extra-focal radiation. The far shutters can be adjusted manually by two rotating knobs located outside the collimator housing. The housing is constructed of suitable material (steel) for maximum radiation protection up to 150 kVp.

The light-beam indicator consists of a mirror and usually a quartz-iodide projection lamp to provide a high-intensity beam. The mirror is angled to reflect the light onto the patient. The light beam must be in perfect alignment with the x-ray beam, otherwise serious problems result in that the area indicated by the light beam may not be the total area irradiated and the patient may receive unnecessary radiation.

Ilumination is controlled by an integrated circuit timer which is activated by a push button in most cases. The lamp is switched off automatically after a fixed period of time, which may vary from about 60 seconds to 90 seconds.

The beam definer is a transparent plastic sheet which has two lines that intersect each other at 90°. The point of intersection marks the position of the central ray (Figure 6:1) of the x-ray beam. This ray is used as a centering pointer in positioning the patient.

All modern collimators have a field coverage indicator, usually in the form of a table. The field coverage reflects the values at which the shutters must be set so that a specific area on the patient will be adequately exposed by the primary beam. Field coverage is based on a number of parameters such as the source-to-image distance, the size of the cassette used for the examination, the distance from the focus of the x-ray tube to the collimator aperture and so on.

Postive Beam Limitation

The term *positive beam limitation* (PBL) refers to automatic field collimation. A PBL device ensures that the primary beam is collimated automatically to the size of the cassette placed in the Bucky tray. Such action may be cassette-controlled or push-button controlled, in which case the technologist selects the appropriate push button which matches the cassette size.

When using the PBL mechanism, the beam is collimated just slightly smaller than the film size, thus indicating evidence of collimation on all four sides of the film. In clinical practice, this is often referred to as "four-cornered collimation."

The principle of automatic field collimation is illustrated in Figure 6:6. Two special circuits (bridge circuits) operate in conjunction with measuring branches to move the shutters which are driven by motors through a control system. Today, such operation is controlled by microprocessors.

Other Aspects of Collimation

The main purpose of collimation is to protect the patient from unnecessary radiation since it limits the primary beam to the area of interest. In discussing the physical and technical factors influencing radiation protection of the patient, the International Commission on Radiological Protection (1976) points out that "the most important is the strict limitation of the size of the x-ray beam to the region of interest. . . ."

Apart from improving contrast, collimation also improves image detail. Because less scatter reaches the film, there are less divergent rays contributing to penumbral effects (the less the penumbral effect, the sharper the image).

Finally, collimation itself provides some filtration (Chapter 10) of the primary beam due to its construction. The mirror, for example, provides some filtration as the beam passes through it. The total added filtration provided by the entire collimator is equivalent to about 1 mm A1.

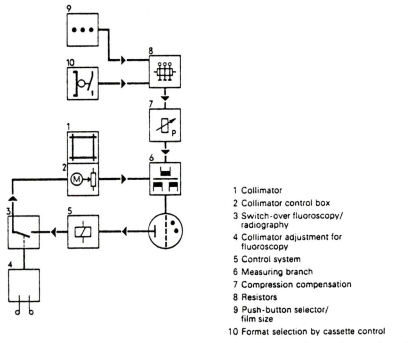

1 Collimator
2 Collimator control box
3 Switch-over fluoroscopy/
   radiography
4 Collimator adjustment for
   fluoroscopy
5 Control system
6 Measuring branch
7 Compression compensation
8 Resistors
9 Push-button selector/
   film size
10 Format selection by cassette control

Figure 6:6. The principle of automatic field collimation. See text for further explanation. (courtesy of the Siemens Corporation.)

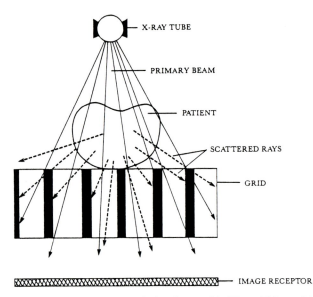

Figure 6:7. The removal of scattered radiation by a grid. The grid is positioned between the patient and the image receptor to absorb scattered rays.

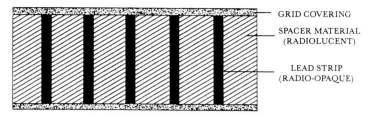

Figure 6:8. The basic construction of a grid.

THE SCATTERED RADIATION GRID

One of the most widely used anti-scatter devices is the scattered radiation grid; therefore, it will be discussed in detail in this section.

Definition and Historical Note

The *scattered radiation grid* is a device which is placed between the patient and the image receptor for the purpose of improving image contrast by absorbing scattered rays. The removal of scattered rays is illustrated in Figure 6:7.

The grid was developed by Dr. Gustave Bucky in 1913. His idea was based on the construction of a device that would absorb scattered rays and allow maximum transmission of the primary beam. The construction featured a special arrangement of a series of very then strips of radio-paque material (*absorber, lamellae* or *septa*) alternating with thin strips of radiolucent material (*interspace material* or *radiolucent slits*) as shown in Figure 6:8. Today, grids are based on the same design parameters except for a few refinements which contribute to better performance than the earlier grids.

Grid Design Parameters

Properties of the Lamellae

The requirements of the lamellae which are important to the overall design and performance of the grid are:

(a) high radiation absorption characteristics.
(b) high density.
(c) high atomic number.

One material which meets these requirements is lead (Pb), although other elements such as gold (Au) and tungsten (W) have been used in the construction of grids.

The atomic number of Pb is 82 and its density 11.35 gm/cm³. These two properties make Pb an effective absorber of scattered rays. Pb is relatively inexpensive and it can be shaped into extremely thin strips, an important feature in the design of the grid.

The thickness of the Pb lamellae or septa should be equivalent to 0.1 mm (100 μm) for effective attenuation, but the thickness equivalent common to most grids is 0.05 mm (50 μm), although thinner strips are used in more recent *high-strip-density* grids (to be discussed subsequently). The height of the lamellae is around 3 mm.

Lamellae Arrangement

The arrangement of the Pb lamellae can assume several forms in order to allow for maximum primary beam transmission. In the first design, the Pb lamellae are arranged so that the are parallel to each other (Figure 6:7). Such a grid is referred to as a *parallel linear grid*.

One of the problems of the parallel-type grid is that in certain defined circumstances it absorbs the primary beam. This phenomenon is referred to as *grid cutoff* and it is unacceptable in clinical work, since it results in decreased density (partial cutoff) or in some cases no density at all (total grid cutoff) on the film.

Another important feature of the parallel grid relates to the source-to-image receptor distance (SID) at which it can be used. These grids are made to be used at specific source-to-image receptor distances, and if they are not used at these distances, severe grid cutoff occurs.

The parallel grid is best utilized at a large SID and with small film sizes, and the x-ray tube can only be angled along the length of the Pb lamellae and not across them.

To overcome the problem of grid cutoff, another arrangement was developed in which the Pb lamellae are angled progressively towards the edges of the grid. Such a grid is called a *focussed grid*, and the arrangement of the lamellae is such that they are in perfect alignment with the oblique rays of the primary

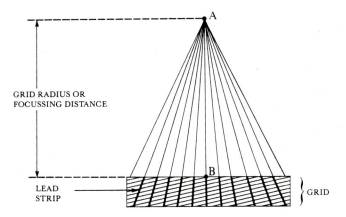

Figure 6:9. A focussed grid. The lead strips and the oblique rays are in perfect alignment. The focussing distance is AB.

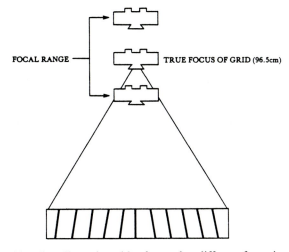

Figure 6:10. The grid radius allows the grid to be used at different focussing distances. (courtesy of the Liebel-Flarsheim Company, Ohio.)

beam. The *focussing distance, AB,* (Figure 6:9) is referred to as the *grid radius,* and the x-ray tube acts as the center of a circle described by this radius. The grid radius is variable, thus allowing the grid to be used at different focussing distances as shown in Figure 6:10.

The *focal range* is the distance at which the focussing distance can be adjusted without causing any detrimental effect (such as cutoff) on the film. The focussing distance may range from about 85 cm (34 inches) to 112 cm (44 inches), with the true focus of the grid being 95 cm (38 inches). The focussing distance is always indicated on the grid.

With focussed grids, the x-ray tube can only be angled along the length of the Pb lamellae but not across them. The central ray of the beam must be in the center of the grid for optimum results.

Later, the *cross-hatched* or *criss-cross grid* appeared. The arrangement of the lamellae is such that two parallel grids are placed one on top of the other so that their lamellae are perpendicular to each other. The cross-hatched grid will remove more scattered rays than the parallel or focussed grid, since it absorbs rays scattered in at least two directions and because of its higher lead content. These grids are not commonly used in imaging departments since their disadvantages outweigh their advantages. For example, tube angulations are not possible and the central ray must always be positioned in the exact center of the grid.

Interspace Material

The interspace material serves to support the Pb lamellae and hold them firmly and securely in position. The materials used for this purpose are very thin (about 350 μm) and radiolucent. It is also highly recommended that they be non-hygroscopic (do not absorb moisture). In this regard, aluminum and plastic fibre are most often used.

Aluminum has the advantages of being non-hygroscopic, reduces the visibility of grid lines on the film and absorbs scattered rays, compared to plastic fibre. A grid made of plastic fibre requires less radiation (than an aluminum grid) to produce the image because aluminum tends to absorb primary radiation as well, thus requiring an increase in exposrue factors especially at lower kilovoltages, in which case the patient dose is about 20 percent higher (Bushong, 1980). Therefore, grids made of plastic fibre interspaces are often more popular than those with aluminum interspaces.

The lamellae and interspace material are enclosed in a casing, which is usually made of aluminum, to give it mechanical rigidity. Other grid strips (lamellae and interspace material) such as those used in mammography are encased in carbon fibre/resin material, which allow a higher primary transmission than the aluminum casing.

The Grid Principle

In the previous discussion, the elements of grid construction were described. It was pointed out that the purpose of a grid is to improve image contrast by absorbing scattered rays.

Table 6-2

CLEAN-UP EFFICIENCY FOR LINEAR AND CRISS-CROSS GRIDS OF DIFFERENT RATIOS

(Courtesy of the Liebel-Flarsheim Company)

CLEAN-UP	TYPE	POSITIONING LATITUDE	RECOMMENDED UP TO	REMARKS
Super-lative	6:1 Criss-Cross	Good	110 kVp	table tilt limited to 5°
Excellent	12:1 Linear	Very slight	110 kVp (Suitable for higher kilovoltages)	extra care required for proper alignment. Usually used in fixed mount
	5:1 Criss-Cross	Extreme	100 kVp	table tilt limited to 5°
Very Good	10:1 Linear	Slight	100 kVp	reasonable care required for proper alignment
Good	8:1 Linear	Fair	100 kVp	for general stationary grid use
Moderate	6:1 Linear 5:1 Linear	Extreme	80 kVp	very easy to use

The grid is placed between the patient and the image receptor and must allow maximum primary transmission (fraction of incident primary radiation transmitted by the grid). Since primary rays are less oblique than scattered rays, most of them pass through the interspace material, however, some are absorbed by the lamellae, thus resulting in grid cutoff. This is one of the reasons why exposure factors must be increased for examinations requiring a grid.

Scattered rays are more oblique than primary rays and therefore will fall on the lead strips of the grid and will be absorbed. However, depending on the energy of the primary beam, these scattered rays may have enough energy to penetrate the lead septa.

If the lead strips are placed closer together, the angle at which two scattered rays are allowed to pass through the strips (*effective solid angle*) decreases and this factor influences the amount of scattered rays removed by the grid. This removal of scattered rays is referred to as the *cleanup efficiency* of the grid. A properly designed grid will exhibit about 80-90 percent cleanup efficiency. The fraction of the incident scattered rays transmitted is referred to as the scatter transmission of the grid. The cleanup efficiency for linear and crossed grids of different ratios is given in Table 6:2.

Types of Grids

In the design of a grid, the lamellae and interspace material are arranged so that they describe parallel, focussed and cross-hatched grids. These grids can either be stationary or moving.

Stationary Grids

A *stationary grid,* whether it be parallel, focussed or cross-hatched, is always fixed onto the image receptor and does not move during the x-ray exposure. This results in the Pb septa appearing in the form of *grid lines* on the film as a result of absorption of primary rays by the Pb septa. The interspace material shows up as thin dark lines. These lines act as distractors when viewing images and are therefore a serious limitation of stationary grids.

The stationary grid is very useful in portable radiography. It may be available as a separate unit, which may be placed over the cassette, or it may be affixed permanently (built in) on the cassette in which case the unit is referred to as a *grid cassette.* Apart from being used in portable work, stationary grids may be used in the operating room and they are also available on some fluoroscopic machines.

Moving Grids — The Potter-Bucky Diaphragm

The problem of grid lines imposed by stationary grids can be eliminated by moving the grid during the exposure. This concept was introduced in 1920 by Dr. Hollis Potter. He used a drive mechanism which was activated in such a way as to move the grid at right angles to the Pb septa during the exposure and to stop the motion after the exposure is terminated. The motion of the grid causes blurring of the Pb septa and completely eliminates grid lines.

The moving grid has become to be known as the *Potter-Bucky Diaphragm* (or Bucky, for short). The Bucky is an integral component of almost all fixed radiographic and radiographic/fluoroscopic units. For radiographic units, the Bucky is mounted just underneath the tabletop and it is fitted onto a rail system that allows the technologist to move it along the length of the table.

The essential features of the Bucky assembly are:

    (a) a scattered radiation grid.
    (b) an electronic motor which provides the mechanism to move the grid.
    (c) a device for controlling grid travel.
    (d) a cassette tray.

To set a grid in motion is not a simple task, since there are a number of points that must be considered to ensure optimum results. For example, the motion must be smooth and the assembly must be free from vibrations which may cause image blurring. The rate of grid travel must be uniform throughout the exposure. This is very critical, and usually the grid is set in motion prior to the exposure to attain some maximum speed of travel. The exposure is released at this point and, finally, the speed gradually decreases to zero after the exposure terminates.

Types of Grid Motion

Three mechanisms are available to move the grid in the Bucky assembly. In the past, the *single-stroke* motion (*single-action hydraulic mechanism*) was common. This mechanism involves motion of the grid in one direction only, that is, the grid travels only once (2-3 cm) across the film during the x-ray exposure. The mechanism requires that the technologist preset a tension on a spring of a piston which acts on a column of oil to ensure a smooth motion of the grid during the exposure. This process was repeated for each exposure. Today the single-stroke mechanism has become obsolete.

Another method of moving the grid is the *reciprocating* mechanism. In this method (also referred to as a two-speed reciprocating Bucky system), an electric motor is used, in conjunction with the x-ray exposure timing circuit, to move the grid across the film at a fast and constant speed, reversing the direction and then moving the grid back at a slower speed. This mechanism still exists on some radiographic units, but it is rapidly being replaced by a more sophisticated and popular type of mechanism, the *oscillating* mechanism, which renders an accelerated motion of the grid.

The oscillatory mechanism is simple in operation compared to the reciprocating grid. It allows the grid to move in a circular fashion during the x-ray exposure. The grid mechanism is shown in Figure 6:11. It consists of a

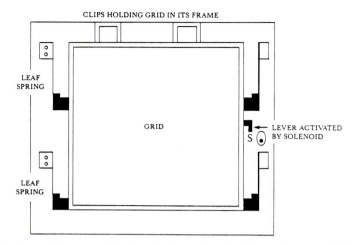

Figure 6:11. An oscillating or vibrating Bucky mechanism (from Chesney, M.D. and Chesney, D.N.: *X-ray Equipment for Student Radiographers.* Blackwell Scientific Publications, Oxford. 1971).

framework to support the grid by means of leaf springs. When the x-ray exposure switch is activated, a solenoid strikes the metal extension, S, and this action sets the grid in motion such that it moves very quickly at first and slows down after about 30 seconds. This time period enables the oscillating grid to be used in examinations requiring long exposures.

The Stroboscopic Effect

In some instances during radiography, although the mechanism to move the grid is activated (that is, the Bucky selector on the control panel indicates that the Bucky is in use), grid lines still appear on the film. This phenomenon is generally referred to as the *stroboscopic effect* and it occurs when the motion of the grid is synchronized with the pulsation of the x-ray generator. This is an important consideration in the design of a mechanism to move the grid.

Apart from the stroboscopic effect, the other causes of grid lines when the moving grid principle is used are:

(a) disrupted motion of the grid during travel,
(b) commencement of the exposure before the grid achieves some maximum speed,
(c) poor centering of the central ray to the center of the grid, and
(d) continuation of the exposure when the grid slows down or comes to rest.

Performance Characteristics

The ability of a grid to remove scattered rays depends on several factors. These factors have been introduced for the purpose of quantitative analysis in the study of grid techniques. The factors are the grid ratio, grid frequency, selectivity, contrast improvement factor, Bucky factor and the relative patient exposure. Each of these will now be described briefly.

The Grid Ratio

In the design of a grid, the lead septa are separated by radiolucent spacers. In Figure 6:12 the dimension of the lead septa such as the thickness, (d), and the height, (h), are shown, while the thickness of the spacer material is shown as D. The *grid ratio* (*GR*) is defined as the ratio of the height of the lead septa to the distance between the septa. This ratio can be expressed as:

$$GR = \frac{h}{D}$$

If the height of a lead strip is 3.2 mm and the distance between two strips is 0.2 mm (thickness of the interspace material), then the grid ratio is:

$$GR = \frac{3.2}{0.2}$$

$$= \frac{32}{2}$$

$$= 16$$

It follows that since the spacer material is 16 times as high as it is wide (not to be confused with the length), the grid ratio is said to be 16:1. When the spacer material is 12 times as high as it is wide, the grid ratio is 12:1 and so on. Grid ratios common to imaging departments are 5:1, 6:1, 8:1, 10:1, 12:1 and 16:1, with the 12:1 being the most commonly used in Bucky mechanisms.

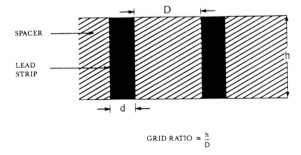

Figure 6:12. The grid ratio is defined as the ratio of the height of the lead strip to the distance between the strips.

The grid ratio relates to the cleanup efficiency such that the higher the ratio, the greater the cleanup efficiency as is indicated in Table 6:1. High-ratio grids remove more scatter than low-ratio grids, because they (high-ratio grids) have smaller effective solid angles — that is, they allow only rays scattered at smaller angles to pass through them, compared to low-ratio grids. However, as the grid ratio increases, the relative patient exposure increases.

Relative Patient Exposure

The *relative patient exposure* is defined as the amount by which the exposure with a grid must be increased to obtain the same exposure at the film without a grid. The patient exposure increases with grids. A moving grid requires at least 15 percent more radiation compared to a stationary grid of the same design features. Higher grid ratios also require more radiation than grids of low ratios.

Grid Frequency

The number of lamellae or grid septa is also expressed as the number of lines per centimeter, or simply the *grid fequency* (also referred to as the *grid lattice* or *strip density*).

This factor plays a role in the performance of the grids in such a way that the higher the frequency, the greater the removal of scatter, and grid lines appear less visible on the film. As the number of lead strips increases, there must be an increase in the grid ratio to produce the same effect as a grid with less strips. A 12:1 high-frequency (fine line) grid will not produce the same effect compared to a 12:1 high frequency grid.

Grid frequencies normally range from about 24 to 43 lines per cm, although higher strip-density grids are available. The relative patient exposure increases with higher strip-density grids since there is more lead to absorb primary radiation.

Contrast Improvement Factor

The main purpose of a grid is to improve image contrast. To measure contrast improvement, a factor was introduced for quantitative work. This factor is the *contrast improvement factor* (K), which is defined as the ratio of contrast with the anti-scatter device to the contrast obtained without the device. For a scattered radiation grid, K is the ratio of contrast with the grid to that of contrast without the grid. K depends on several factors, including the thickness of the patient, the field size, and the physical characteristics of the primary beam.

In Table 6:3, the contrast improvement factors for several grids with different ratios, but of the same thickness of lead and interspace material, are shown. Where K is equal to 1, there is no contrast improvement. Values higher than 1 indicate better contrast improvement.

Table 6-3

THE CONTRAST IMPROVEMENT FACTOR FOR GRIDS OF DIFFERENT RATIOS
BUT WITH THE SAME THICKNESS OF LEAD STRIPS AND
INTERSPACE MATERIAL

(Courtesy of the Liebel-Flarsheim Company.)

RATIO	AT 70 kVp	AT 95 kVp	AT 120 kVp
No grid	1.0	1.0	1.0
5:1	3.5	2.5	2.0
8:1	4.75	3.25	2.5
12:1	5.25	3.75	3.0
16:1	5.75	4.0	3.25
5:1 Crossed grid	5.75	3.5	2.75
8:1 Crossed grid	6.75	4.25	3.25

Selectivity

The *selectivity,* represented by the Greek letter sigma (Σ), is the ratio of transmitted primary radiation (T_p) to the transmitted scattered rays (T_s). This can be expressed as:

$$\Sigma = \frac{T_p}{T_s}$$

Grid selectivity not only depends on the grid ratio but also on the amount of lead used in grid construction. By making the grid septa wider, one can increase the total amount of lead without changing the grid ratio. This also increases the cleanup efficiency and the contrast improvement factor, however, the thickness of the septa must be kept within reasonable limits.

Bucky Factor

The *Bucky factor* (BF) is of importance to the technologist, since technique charts (exposure factors) are made up for Bucky and non-Bucky techniques.

Table 6-4

CONDITIONS CAUSING GRID CUT OFF WITH A FOCUSED GRID

CONDITIONS PRODUCING GRID CUT-OFF	EXPLANATION	EFFECT ON FILM DENSITY
Grid turned upside-down (tube side not facing tube)	Oblique primary rays are absorbed by the lead strips at the periphery of the grid. Some primary rays pass through center of grid	Narrow strip of density in the middle of the film
Lateral decentering (central ray not centered to middle of grid)	Primary rays absorbed uniformly by all grid strips resulting in cut off over the entire film	Loss in density (light film) over the entire film
Grid not used at the correct source-to-image distance (SID) (off-focus)	(a) Closer than specified SID. — cut off of primary rays (b) Greater than specified SID — more cut off of primary rays than in (a) above	(a) Loss in density at periphery of film (b) Effect same as in (a) but less pronounced loss in density at periphery compound to middle of film
Lateral decentering with incorrect focussing distance	(a) Lateral decentering with smaller focussing distance — cut off of phenomenon (b) lateral decentering with greater focussing distance — cut off of phenomenon	For both, the effect is the same, that is, there is a loss in density on one side compared to the other side of the film which is much darker

The BF for any anti-scatter technique is defined as the ratio of incident to transmitted radiation. For a grid, the BF is expressed as

$$BF = \frac{\text{technique factors (mAs) with grid}}{\text{technique factors (mAs) without grid}}$$

In general, grids with high frequencies and high ratios have higher Bucky factors. For example, a 16:1 ratio grid with 57 lines per cm has a slightly higher

BF than a 12:1 ratio grid with 33 lies per cm (Doi et al, 1983).

Other definitions of the BF state that it:

(a) "is equal to the ratio of radiation emerging from the patient to that transmitted by the device divided by the fractional field of coverage" (Barnes, 1978).

(b) "is the increase in tube loading required to employ the scatter reduction technique at the same kVp" (Barnes, 1978).

The Bucky factors for a 12:1 and 16:1 grid used at 70 kVp are 4 and 4.5, respectively. This means that image quality is slightly better than the 16:1 grid, however, a higher BF also implies greater patient dose, and since the increase in BF from 12:1 to 16:1 is not significant, a 12.1 grid is preferable for routine clinical work.

Conditions for Grid Cutoff

Cutoff problems are not often encountered with Bucky techniques, however, in some instances cutoff may occur if the central ray is centered to the grid. Most problems are encountered when the stationary grid is used, particularly in portable work. Table 6:4 lists the more common problems encountered with the use of stationary focussed grid.

In using cross-hatched grids, precise relationships between the central ray and the grid must be maintained. If the tube is angled or the grid is not used at the correct focussing distance, grid cutoff results.

The focussed grid was developed to minimize grid cutoff. Such factors as reduced grid ratio (cutoff is directly proportional to grid ratio) and construction of the grid so that it is thinner at the edges compared to the center will also minimize grid cutoff.

Finally, when a stationary grid is used by a technologist in a portable examination, the following points must be taken into consideration:

(a) check the grid ratio, since this will affect the choice of exposure factors.

(b) check for the tube side of the grid and ensure that this side faces the x-ray tube during the exposure.

(c) check the direction in which the lead septa lie, that is, whether they lie along the length of the grid or across the width. This will assist you during angled beam techniques.

(d) check for the correct focussing distance of the grid and use a measuring tape to measure this distance.

(e) check that the grid is not angled.

(f) position central ray to center of the grid.

New High Strip-Density Grids

Recall that conventional stationary grids cast grid lines on the film which may be disturbing when viewing images. The introduction and development new *high strip-density* (HSD) grids have gained popularity in some imaging departments.

The purpose of HSD grids is to reduce the line pattern interference imposed by conventional low strip-density (LSD) grids and in some cases eliminate the need for Bucky mechanisms, which may produce geometric and motion unsharpness and are also very costly.

Design Features

The characteristic features of HSD linear grids are the grid lattice, thickness of the lead septa, and the interspace material.

HSD grids are made of lead septa which are 45 microns thick, separated by spacers, each of which is 130 microns thick, compared to LSD conventional grids in which the lead septa are 50 microns thick and 200-250 microns thick aluminum spacers. The grid frequency of HSD grids is about 57 lines per cm compared to 33 to 40 lines per cm for conventional LSD grids.

Performance

An interesting study carried out by Doi et al. (1983) indicates that:

(a) the contrast improvement factor and the Bucky factor for HSD grids are either comparable or somewhat less than LSD conventional grids.

(b) when the grid is stationary, grid lines cannot be seen.

(c) the conventional Bucky mechanism can be removed and the HSD grid may be used instead for both radiography and fluoroscopy.

(d) removal of the Bucky provides sharper images due to better beam geometry in image formation (shorter object-film distance) and elimination of grid motion.

(e) there is "potential for decreased patient dose and the elimination of grid decentering."

(f) exposure times can be reduced because the stroboscopic effect is eliminated.

HSD grids are available commercially and they can be used in all radiography work, particularly in portable examinations and in the operating room.

Considerations in Grid Selection

The selection of a grid for clinical radiography depends on three factors:

(a) the amount of scattered rays produced by the patient. For thicker body parts, higher ratio grids are more efficient than those with lower ratios.

(b) kilovoltage technique. The use of high kVp (reduced patient dose) requires higher ratio grids. When techniques are below 90 kVp, 8:1 ratio grids provide acceptable contrast. In general, 12:1 ratio grids are

Table 6-5

CONSIDERATIONS IN THE SELECTION OF A GRID

(Courtesy of the Leibel-Florsheim Company.)

TYPE OF GRID	FEATURES AND USES
4:1 ratio linear (Low dose)	Special grid for use in image intensification and spot filming. Adequate clean-up for small coned-down areas combined with relatively small patient dosage.
5:1 ratio linear	Moderate clean-up. Extreme latitude in use. Use at lower kilovoltages (up to 80 kVp), wherever wide latitude is desired. Very easy to use.
5:1 ratio crossed	Very high clean-up, especially at lower kilovoltages. Extreme latitude in use. Use up to 100 kVp, wherever wide and excellent clean-up are desired. Very easy to use. Not recommended for tilted-tube techniques.
6:1 ratio linear	Clean-up slightly better than the 5:1 ratio linear, but with approximately the same positioning latitude.
6:1 ratio crossed	Better clean-up than the 5:1 crossed. Very easy to use. Not recommended for tilted-tube techniques.
7:1 ratio linear	Better clean-up than 6:1 linear. Fair distance latitude. Little centering and leveling latitude. Use up to 100 kVp where wide latitude is not required.
8:1 ratio crossed	Extremely high clean-up. Superior to 16:1 ratio linear grid at kilovoltages up to 125. Positioning latitude equivalent to 8:1 ratio linear. Not usable for tilted-tube techniques.
12:1 ratio linear	Better clean-up than 8:1 linear. Very little positioning latitude. Use for both low and high kilovoltage techniques (up to 110 kVp or slightly higher). Extra care is required for proper alignment. Usually used in fixed mount or Potter-Bucky Diaphragm.
16:1 ratio	Very high clean-up. Practically no positioning latitude. Intended primarily for use above 100 kVp in Potter-Bucky Diaphragm. Excellent for high kVp radiographs of thick body sections.

used in techniques above 90 kVp. For high voltages (greater than 100 kVp), 16:1 grids may be used to the best advantage.

(c) x-ray generator capacity. In general, a 16:1 grid is most efficient with generators which can yield more than 100 kVp.

In Table 6:5, the general features and uses of grids which may assist in the selection process are presented.

Limitations of Anti-Scatter Grids

In the foregoing discussion, several problems associated with grids are identified. Among these are the higher patient doses (although lower doses can be obtained with more sensitive image receptors such as rare-earth screens). The main shortcoming of the grid is that it does not transmit the primary beam very efficiently. This is due to absorption of the beam by the lead septa, the spacers and the casing material.

SCANNING SLIT TECHNIQUES

To overcome the problems imposed by grids, attention has been focussed recently on *scanning slit assemblies*. The technique essentially involves a series of slits (a slit is a long and narrow aperture cut into a thin metal plate) placed before and after the patient, define the primary beam and absorb most of the rays scattered out of the primary beam, respectively.

Historical Note

The idea of scanning slits as an anti-scatter device is not new. The method was first suggested by the Swiss radiologist, Pasche, in around 1902 and the results were published in 1903. Later, in 1913, Wahl, a German researcher, rediscovered the concept. In 1921, Cole applied for patents for the scanning apparatus. In 1952, Vallebona studied the technique once again. In 1975, Jaffe and Webster revived the technique and published their findings in *Radiology,* Journal of the Radiological Society of North America (RSNA). Since then, several papers describing scanning slit assembilies and their usefulness in clinical practice have been published in other recognized journals of physical and clinical imaging.

The Dual Scanning Slit Assembly

A *dual scanning slit assembly* is shown in Figure 6:13. It consists of two scanning slits: a *fore slit* which serves to define the primary, and an *aft slit* which prevents scatter from reaching the image receptor. The fore slit is positioned between the x-ray tube and patient, while the aft slit is placed between the patient and image receptor.

In producing an image, the two slits move in the same direction and at the same time to scan the area to be imaged. Since the beam is highly collimated (a small defined beam of radiation), very little scatter is produced in the patient. The scattered rays do not fall on the image receptor because of the position of the aft slits.

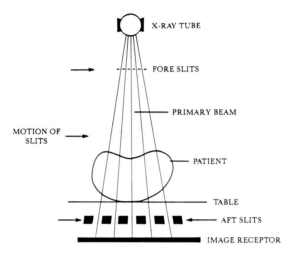

Figure 6:13. Schematic representation of the scanning multiple slit assembly. See text for further explanation.

The dual scanning slit technique has not found widespread use in clinical practice because of the long exposure time required and the increased loading on the x-ray tube. Although the technique provides significant contrast improvement over cnventional anti-scatter grids, the Bucky factor is too large. This is due to the fact that the fractional area of interest irradiated at any given time during the exposure is too small.

In the dual scanning slit assembly, it is important that the fore and aft slits be aligned carefully in order to provide maximum primary transmission.

The Multiple Scanning Slit Assembly

The problems associated with dual scanning slits (for example, the Bucky factor) can be reduced by using multiple slits. One such recent device is the *scanning multiple slit assembly* (SMSA), which was developed by Barnes, Brezovich and Witten (1977) for use in abdominal radiography at the University of Alabama in Birmingham.

The SMSA is illustrated in Figure 6:13. Essentially, it consists of an array of beam-defining fore slits which are in perfect alignment with an array of *aft slots.* The fore slits and aft slots are also coupled and move synchronously during the exposure. Barnes et al. (1977) make a distinction between a slit and a slot. They state that "a slit refers to a long and narrow cut in a plate about 1.6 mm thick or less, whereas a slot refers to a similar cut in a much thicker piece of material."

When an exposure is made (the rotor of the x-ray tube is allowed to attain some maximum speed), the slit assembly begins to move for about 5 cm when the x-ray generator is turned on. The movement is such that the aft slots travel a little faster than the fore slits. The aft slots are responsible for the elimination of scatter and the motion also eliminates grid cutoff.

The SMSA features relatively thick and dense slots to prevent scatter penetration. Other features, such as the narrowness of the slits and slots, allow the assembly to approximate an "ideal" grid. In this regard, Barnes et al. (1977) have reported that the device produces a marked improvement in contrast compared to conventional grids for the same patient exposure. The device has been found to be the most efficient and practical method for reducing scatter in large field (such as in abdominal radiography) examinations.

The SMSA has also been applied to mammography, an area where the grid poses a problem because of its poor transmission of soft rays. King, Barnes and Yester (1978) have used a SMSA in mammography and have reported that the device virtually eliminates all scatter and provides images that are comparable to conventional anti-scatter techniques at reduced doses.

The use of scanning slit assemblies to reduce scatter has been under investigation for some time. The results to date indicate that the SMSA is a practical alternative to the grid, since it provides a very efficient means of scatter elimination despite a few limitations.

Limitations of SMSA

The SMSA is restricted for use in static x-ray imaging because of the longer exposure times required during operation in comparison to conventional grid techniques. The device cannot be applied to dynamic imaging such as in cine-fluorography, fluoroscopy and spot film imaging. The SMSA must be used at the specified source-to-image distance (100 cm), otherwise its efficiency decreases. Finally, the tube loading is increased when these devices (SMSA) are used, although such loading can be reduced by increasing the kVp.

In the future, one may see the appearance of rotating aperture wheel anti-scatter devices. One such unit (see following Research Studies section in this chapter) is presently under development.

RESEARCH STUDIES

A New Grid

STUDY 1. A new type of grid. Brezovich, I.A., and Barnes, G. T. Medical Physics, 4 (5), September/October, 1977.

In this study the authors discuss their research on a new type of grid in which the lead septa are arranged in a "zigzag" pattern. Their results indicate that, compared to a conventional linear grid having the same lead content and lead septa of the same width and height:

   (a) the zigzag grid is much better in eliminating scatter.
   (b) the contrast improvement factor for the zigzag grid is better.
   (c) the Bucky factor is larger.
   (d) a more sophisticated motion to blur out moire patterns resulting from the linear motion of the zigzag grid would have to be developed.

Tantalum Air-Interspace Grid

STUDY 2. Tantalum air-interspace crossed grid. Design and performance characteristics. Sorenson, J.A., Niklason, L. T., Jacobsen, S.C., Knutti, D.E., and Johnson, T.C. Radiology, 145, 485-492, November, 1982.

This study examined a more efficient grid design compared to conventional linear and crossed grids. The authors also investigated a design which could provide scatter elimination comparable to a slit scanning device "but with more acceptable tube loading and exposure time requirements."

They constructed a crossed grid made of 0.1-mm thick tantalum strips supported between 1-mm thick carbon fibre plates with air as the interspace material. They then compared the performance characteristics of the tantalum air-interspaced grid to a 12:1 linear grid, a 6:1 crossed grid and a slit scanning device with a 6:1 conventional grid.

Their results indicated that "the tantalum crossed grid provided a high level of scatter clean-up (comparable to some slit methods), but had a tube loading and exposure time requirement similar to those of conventional anti-scatter grids."

The Use of Grids in Digital Subtraction Angiography

STUDY 3. Effectiveness of Anti-scatter grids in digital subtraction angiography. Kruger, R.A., Sorenson, J.A., and Niklason, L. T. Investigative Radiology, 18 (3), May/June, 1983.

In this study, the researchers analyze the benefit of the use of anti-scatter grids for digital subtraction angiography (DSA — Chapter 18). The theory and methodology of their work is not within the scope of this text, however, the authors found that:

"According to this analysis, conventional grids offer a small improvement in image quality for DSA exams. The use of magnification reduces the detected scatter-to-primary ratio and has a 100 % primary transmission, but is not a dose efficient means of scatter rejection. Because patient exposure increases as the square of the magnification, gains in scatter rejection are almost completely offset by increased patient exposure. For DSA studies, there exists the possibility of reducing dose by 20% to 45% compared with conventional grids by employing grids with higher primary transmission and modest selectivities. Such grids currently are being constructed in our laboratory and will be tested for DSA application in the near future."

Rotating Aperture Wheel Anti-Scatter Device

STUDY 4. Fore-and-Aft Rotating Aperture Wheel (RAW) device for improving radiographic contrast. Rubin, S. Society of Photo-optical Instrumentation Engineers (SPIE) Volume 173. Application of Optical Instrumentation in Medicine, VII. 1979.

This study describes the theory of RAW technology and presents preliminary results using the device. The authors' abstract states:

A Rotating Aperture Wheel (RAW) techology is under development which involves replacing a grid for scatter elimination with an assembly of one fore and two aft lead aperture wheels which are rotated so as to maintain the alignment between the split or aperture pattern of each. Such a design has the unique feature that its motion can be made independent of the x-ray exposure time and duration allowing for the first time the practical use of a moving slit anti-scatter technique in rapid sequence and dynamic radiographic procedures. The technology is flexible so as to lend itself toward use with varying source to image receptor distances such as is involved in fluoroscopy.

SUMMARY

1. When a beam of x-rays interacts with an object, a portion of it is absorbed and a fraction of the other portion is transmitted through the object. The other fraction is scattered at various angles.
2. The effect of scattered rays is detrimental to image quality and, therefore, it must be controlled or eliminated.
3. The factors influencing the production of scattered rays are patient thickness, field size or the area irradiated and the kilovoltage. The sources of scatter, on the other hand, include the x-ray tube housing, the collimator, the table, the film cassette, the floor and, most importantly, the patient.
4. Anti-scatter techniques include reducing the kVp, the use of compression, the air gap technique, limitation of the field size, the scattered

radiation grid technique and the scanning slit method.

5. Lowering the kVp reduces the production of scatter and improves image contrast.

6. Compression decreases patient thickness, hence, decreases the amount of scattered rays reaching the film. Compression also ensures that the exposure at the image plane is more uniform and image sharpness is improved since the object is now closer to the film.

7. The air gap technique ensures that a space of about 15 cm is left between the object and the image receptor. Most of the scattered rays fall out of this gap before they reach the film. Other considerations, such as the problem of magnification, are discussed.

8. Restriction of the x-ray field size is accomplished through the use of beam limiting devices or beam restrictors. These include cones, cylinders, diaphragms and a specially constructed unit called a collimator. Reducing the field size only to the area of interest reduces the amount of scattered rays reaching the film.

9. The scattered radiation grid is one of the most widely used antiscatter techniques. The grid consists of a series of very thin strips of radio-opaque material, such as lead, alternating with thin strips of radiolucent material such as aluminum or plastic fibre.

10. The grid is positioned in between the patient and the image receptor to absorb scattered rays before they reach the film. This process improves image contrast.

11. The main purpose of an anti-scatter technique such as the grid principle is to improve contrast.

12. The strips are arranged in a definite fashion to describe at least three types of grids: a parallel grid, a focussed grid and a criss-cross grid. Each of these are described and their limitations identified.

13. The main purpose of a focussed grid is to minimize grid cutoff (absorption of the primary beam).

14. Grids may be stationary or moving. A stationary grid does not move during the exposure and hence causes the appearance of grid lines (shadows of the lead strips) on the image. A moving grid consists of some mechanism to move the grid during the exposure, thus eliminating grid lines.

15. The Potter-Bucky diaphragm consists of a grid, a motor to move the grid, a device for controlling grid travel and a cassette tray.

16. Three types of grid motion are identified and discussed. These include the single-stroke action, the reciprocating mechanism and the oscillating mechanism.

17. The stroboscopic effect occurs when the motion of the grid is synchronized with the pulsation of the x-ray generator. This effect causes the appearance of grid lines on the image. Other causes for the appear-

ance of grid lines are identified.

18. The performance of a grid is influenced by the grid ratio, grid frequency, selectivity, contrast improvement factor, Bucky factor, and the relative patient exposure. A definition of each of these is given and their influence on the ability of the grid to remove scattered rays are discussed.

19. The purpose of a high strip-density (HSD) grid is to reduce the line pattern interference imposed by conventional low strip-density grids. HSD grids have more lines per centimeter and are made of much thinner lead strips and interspace material compared to conventional grids.

20. Three factors influence the selection of a grid. These are the amount of scattered rays produced by the patient, the kVp technique and the x-ray generator capacity.

21. The main limitation of an anti-scatter grid is that it does not transmit the primary beam efficiently.

22. Scanning slit assemblies are intended to overcome the problems imposed by grids. A scanning slit assembly consists of two sets of scanning slits: a fore slit and an aft slit. The fore slit defines the primary beam, while the aft slit prevents scatter from reaching the film. Two types of assemblies are available: the dual slit and multiple slit scanning assemblies. The characteristic features of each of these are described and their limitations identified.

23. Several research studies are described very briefly with respect to a new grid, tantalum air-interspaced crossed grid, grids in digital subtraction angiography, and a rotating aperture wheel anti-scatter device.

CHAPTER 7

THE X-RAY MACHINE — PART II

IN Chapter 2, the x-ray machine was discussed in terms of the main components relating to the generation and control of x-rays. While the overall goal of that chapter was to provide an overview of several parameters influencing x-ray exposure, other concepts (for example, rectification) were introduced to draw the student's attention to the general complexity of the x-ray machine.

The purpose of this chapter is to describe such complexity by providing a more complete discussion of alternating current (AC), rectification of AC, and x-ray generators.

ALTERNATING CURRENT

The electrical power supplied to houses, large buildings (including hospitals) is AC. With AC, the voltage and current across a resistor change values as a function of time. If these values are plotted (on graph paper) with respect to time, a waveform (Figure 7:1) results. Two points to note about Figure 7:1 are:

(a) Voltage and current are in phase.
(b) There are positive and negative half cycles.

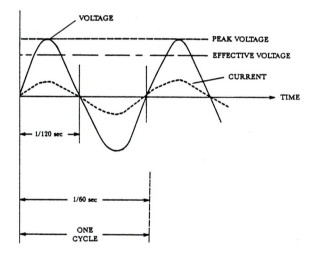

Figure 7:1. The waveform of an alternating current which shows that the voltage and current are in phase and that there are positive and negative half cycles.

Frequency of AC

The frequency of AC can be defined as the number of complete cycles per second. In the United States and Canada, electric power companies produce AC with a frequency of 60 cycles per second. This means that each cycle of AC takes 1/60 second for completion.

In discussing AC, the following points are considered important, since they will help the student understand further concepts such as rectification, testing x-ray exposure timers, and so on:

(a) The unit of frequency is the Hertz (Hz).
(b) 1 Hertz = 1 cycle per second.

(c) 1 cycle per second = 2 impulses per second.
(d) 60 cycles per second = 60 × 2
                        = 120 impulses per second.

Single-phase AC

The alternating waveform shown in Figure 7:1 represents *single-phase power,* since it is produced by a generator having a single circuit or phase as shown in Figure 7:2. This kind of power is available in radiology departments, and there are x-ray machines which operate on single phase. However, single-phase units are limited in their efficiency of x-ray production and exposure times. This has lead to the development and introduction of x-ray machines which operate on three-phase power.

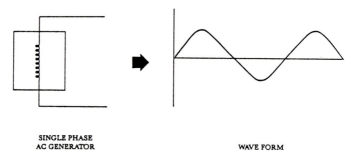

SINGLE PHASE
AC GENERATOR   WAVE FORM

Figure 7:2. A single-phase alternating current generator and associated waveform.

Three-phase AC

In three-phase generation of electrical power, specially designed generators (which can be of two types) produce waveforms as shown in Figure 7:3 a-b. These waveforms have the same frequency and magnitude, but instead of being in phase with each other, they are now out of phase by one-third of a cycle (or *120°*). In this arrangement, the peak voltage for each phase is produced at different times. Therefore, the overall effective voltage will be very close to the value of the peak voltage. This point has implications for producing x-rays more efficiently, compared to single-phase power. For example, the quality and quantity of x-rays produced with three-phase equipment is higher than with single-phase units.

Advantages of AC

The advantages of AC from the standpoint of x-ray equipment operation include:

(a) Transformers operate on AC power rather than with direct current.

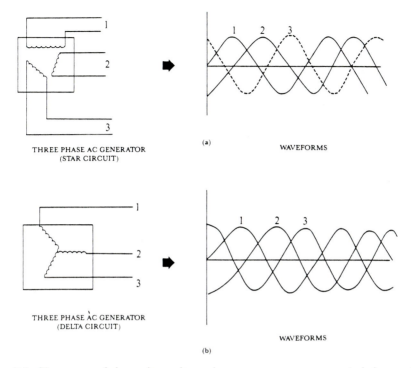

THREE PHASE AC GENERATOR
(STAR CIRCUIT)

(a) WAVEFORMS

THREE PHASE AC GENERATOR
(DELTA CIRCUIT)

WAVEFORMS

(b)

Figure 7:3. Two types of three-phase alternating current generators and their associated waveforms. Each waveform is out of phase by one-third of a cycle or 120°.

  (b) The motor (induction motor) used to rotate the disk in a rotating-anode x-ray tube operates on AC.
  (c) Other components in the x-ray unit operate on AC.

RECTIFICATION OF AC

If AC is supplied to the x-ray tube, the following occurs:

  (a) During the positive half of the AC cycle, the anode is positive and the cathode negative. Therefore, electrons flow from cathode to anode (the tube conducts).
  (b) During the negative half cycle, the cathode is positive and the anode negative. Therefore, electrons will try to flow from anode to cathode.

The action in (b) is predominantly unacceptable and hence some process is required to suppress the negative half cycle (inverse voltage), thus changing a pulsating AC to a pulsating direct current. The process of accomplishing this is referred to as *rectification,* and the devices in the x-ray circuit used for this purpose are called *rectifiers.*

Rectifiers

Rectifiers are of two types:

(A) Thermionic high-vacuum tube rectifiers or *"valve tubes"* which are akin to the x-ray tube in basic construction .

The design and operation of the valve tube is such that it allows electrons to flow only from cathode to anode, thus converting the AC voltage from the high tension transformer (Chapter 2) to a direct current. This voltage can now be used by the x-ray tube without the fear of reverse voltage across the x-ray tube.

The valve tube will only conduct during the positive half of the AC cycle. During the negative half cycle, the anode is maintained at a low voltage and, therefore, electrons cannot flow.

Since valve tubes are located in the high-voltage section of the x-ray machine, they are immersed in oil for insulation purposes. In the past, valve tubes were used in x-ray circuits, but recent developments in solid-state electronics have made them obsolete. Today, more and more efficient solid-state rectifiers are being used in x-ray machines.

(B) *Solid-State Rectifiers*

Solid-state rectifiers are made of semi-conducting materials. Semiconductors are materials such as germanium, silicon, lead telluride, selenium and so on, which conduct only when a certain amount of energy is applied to them. Semiconductors exhibit two types of conductivity.:

(a) *n-type conductivity,* in which an impurity (phosphor) is added to give the semiconductor a surplus of negatively charged electrons. This type of material is called an n-type conductor.

(b) *p-type conductivity,* in which an impurity (aluminum) is added to accept electrons from the semiconducting material. The "holes" or vacancies left by these electrons (which move to the acceptor, aluminum) act as though they are positive charges and move readily about the semiconductor. This type of material is referred to as a p-type conductor.

The basis of a solid-state rectifier (semiconductor diode) is a semiconductor junction called a *p-n junction,* shown in Figure 7:4. In A, the current is very large because the electron exchange across the junction is aided by the battery such that the electrons are driven from n to p. In B, since the polarity connection of the battery is now reversed, a minute current flow is generated because of a certain amount of resistance to the exchange of electrons from p to n. Apart from being more efficient than valve tubes, solid-state rectifiers have other advantages, such as:

(a) Since they do not have filaments:
  (1) they do not require a special filament transformer.
  (2) there is very low heat loss.
  (3) they have a longer life span.

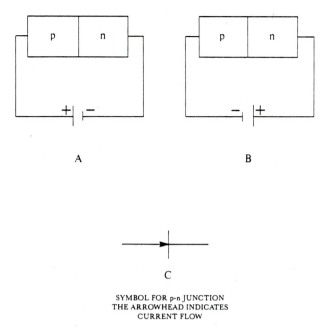

Figure 7:4. The semiconductor junction (p-n junction) of a solid-state rectifier. See text for further explanation.

  (b) They produce more consistent radiographic output, since they do not produce gas which may cause momentary instability in the output.
  (c) They have a smaller transformer enclosure because of the exclusion of filament transformers.
  (d) They do not present a radiation hazard (a problem with valve tubes) and, therefore, do not require special shielding considerations.

Rectification

The type of rectification used in x-ray machines can be any of the following:
  (a) Self-rectification.
  (b) Half-wave rectification.
  (c) Full-wave rectification.

Self-Rectification

In a *self-rectified* circuit (Figure 7:5), the x-ray tube acts as its own rectifier. During the positive half cycles, a current flows, since the cathode is negative with respect to the anode. During the negative half cycles, when the anode is negative, no current flows.

With self-rectified circuits the exposure output is limited to about 100 kVp and 100 mA, and hence, they are commonly used in low-powered mobile and dental units. Another drawback of this type of circuit is that if for some reason

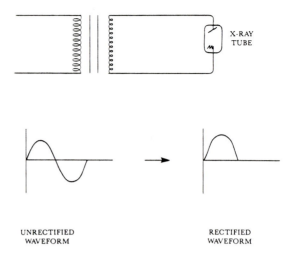

UNRECTIFIED
WAVEFORM

RECTIFIED
WAVEFORM

Figure 7:5. A self-rectified x-ray circuit. In this situation, the x-ray tube acts as its own rectifier. The voltage waveforms before and after rectification are also shown.

(overloading) the anode temperature becomes exceptionally high, the anode emits electrons which are accelerated towards the cathode during the negative half cycle (anode negative). This phenomenon is referred to as *inverse arc over* and it destroys the filament, thus terminating the life of the tube.

Half-wave Rectification

Figure 7:6 shows two half-wave rectified circuits, one which makes use of two rectifiers and the other, one. These arrangements prevent a reverse current flow if the anode becomes overheated by maintaining the cathode and anode at negative and positive voltage, respectively.

In Figure 7:6a, there are two cables going to the x-ray tube. The insulation of the one going to the tube from the transformer may breakdown due to certain influencing factors. By using two rectifiers (Figure 7:6b), this breakdown of cable insulation can be prevented.

Half-wave rectified units are not common in modern radiology departments (although they do exist).

Full-wave Rectification

The circuit shown in Figure 7:7 is based on full-wave *rectification*. The circuit arrangement (bridge circuit or Graetz circuit) makes use of four rectifiers to ensure that the cathode of the x-ray tube is always maintained at a negative potential by reversing and using the negative half of the AC cycle.

Since this type of circuit is common in radiology departments, it is mandatory that the technologist understand how it works. Consider the following with reference to Figure 7:7.

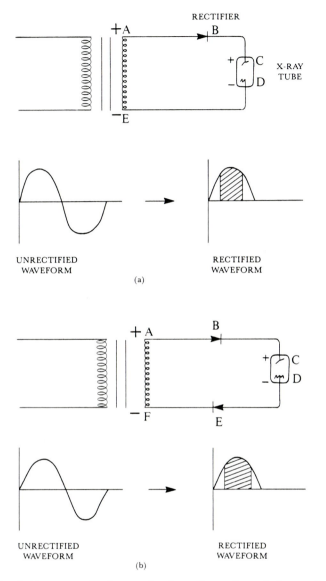

Figure 7:6. Two half-wave rectified x-ray circuits and waveforms before and after rectification. In (a) only one rectifier is used and the cable from the high tension generator may break down. This breakdown is prevented by using a two rectifier circuit.

(a) During the positive half cycle when the transformer terminal A is positive, current flows through the path ABCDEFGHI. No other path is possible, because current flow is from the positive pole of the transformer to the negative pole.

(b) During the cycle when the polarity of the transformer terminals is reversed, current flows through the path IHCDEFGBA to terminal A of the transformer, which will now be negative. The full-wave rectified voltage waveform now consists of 120 impulses per second produced by a half-wave rectified circuit. This simply means that with a full-wave rectified circuit, the production of radiation can be achieved more efficiently and shorter exposure times are possible.

TYPES OF X-RAY GENERATORS

The term *x-ray generator* refers to all electrical elements of the machine which play a role in energizing the x-ray tube, such as the high tension transformer,

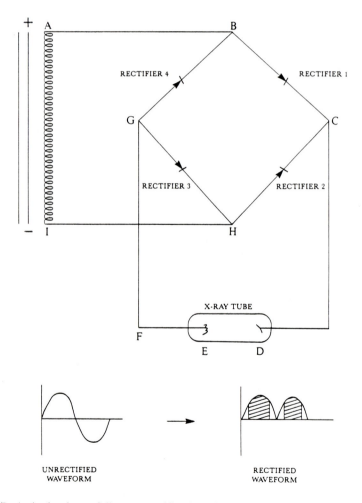

Figure 7:7. A single-phase, full-wave rectification circuit, using four rectifiers. See text for further explanation. Note that only a portion of this circuit is shown.

Table 7-1
CHARACTERISTICS OF FOUR TYPES OF X-RAY GENERATORS

TYPE	CIRCUIT (No. of pulses per cycle (1/20 sec.)	SYMBOL	RECTIFIERS	RECTIFIED VOLTAGE WAVEFORM	RIPPLE
1.	Single-pulse single phase (half wave)	$^1\phi^1$	x-ray tube itself		~100%
2.	Two-pulse single (full wave)	$^1\phi^2$	usually 2 rectifiers		~100%
3.	Six-pulse three phase	$^3\phi^6$	6		14%
4.	Twelve-pulse three phase	$^3\phi^{12}$	12		3.4%

the high tension switch and so on.

X-ray generators fall into several categories based on the type of circuitry characteristic of each.

Table 7:1 identifies four categories and lists essential features of each. The basic circuit diagrams for the three-phase, six-pulse and three-phase, twelve-pulse generators are shown in Figures 7:8 and 7:9, respectively.

Constant Potential Generator

With the most advanced technology, constant DC voltage is possible with almost zero *ripple* (variation of voltage throughout the cycle). This is accomplished by placing capacitors between the rectifiers and the x-ray tube as shown in Figure 7:10. Once the voltage approaches its peak, electrons from the rectifi-

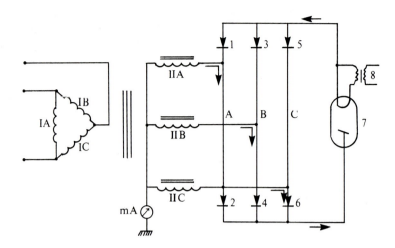

Figure 7:8. A three-phase, full-wave rectification, six-pulse circuit. Using the principle shown in Figure 7:7, trace the flow of current from transformer to rectifier to x-ray tube and back to the transformer (from Van der Plaats, G.J.: *Medical X-ray Techniques in Diagnostic Radiology.* The Netherlands. Martinus Nijhoff Publishers, Fourth Edition, 1980).

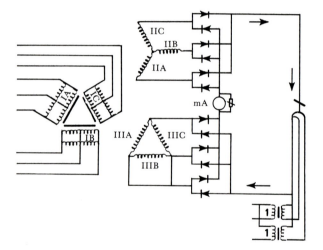

Figure 7:9. A three-phase, full-wave rectification twelve-pulse circuit. Note the flow of current from transformer to rectifiers to the x-ray tube and back to the transformer (from Van der Plaats, G.J.: *Medical X-ray Techniques in Diagnostic Radiology.* The Netherlands, Martinus Nijhoff Publishers, Fourth Edition, 1980).

cation circuit flow to the tube and to the capacitors. As the voltage from the rectification circuit starts to drop, electrons move from the capacitor to the x-ray tube. This process provides a constant voltage across the tube.

Falling Load Generator

With the introduction of automatic exposure timers where the exposure

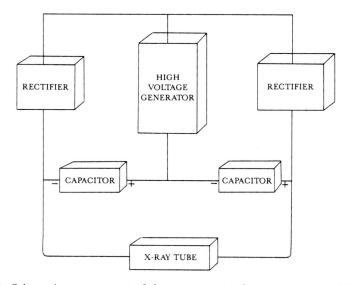

Figure 7:10. Schematic arrangement of the components of a constant potential generator (Greinacher). The voltage approaches its peak electrons from the rectifiers flow to the tube and capacitors. As the voltage starts to drop, electrons flow from the capacitors to the tube. This process provides a constant voltage (zero ripple) across the x-ray tube.

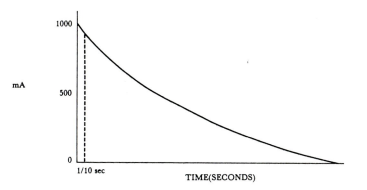

Figure 7:11. The principle of the falling load x-ray generator ensures that every exposure commences at the maximum permissible mA so that the shortest possible exposure time can be used.

time is unknown before the exposure commences, the falling load generator was developed.

In theory, the falling load generator ensures the shortest possible exposure each time by using the maximum permissible mA allowable by the tube — that is, every exposure commences at maximum mA. This process is accomplished through the use of the cooling curve of the anode of the x-ray tube as shown in Figure 7:11.

For automatic exposure control, the falling load generator would appear to

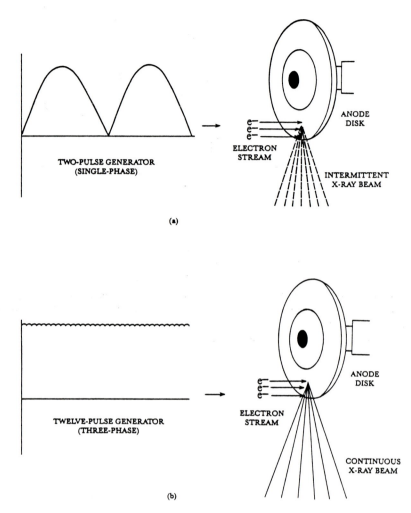

Figure 7:12. A diagramatic representation of one of the advantages of three-phase x-ray generators. In (b) the radiation emitted from the x-ray tube is constant and therefore shorter exposure times are possible compared to the scheme shown in (a).

be more advantageous in terms of providing the shortest possible exposure time for each exposure, however, there are a few drawbacks. For example, as more and more exposures are made in rapid sequence, the exposure time increases, since the next exposure (mA) will start out at the value of the previous exposure (mA) and so on. The exposure will increase in time and decrease in mA as more and more heat is developed in the anode. In practice, it is very difficult to duplicate the technical factors (exposure) for the technologist if she/he encounters problems with exposure factors.

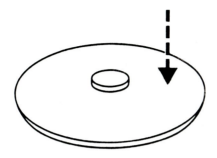

With the two-pulse generator, the maximum heat capacity per surface unit of the anode material can only be used point by point on the focus track.

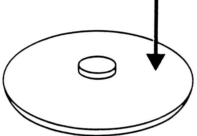

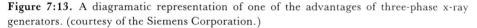

With the six-pulse generator, the maximum heat capacity per surface unit of the anode material is used without interruption on the focus track.

Figure 7:13. A diagramatic representation of one of the advantages of three-phase x-ray generators. (courtesy of the Siemens Corporation.)

Advantages of Three-Phase Generators

X-ray generators have an influence on radiogrpahic quality, tube loading, spot film techniques, angiographic techniques, and power requirements. The advantages of three-phase generators are several, such as:

1. In a single-phase generator, the electrical energy is taken from one phase of a three-phase supply and, therefore, the load on the three-phase supply is unequal. This is not advantageous for the power station as well as for the user, since the supply of energy to a system is much more important than the way it is converted. By using all three phases, equal loading is possible with high power consumption.
2. In single-phase, two-pulse generators, x-rays are produced during the maximum voltage. This results in an intermittent production of x-rays (Figure 7:12a). In a three-phase, six-pulse generator, on the other

hand, the radiation emitted from the tube is constant (Figure 7:12b) and more x-rays are produced per unit time; therefore, shorter exposure times are possible.

3. In a three-phsae generator, the anode of the x-ray tube is heated consistently and uniformly because of the almost constant voltage through the tube. This provides a higher heat-loading capacity of the tube compared to single-phase generators, where the heat is not uniformly distributed on the anode (Figure 7:13).

4. Three-phase generators produce less ripple. The ripple is always stated as a percentage. For example, the ripple of a six-pulse, three-phase circuit is 14 percent and for a twelve-pulse, three-phase it is 3.4 percent. This means that the kVp to the x-ray tube is maintained at about 86 percent (14° ripple) and 96.6 percent (3.4° ripple) of the maximum value compared to a single-phase, two-pulse circuit, where the kVp varies from zero to its maximum value. The low values of kVp as the cycle or pulse rises and falls to zero produce softer radiation, which increases patient dose and does not play a role in formation of images, a phenomenon not characteristic of three-phase circuits.

NEW CONCEPT IN X-RAY GENERATORS

More recently, new x-ray generators have become available for use in radiology. These generators are designed to meet the demands of more and more specialized clinical techniques. For example, higher output and shorter exposure times are needed to image rapidly moving structures, high mA and low kVp values are required to image low contrast objects, and, for optimum fluoroscopic images, electronic dose rate regulation is required.

In this section only one generator prototype, the Pandoros Optimatic® (Siemens), will be described here, since it meets the requirements of the problems identified in the previous paragraph.

The essential characteristics of the new generators are related to their operation, design, installation, and maintenance. For example, with respect to design, the electronic building blocks are located in wall cabinets instead of in the generator housing (for easy accessibility). Auxillary circuits are made on plug-in printed circuit boards.

In Figure 7:14, the circuit principle of the Pandoros Optimatic® (Siemens) is shown. The following points are of interest in terms of innovations:

(a) The high tension transformer is connected directly to the mains supply, thus eliminating the need for a regulating transformer for radiographic and fluoroscopic kVp.

(b) Two control triodes are positioned between the tube and high tension generator to switch the high voltage to the x-ray tube, on and off, and also to set the radiographic and fluoroscopic voltage.

(c) "The advantage of this high tension regulation over the conventional method lies in the fact that the voltage cross the x-ray tube can be measured by two voltage dividers at the anode and the cathode sides of the x-ray tube and compared with the desired value. If the value measured deviates from the value set, a correction is made immediately. Furthermore, the x-ray tube voltage can be reproduced over long periods of time. (Schmitmann and Ammann, 1973)

Fluctuations in the mains voltages or changes in the x-ray tube current have no influence on the tube voltage." (Schmitmann and Ammann, 1973)

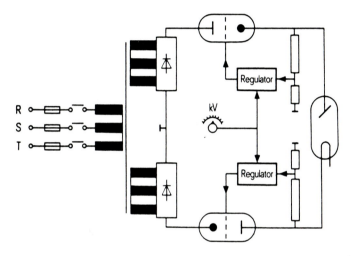

Figure 7:14. The circuit principle of the PANDOROS OPTIMATIC® (Siemens) x-ray generator. See text for further explanation. (From Schmitmann, H. and Ammann, E.: Pandoros Optimatic — An x-ray generator with new possibilities. *Electromedica* 4-5, 1973).

The principle of this circuitry allows for:

(a) A short generator switching time of 0.3 milliseconds (no mechanical switching is used to control the voltage to the x-ray tube at the secondary of the high tension generator).

(b) Constant direct potential

(c) Shortest exposure time for automatic timing is 1 ms with the appropriate film density.

(d) High exposure output (150 kilowatts at 150 kV at 2000 mA).

(e) A switching rate of up to 50 exposures per second in pulsed operation without the use of a grid-controlled x-ray tube.

(f) A constant image for fluoroscopy as a result of electronic stabilization of voltage and current.

(g) Bi-plane applications, and so on.

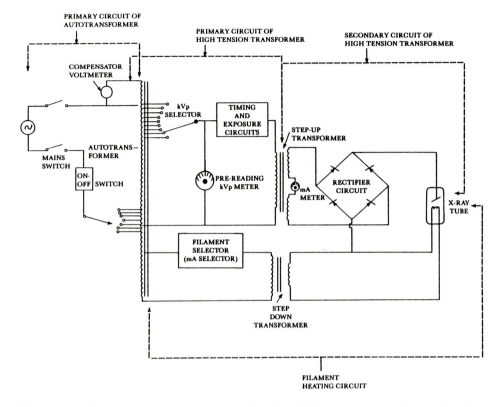

Figure 7:15. A basic x-ray generator circuit. This circuit is by no means complete. Other elements have been omitted on purpose to render the diagram less confusing.

These advantages make the new generator system very versatile with special fields of application, such as cardioangiography, functional analyses, chest radiography, radiological research, sports medicine, pediatric radiology, orthopedics, general cineradiography and coronary angiography.

THE BASIC X-RAY GENERATOR CIRCUIT

A basic x-ray generator circuit is shown in Figure 7:15. The circuit is by no means complete, and other elements have been omitted on purpose to render the diagram less confusing. The other circuits, however, are covered in some detail in any radiography physics text.

The circuit can be divided up into four parts:

1. The PRIMARY CIRCUIT OF THE AUTOTRANSFORMER, which consists of the following components:
    (a) mains switch (located on the wall).
    (b) on-off switch (located on the control panel).

(c) circuit breaker.

(d) mains voltage.

(e) compensator voltmeter.

2. The PRIMARY CIRCUIT OF THE HIGH TENSION TRANS-
FORMER, which consists of the following components:

(a) Autotransformer.

(b) kVp selector.

(c) kVp meter.

(d) exposure switch.

(e) exposure timer.

3. The SECONDARY CIRCUIT OF THE HIGH TENSION
TRANSFORMER, which consists of the following:

(a) Rectifiers.

(b) mA meter.

(c) Anode of the x-ray tube.

(d) High tension switch (located in the high tension tank).

4. The FILAMENT HEATING CIRCUIT OF THE X-RAY TUBE,
which consists of the following:

(a) Step-down transformer.

(b) Line voltage compensator.

(c) Space charge compensator.

(d) Voltage stabilizer.

(e) mA selector (could be a choke coil or other mechanism).

(f) Autotransformer.

(g) Cathode of the x-ray tube.

Meters

The mA or tube current meter is a DC milliammeter which is actually located in the high-voltage circuit. This part of the circuit (mA meter location) is at ground potential, and, therefore, the mA selector is positioned on the control console without using much insulation. This is one of the reasons why the high-voltage transformer is tapped at the center. This also allows the high tension cables to carry only half the voltage and puts the center of the x-ray tube at ground potential.

There are two currents with respect to the x-ray tube: the filament current and the tube current. The filament is heated by current from the step-down transformer which in time affects the tube current (cathode to anode), or mA. It is important that the filament be kept at a low temperature when not in use in order to avoid evaporation of the filament due to high temperatures. For this reason, the filament temperature is increased to generate the desired mA, just prior to the exposure. This can be achieved by the rotor switch of the rotating-anode x-ray tube.

The kVp meter is a standard AC meter positioned across the primary of the high tension transformer before the high-voltage switch. Since the kVp influences the mA value such that an increase in kVp decreases the space charge (electron cloud around the filament at low kVp), a space charge compensation circuit is added to the x-ray generator circuit to provide a constant tube current as the kVp is varied. The circuit is designed to increase the filament temperature at low kVp and decrease it at high kVp settings.

The High Tension Switch

Some x-ray rooms may have two or more x-ray tubes under the control of one generator, and, hence, a means must be provided to allow for tube selection. This is accomplished by the *high tension switch* (tube selector switch), which is positioned in the transformer tank and immersed in oil. Whenever a tube is selected by the technologist, the high tension switch is closed and passes high voltage from the high-voltage transformer to the specific x-ray tube. Apart from tube selection, the switch is also designed to connect the filament leads. It does not select mA or focal spot size. The switch has nothing to do with exposure switching.

Exposure Switching

Exposure switching is a very complicated topic. Since it is important for the technologist to be familiar with the switching mechanism, a brief identification of these systems is in order.

Exposure switching involves:

(a) *Primary switching* where high currents are switched at mains voltage.
(b) *Secondary switching* where low currents (x-ray tube current) are switched at high voltage (the x-ray tube voltage).

Exposure switching can be achieved by any of the following:

(a) *Mechanical devices* (contactors) which operate on the principle of electromagnetism. It is for this reason that they are also referred to as electromagnetic contactors. These were used in earlier machines.
(b) Use of *thyratrons* (gas-filled three-electrode valve tubes) in the circuits. The thyratrons act as switches.
(c) *Electronic devices.* Today, these devices are used, instead of mechancial and thyratron tubes, because of the high output and short exposure times required by present clinical techniques. One major advantage of electronic devices is that they can be made to make or break contact at the zero crossing (sine wave), thus reducing the heavy surge of power found at the maximum pulse height. More recently, *solid-state devices* such as *silicon-controlled rectifiers* and *thyristors* are used. Their operation is based on the principle of semiconductors.

Exposure switching can be accomplished by two methods, namely, through the *electronic timer* and by *automatic exposure control* (Chapter 2).

The electronic timer makes use of a preset time that is determined by a resistance/capacitance (RC) network. The exposure terminates at the end of he preset time. These times can be selected by the technologist and usually range from 1 millisecond to 4 seconds.

The automatic exposure timer (control) is designed so that the exposure terminates once a predetermined film density is obtained (amount of radiation measured by special detectors).

Exposure timers are important tools for the technologist and, hence, they were discussed further in Chapter 4.

SUMMARY

1. The electrical power supplied to hospitals is alternating current (AC).
2. In an AC waveform, voltage and current are in phase and there are positive and negative half cycles.
3. The frequency of AC can be defined as the number of complete cycles per second and is often expressed in Hertz, where one Hertz is equal to one cycle per second.
4. Both single-phase and three-phase AC are available in the radiology department. X-ray units which operate on single-phase power are limited in x-ray production and exposure times. Three-phase operated units produce x-rays more efficiently.
5. The advantage of using AC in terms of x-ray equipment operation is that numerous components in the imaging scheme operate on AC power rather than direct current (DC).
6. Rectification of AC refers to changing the pulsating AC to a pulsing DC. This process is acomplished by rectifiers. It is necessary to rectify AC, because the x-ray tube operates more efficiently with a pulsating DC.
7. There are two types of rectifiers: valve tubes and solid-state rectifiers. Valve tubes are thermionic high-vacuum tubes similar to the x-ray tube in construction. Solid-state rectifiers are made of semiconductors and are more efficient than valve-tube rectifiers.
8. X-ray machines may operate on one of three types of rectification. In self-rectification, the x-ray tube acts as its own rectifier and produces x-rays only during the positive half cycle. In general, a half-wave rectification circuit utilizes two rectifiers to prevent reverse current flow and maintain the cathode and anode of the x-ray tube at negative and positive voltage, respectively.
9. A typical full-wave rectification circuit uses four rectifiers to ensure that the cathode of the x-ray tube is always maintained at a negative

potential by reversing and using the negative half cycle. Full-wave rectification ensures more efficient production of radiation and the use of shorter exposure times as compared to self- and half-wave rectification.

10. The x-ray generator refers to all electrical components which play a role in energizing the x-ray tube, such as the high tension transformer, for example.

11. X-ray generators are categorized according to the type of circuitry used. Four types of circuitry are identified and described briefly.

12. Constant potential generators are used to provide a constant voltage across the x-ray tube by placing capacitors between the rectifiers and the x-ray tube.

13. The falling load generator is designed to permit the use of the shortest possible exposure time through the use of the maximum permissible mA allowable by the tube.

14. The advantages of three-phase x-ray genertors are several and they are discussed briefly.

15. New concepts in x-ray generator design, operation and installation are identified and described with respect to one prototype unit. In terms of innovations, the high tension transformer is connected directly to the mains supply, hence eliminating the need for a regulating transformer and so on.

16. Finally, the complete x-ray generator circuit is described with respect to four divisions:
    (a) the primary circuit of the autotransformer
    (b) the primary circuit of the high tension transformer
    (c) the secondary circuit of the high tension transformer
    (d) the filament heating circuit of the x-ray tube

17. The two meters which are of importance to the technologist are the mA meter and the kVp meter. The mA meter is located in the high-voltage circuit, and this part of the circuit is at ground potential to facilitate positioning of the mA selector on the control console without the use of significant insulation.

18. The kVp meter is a standard AC meter positioned across the primary of the high tension transformer before the high-voltage switch.

19. Apart from tube selection, the high tension switch is also designed to connect the filament leads. It does not select mA or focal spot size and has nothing to do with exposure switching.

20. Exposure switching may be accomplished by mechanical devices (contactors), thyratrons (gas-filled three-electrode valve tubes), or by electronic devices, which have replaced the former two devices. More recently, solid-state devices (silicon-controlled rectifiers and thyristors) are used.

CHAPTER 8

GEOMETRIC TOMOGRAPHY

IN radiography, all structures in the patient are superimposed on film. In some instances, the image may not clearly demonstrate distinct features of a particular area that may be of interest to the radiologist. Fortunately, the technique of *body-section radiography* (BSR) can be used to demonstrate this area with a greater degree of contrast and detail than conventional techniques. In short, BSR is a procedure whereby specific layers or planes of the body can be x-rayed by blurring out those structures laying above and below the layer or plane of interest.

In the developmental stages of BSR, other techniques were introduced to produce the same kind of imaging. These techniques (*planigraphy, laminography,* and *stratigraphy*) are all based essentially on the same principle.

Today, the general consensus is the use of the word *tomography*, from the Greek *tomos* (section) and tomé (cut), to refer to any kind of imaging technique which demonstrates sections or "cuts" of the body.

More recently, another term, *geometric tomography* (McCullough and Coulam, 1976), has been used to describe the fundamental principles of body-section radiography and particularly to distinguish it from *computed tomography* (a new technique to image cross sections of the body using a computer).

HISTORICAL PERSPECTIVES

Students who are interested in complete historical notes on BSR may refer to excellent reviews presented by J.R. Andrews (1936, 1937).

The following is a brief outline of the early history of BSR.

1921	Bocage described principles of BSR in a French patent by listing three practical methods:
	(a) Movement of film and tube in a straight line and in opposite directions.
	(b) Movement of tube and film in parallel planes and in circles, spirals, etc.
	(c) Movement of tube and film is rotational about an axis which lies in the plane of the projected section.
1921-22	Ziedes des Plantes, working in the Netherlands, also developed the method independently.
1922	Portes and Chausse received patent. They suggested that the principle be applied to therapy problems.
1930	Professor Vallebona in Italy used the skull to provide clinical results from his basic technique which he referred to as *stratigraphy* (from stratum, meaning layer).
1931	Ziedes des Plantes published the results of his extensive study of BSR and gave practical applications of the method. He also discussed the principle of *multisection radiography.*
1935	Grossman pointed out refinements of the linear method. He called the procedure *tomography.*
1934	J.R. Andrews, in Philadelphia, started work on tomography by adapting conventional x-ray equipment to perform BSR.
1936-37	Jean Kieffer, in America, received a patent for the *laminograph.*

1937   J.R. Andrews provided mathematical basis for BSR.
Watson, in England, developed *transverse axial tomography.*

Following these developments, a number of workers introduced other body-section imaging techniques. For example:

      Amisano and Abrea developed transverse axial tomography.

      Paatero developed the technique of *pantomography* to image curved outer surfaces (for example, the mandible).

1950   Ziedes des Plantes described *automography* by rotating the skull while the tube and film remained stationary.

Geometric tomography can perhaps be described in terms of:

  (a) Longitudinal tomography.
  (b) Transverse axial tomography.

PRINCIPLES OF LONGITUDINAL TOMOGRAPHY

The term *longitudinal* is used in this context to specify the section of the body to be imaged, that is, a longitudinal section or layer. This layer is parallel to the film. If the patient is in the prone or supine position, then the section is said to be *coronal* in direction. On the other hand, if the patient is in the lateral position (for a tomographic procedure), then the section is said to be *sagittal* in direction.

The principle of longitudinal tomography is illustrated in its most fundamental form in Figure 8:1. The important point in the figure is the relative positions of the projected structures on film. When the x-ray tube is in position 1, the rib structure is projected on the right side of the film. When the tube moves to position 2, the rib is now projected on the left side of the film. The same applies to the kidney; that is, in tube position 1, the kidney is projected on the left side of the film, while in tube position 2, it is now projected on the right side of the film. The spine is the only structure which maintains the same position on the film regardless of the position of the tube and film. This indicates that the spine would be imaged sharply and all other structures lying in the same plane as the spine would be imaged with equal clarity. The spine, then, is said to be in the "*plane of focus.*" All other structures which lie above and below the plane of focus are blurred.

The principle of longitudinal tomography involves simultaneous movement of the x-ray tube and film in opposite directions. This movement forms the basis of all tomography and determines the blurring characteristics and thickness of the section that can be imaged.

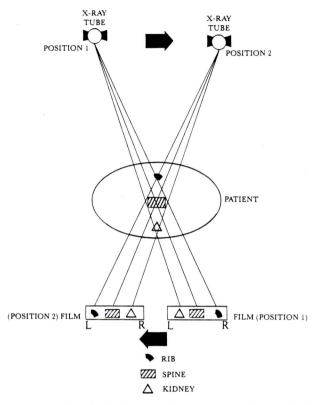

Figure 8:1. The principle of longitudinal geometric tomography. See text for further explanation.

A discussion of tomography would be incomplete without careful consideration of the following:

    (a) *Fulcrum.* This is the point of rotation, or the point at which the x-ray tube and film pivot. The fulcrum corresponds to the layer or section (which lies in the plane of focus) to be imaged.

Two types of fulcrum are shown in Figure 8:2: the *variable fulcrum* and the *fixed fulcrum.* With a varible fulcrum, the level of the section can be changed by adjusting the fulcrum. The height of the layer can be set by moving the fulcrum between the film and the tube focus, in relation to the patient, while the tabletop (patient) remains in a fixed position. Hence, the *focus-fulcrum distance* and the *fulcrum-film distance* will vary with the layer height. The *image enlargement E,* which results from varying the layer height, can be computed from the following relationship:

$$E = \frac{\text{Focus-film distance}}{\text{Focus-fulcrum distance}}$$

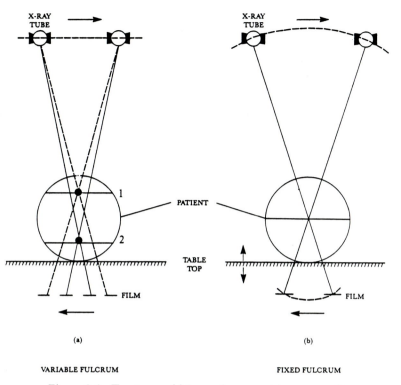

X-RAY TUBE →

PATIENT

TABLE TOP

FILM

(a)

VARIABLE FULCRUM

X-RAY TUBE →

FILM

(b)

FIXED FULCRUM

Figure 8:2. Two types of fulcrum for geometric tomography.

The second type of fulcrum is the fixed fulcrum, in which the level of the section can be adjusted by moving the patient (and hence the tabletop) towards or away from the fulcrum. The tube-fulcrum and the fulcrum-film distances will remain constant. The enlargement will also remain constant.

Today, both types of fulcrum are available. The student should note that the fulcrum is one aspect of the machine and that it corresponds to the layer of interest.

(b) *Focal plane.* This is sometimes refered to as the *"body-section plane."* It is the level of the patient which is in maximum focus.

(c) *Focal-plane level* is the height of the focal plane above the tabletop.

(d) *Blurring.* This term refers to blurring of those objects outside the focal plane due to motion unsharpness. The effectiveness of the blurring depends on the distance of the layer from the film, the direction of the tube travel, and the amplitude of the tube travel.

(e) *The amplitude* of the tube travel is the distance moved by the x-ray tube (with reference to the fulcrum) to form a certain angle of movement. This angle is popularly referred to as the *tomographic angle.* The amplitude affects the thickness of the section in a certain way. As the amplitude increases, the effective tomographic angle increases and thinner

Table 8-1

THE THICKNESS OF CUT OBTAINED FOR SEVERAL TOMOGRAPHIC
ANGLES USING LINEAR TOMOGRAPHY

(From Bushong, S.C.: Radiologic Science for Technologist. St. Louis, 1975.
The C.V. Mosby Company.)

TOMOGRAPHIC ANGLE	THICKNESS OF CUT
0°	Infinity
2°	31 mm
4°	16 mm
6°	11 mm
10°	6 mm
20°	3 mm
35°	2 mm
50°	1 mm

sections can be imaged. This is shown in Table 8:1.

(f) *Thickness of cut.* This is the width of the layer which is in focus.

(g) *Direction of tube travel* is the motion of the tube travel with respect to the long axis of the object being tomographed. Table 8:2 shows motions frequently used in longitudinal tomography. The motions have resulted in the use of two terms that are frequently encountered in the literature. These are *linear* tomography and *multidirectional* (pluridirectional) tomography.

Linear Tomography

In linear tomography, the x-ray tube and film travel in a linear (straight line) fashion. It is the simplest and most often used of all tomographic motions.

In linear tomography, the thickness of the cut is related to the tomographic angle. This angle can be adjusted from 10° to about 50° to provide excellent tomograms in cases where short exposures are required. Exposure times can range from about 0.5 seconds to 0.9 seconds for 10° and 50° respectively.

Linear tomography is particularly useful in examinations of the larynx and chest.

Table 8-2

MOTIONS FREQUENTLY USED IN LONGITUDINAL TOMOGRAPHY

MOTION	SHAPE OF TUBE TRAJECTORY

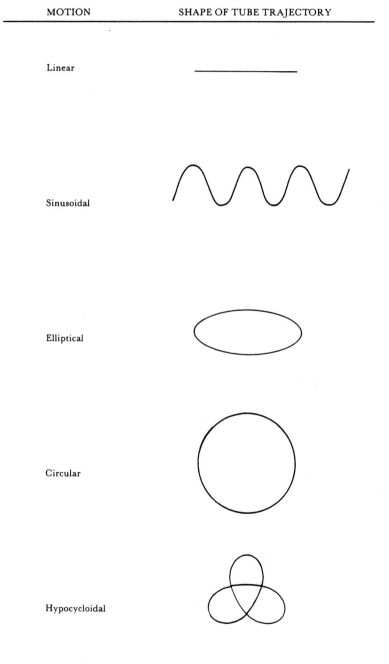

Linear

Sinusoidal

Elliptical

Circular

Hypocycloidal

Multidirectional Tomography

One of the major disadvantages of linear tomography is that it produces streaks on the film. This occurs because those structures which are oriented parallel or along the direction of the tube motion are not completely blurred out. This observation has led to the development of special x-ray units capable of performing both linear and multidirectional tomography. The basic objective of multidirectional movements is not only to remove the streaks caused by linear motion but also to provide thinner cuts and sharper tomographic images.

Multidirectional movements include: *elliptical, circular* and *hypocycloidal*. Table 8:3 summarizes the type and pattern of motion, tomographic angles and thickness of cut for both linear and multidirectional movements of the *Polytome unit* (Philips, Eindhoven, Netherlands).

Table 8-3

TUBE MOVEMENTS AND OTHER PARAMETERS USED IN LINEAR
AND MULTIDIRECTIONAL TOMOGRAPHY FOR A PHILIPS POLYTOME*

TUBE MOVEMENT	SHAPE OF TRAJECTORY	ANGLE OF SWING	MAXIMUM EXPOSURE TIME FOR COMPLETION	THICKNESS OF CUT	LENGTH OF TUBE TRAVEL
LINEAR TOMOGRAPHY					
Linear		29°		2.3 mm	56 cm
		40°		1.6 mm	77 cm
		48°		1.3 mm	92 cm
MULTIDIRECTIONAL TOMOGRAPHY					
1. Elliptical		40°	3 sec.	1.6 mm	186 cm
2. Circular		29°	3 sec.	2.3 mm	176 cm
		36°	3 sec.	1.8 mm	217 cm
3. Hypocycloidal		48°	6 sec.	1.3 mm	451 cm

* Medical Systems Division — N.V. Philips — Eindhoven, Netherlands.

REMARKS:

1. Combines some of the advantages of linear and multidirectional movement.
2. 2 layer thickness may be selected. Simplest of multidirectional movements. It ensures retention of the layer thickness and constancy of detail perceptibility.
3. Most complex of all multidirectional movement, and provides almost perfect blurring hence structures lying in the layer of interest are totally obscured. It enhances the quality of the tomograph.
4. For the shape of the trajectory refer to Table 8:2.

In examining Table 8:3, the following should be noted:

(a) The thickness of cut obtained with linear motion with tomographic angles of 29°, 40° and 48° is the same obtained for circular 29°, elliptical 40° and hypocycloidal 48°, respectively.

(b) With 48° tomographic angle, in the linear mode, the length of the tube travel is 92 cm. Taken over the same angle in hypocycloidal motion (48°), the length of the tube travel is 451 cm.

The blurring efficiency of hypocycloidal motion is hence greater, since it is dependent on the length and direction of the tube travel. Hypocycloidal motion is about five times more efficient than linear motion in terms of image sharpness.

Zonography or Narrow Angle Tomography

This refers to body-section radiography using tomographic angles ranging from 0° to 10°. In practice, it is found that angles of 2° and 3° produce the most satisfactory results. Zonography is especially useful when subject contrast is minimal (for example, the lung is an ideal part to be examined with zonography).

Since tomographic angles used in zonography are small, the thickness of cut obtained is large (thick cut) and entire structures can be imaged with very little background blurring.

Simultaneous Multisection Tomography

Simultaneous multisection tomography ensures the acquisition of several longitudinal layers of the body at the same time. In this procedure each specific layer is in "focus." The principle is based on the use of a *multisection cassette*, which consists of several intensifying screens mounted on plastic foam layers (spacer material), the thickness of which can be varied to suit the needs of a particular examination. The whole arrangement has the appearance of a book in which the intensifying screens form the "leaves" of the book. The screens are positioned so that uniform film density of several layers is obtained using one exposure.

Exposure factors in mulitsection tomography have to be increased due to the nature of the film-screen combination of the multisection cassette. However, the radiation dose to the patient is significantly reduced in view of the fact that usually one exposure produces almost the same information that linear and multidirectional tomography offer using several exposures.

Multisection tomography offers other advantages such as:

(a) Shorter patient examination times than the other methods.
(b) Increased patient throughtput.
(c) Reduced electrical loads on the x-ray tube.

(d) Tomographs of structures that are imaged in the same physiological phase (for example, respiratory phase).

Finally, the quality of multisection tomographic images is poor compared to other tomographic methods and, therefore, the technique is not widely used.

TRANSVERSE AXIAL TOMOGRAPHY

The fundamental objective of *transverse axial tomography* (TAT) is to produce selectively, transverse sections (cross sections) of the body by rotating both patient and film simultaneously and in the same direction.

Figure 8:3 shows a patient positioned on a pedestal which is coupled to a turntable that holds the film. The coupling is such that the turntable and pedestal could rotate through 360° in the same direction. Two points that deserve careful attention in this technique are collimation and scattered radiation. The use of a scattered radiation grid is not practical in TAT (due to the nature of the technique), and hence the x-ray beam must be collimated tightly so that the amount of scatter produced in the patient is minimal. The greater portion of any scatter produced does not reach the film because of the air gap between the patient and film.

The following procedural steps are suggested for use in TAT:

(a) Position patient on pedestal. Some TAT systems are designed to allow the patient to either sit or stand during the procedure.
(b) Select the level of the section to be imaged by raising or lowering the patient.
(c) Angle the x-ray tube about 30° downward. This allows the central ray to pass through the center of the section projecting an image on the middle of the film.

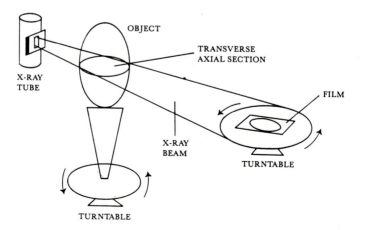

Figure 8:3. The principle of transverse axial tomography.

(d) Make exposure. During the exposure, the patient and film rotate through 360° at the same speed and in the same direction.

TAT has not found widespread use in clinical imaging because of its poor image quality. Such quality can be attributed to geometric unsharpness and patient movement, which is sometimes difficult to control.

EQUIPMENT

Presently, two kinds of equipment are available for longitudinal tomography with linear and multidirectional motion: non-specialized and specialized units.

Non-specialized Units

Conventional radiographic equipment can be converted to a simple "tomographic machine" using suitable accessory devices, such as:

(a) A *linkage device* (steel rod) which is used to couple the x-ray tube and the Bucky so that they can move simultaneously and in opposite directions during the exposure.
(b) A *pivot unit* which is used to change the height of the fulcrum. It consists of a scale that indicates the height of the layer above the tabletop. The pivot unit also serves to commence as well as terminate the x-ray exposure.
(c) A *mechanical drive* which is used to move the tube and film during the exposure.
(d) A separate *control unit* (usually mounted on the wall) which is used to select the rate and amplitude of the tube travel.

This equipment is still used in some departments, however, because of the availability of more and more specialized tomographic machines, routine radiographic equipment adapted for tomography may soon become obsolete.

Specialized Units

The limitations imposed by conventional x-ray equipment adapted for tomography are several, including:

(a) Poor image quality.
(b) The use of linear motion only.
(c) Limitation in the thickness of cut.
(d) Examination of the part only in the horizontal plane.

Specialized units for tomography are available commercially. Although these machines are costly, they overcome the limitations listed above. A complete discussion of specialized units for tomography is not within the scope of this text, however, a brief description of one common prototype is in order. In this regard, a short description of the *Polytome U* (Philips Medical Systems) follows.

The unit shown in Figure 8:4 is capable of both linear and multidirectional tomography. The Polytome U consists of a cast iron base which supports the tabletop and carries a freely moveable parallelogram-type tube support. The support couples the x-ray tube and Bucky diaphragm. The motion of the table-top is variable and has a wide range to facilitate exact centering and positioning of the patient. The height of the tabletop can be adjusted to a point 23 cm above its resting position. The tabletop can also be tilted traveling at a rate of 0.5 cm sec^{-1} (via a motor-drive mechanism) from the horizontal to vertical to 15° Trendelenberg positions.

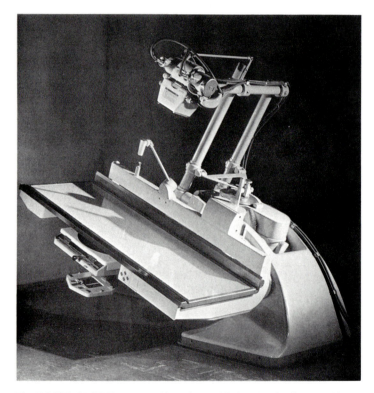

Figure 8:4. The POLYTOME U, a versatile universal Polytome for linear, elliptical, circular and hypocycloidal tomography and circular zonography. (courtesy of Philips Medical Systems.)

For tomography, a choice of blurring movements (linear, hypocycloidal, circular and elliptical) can be obtaied by coupling the parallelogram support to a motor-driven gearbox (mounted on the base) using suitable accessories (cams, bushings, crankpins).

The Polytome U features a main cassette holder to which an anti-scatter, circular focussed grid is affixed and which is driven by the parallelogram support. During tomography the grid always rotates to ensure that the lead strips and the angle of incidence of the radiation beam are in the appropriate orientation pattern. Because the main cassette holder is located some distance below the tabletop, the machine operates at a *constant enlargement factor of 1.3*. This factor can be changed to 1.6 by using a second cassette tray which is positioned below the main cassette holder.

With the Polytome U, television fluoroscopy is possible by attaching a suitable image intensifier to the main cassette holder, in which case the second cassette tray must be removed. In this instance, television fluoroscopy can be used effectively for accurate centering and positioning of the patient.

The unit can also be used for routine Bucky radiography, and hence a Bucky diaphragm is included as an integral part of the system. Tabletop radiograhy is also possible with the unit.

Other characteristic features of the Polytome U are given in Table 8:3. The advantages of a specialized unit for tomography are:

    (a) Choice of different blurring movements.
    (b) A constant enlargement factor.
    (c) Very thin cuts.
    (d) Fluoroscopically controlled patient positioning.
    (e) Efficient and effective examination of any part (for example, skull, mastoids, chest, vertebral column, extremities).
    (f) Magnification techniques.
    (g) Use of several exposures on one film. For example, the Polytome U can provide 4 to 6 exposures on a 24 × 30 cm (10″ × 12″) film.
    (h) Accurate centering
    (i) Mechanical stability.
    (j) Automatic density control.

Tomographic Density Control

In the past, automatic timing could not be used in tomography since the concept of integrated measurements was not possible. "Exposure rate control had to be introduced, known as TDC (*tomographic density control*), to ensure that each segment of the blurring angle was correctly exposed during the tomographic movement. The TDC system presently in use provides proper control of density for exposure times exceeding few tenths of a second; this is done by varying the tube current. Faster variation of the exposure rate is obtained by controlling the x-ray tube voltage with the aid of a tetrode in the high tension circuit" (Medicamundi, 1977).

OTHER METHODS OF TOMOGRAPHY

Conventional tomographic imaging with synchronous movement of x-ray tube and film cassette is a well-established technique in radiology. There are a few limitations imposed by this method (such as low contrast resolution and long exposure times), however, these are not serious since this method of imaging has been used successfully for decades. One such limitation (long exposure time) and others have prompted the need to investigate other forms of tomographic imaging. These methods are discussed below.

Tomosynthesis

The word *tomosynthesis* implies that the tomographic image can be manipulated by electronic means. It is a term that has evolved during the development and study of other forms of tomography. Whereas, a conventional tomographic image is processed chemically by developer and fixer solutions and cannot be changed or enhanced at this point (after wet processing), images obtained by methods of tomosynthesis can be manipulated electronically through the use of suitable image processing operations such as spatial frequency filtration, for example.

The methods of tomosynthesis are few and they have not gained popularity and widespread use; therefore, only brief descriptions will be given here.

The purpose of short exposure tomography can be traced back to the 1950s when Lindblom applied the technique to a machine called the *blomograph*. In 1968, Dummling proposed *televised electronic tomography* using conventional tomographic equipment with an image intensifier and television camera tube. This was followed by another technique called *flashing tomosynthesis* in which 24 stationary-anode x-ray tubes are used and which are all energized at the same time. Specially coded apertures are also used in this method.

Late in 1974, Weiss published a report on a system called *cinetomosynthesis* using the coded aperture principle. The quality of the image obtained with cinetomosynthesis is below acceptable limits and, therefore, it will not be described here.

More recently, another electronic tomographic technique, *tomoscopy*, was described by Sklebitz and Haendle (1983) and their results published in the American Journal of Roentgenology.

Televised Electronic Tomography

This technique is based on the same principle as conventional geometric tomography except that the film cassette has been replaced by an image intensifier and television camera tube. The principle is illustrated in Figure 8:5. In this method, Haendle, Wenz, Sklebitz, Dietz and Meinel (1981) point out that:

> During one tomographic cycle, this television camera produces many television pictures which are recorded on a videotape recorder or a video disk store. The individ-

ual television images correspond to specific projections related to the particular positions of x-ray tube and x-ray image intensifier. The stored television images are finally played back and superimposed on one another in a storage tube with an appropriate spatial displacement. Tomograms of different layer heights are obtained by varying the displacement of the televised images when they are superimposed. With this method, therefore, subsequent selection of any particular tomogram can be made.

Because of the repeated information conversion and associated relatively poor tomogram quality, this tomosynthesis has not so far been successful.

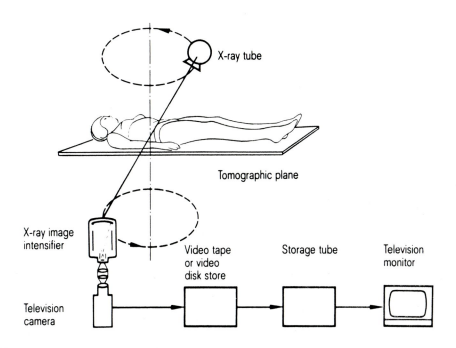

Figure 8:5. The principle of televised electronic tomography. (From Haendle, Wenz, Sklebitz and Meinel: A new electronic tomographic system. *Electromedica* 2, 1981.)

Flashing Tomosynthesis

This technique is described quite clearly by Woelke, Hanrath, and Schlueter et al. (1982), who explain it as follows:

The procedure consists of a recording step and a reconstruction step.

In the recording step (Figure 8:6), the three-dimensional object is recorded on a large film (60 × 60 cm^2) by means of 24 statinary x-ray tubes. During exposure, all x-ray tubes are fired simultaneously. Exposure time is about 50 msec, with a skin dose of approximately 1R (2.58 × 10^{-4} C/kg) at 100 kV. The x-ray image thus produced is coded in a subsequent image processing step (Figure 8:7). The coded recording is placed in front of a light box and imaged by an array of 24 lenses, mounted according to the distribution of the x-ray tubes. Because of this multiprojection, a real-time three-dimensional image of the object is reconstructed in space. If a screen is now inserted in any arbitrary position into the reconstruction volume, the corresponding tomographic layer is isolated from the object. This offers the possibility of continuously "going through the object."

Layer depth is about 1 mm. Due to the optical superimposition of 24 single recordings, image contrast is considerably enhanced, and the reconstructed layer images are less "noisy" than the single cine frames.

By proper choice of layer orientation, an undistorted focussed display of stenotic areas with no superimposition of vessels is obtained. A special device then projects the reconstructed layers onto a TV monitor that can consequently be photographed.

It should be noted here that this technique does not involve synchronous motion of x-ray tubes and detector. This mechanical notion has been eliminated completely.

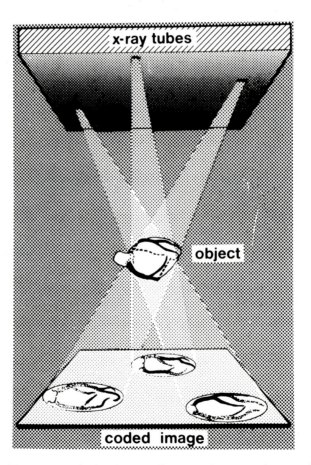

Figure 8:6. Flashing tomosynthesis, the recording step. An array of x-ray tubes projects the object onto different locations on the recording film. During the exposure, all x-ray tubes are fired simultaneously. (From Woelke et al.: Work in Progress. Flashing tomosynthesis- A tomographic technique for quantitative coronary angiography. *Radiology* 145: November, 1982.)

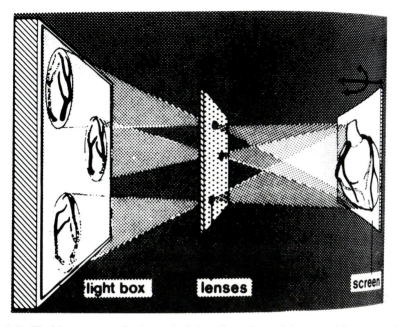

Figure 8:7. Flashing tomosynthesis, optical decoding. A special array of lenses produces a real three-dimensional image of the object in space. Selected object layes can be isolated by proper positioning of a ground glass screen within the reconstruction volume. (From Woelke et al.: Work in Progress. Flashing tomosynthesis- A tomographic technique for quantitative coronary angiography. *Radiology* 145: November, 1982.)

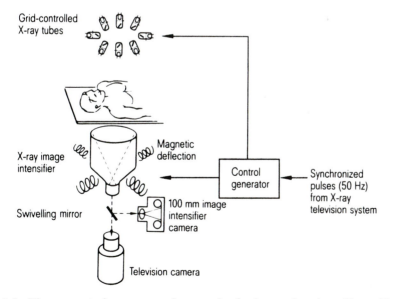

Figure 8:8. The concept of tomoscopy. See text for further explanation. (From Haendle, Wenz, Sklebitz and Meinel.: A new electronic tomographic system. *Electromedica* 2, 1981.)

Tomoscopy

Tomoscopy is an electronic tomographic method which eliminates mechanical motion of x-ray tube, detector and patient.

The word is derived from *tomos*, meaning section, and *skopein*, meaning observe. Tomoscopy provides real-time fluoroscopic tomography through the use of a number of grid-controlled x-ray tubes and magnetic fields and other control units (generator) to produce a tomographic image.

The concept of tomoscopy is shown in Figure 8:8. The x-ray tubes (about 16 are housed in a tube shield and are energized consecutively for about 1 millisecond each. The "beam on" for each tube describes a circle which is analogous to movement of the x-ray tube in conventional imaging.

The image at the output screen of the image intensifier is deflected by means of magnetic coils (electromagnetic deflection). This deflection is analogous to movement of the film cassette in conventional tomography. Since there are 16 x-ray tubes, there are 16 magnetic deflector coils which can produce 16 deflection steps. Each image is deflected to the output screen of the image intensifier tube with each deflection step.

The control unit serves to deflect an image and energize the associated focal spot at the same time so that complete operation occurs in the time taken for one television field, which is about 0.020-0.017 seconds. By repeating this process rapidly, real-time tomofluoroscopy is possible. All of these images are superimposed on the output screen. They are then picked up by the television camera tube and are displayed on the television monitor as a tomographic slice.

The *tomographic angle* and the *thickness of cut* (layer height) depend on several factors such as the image intensifier imaging ratio, the radius of the circle traced by the focal spots of all tubes and the distance between the x-ray tube (focal plane) and the image intensifier (input plane), as well as the amount of deflection of the image at the intensifier (Sklebitz and Haendle, 1983). The maximum tomographic angle that can be achieved with this design is about 20°.

The quality of images is reasonable and has been reported to be 3 line pairs per millimeter on a high-resolution television screen and about 4 line pairs per millimeter with cut film.

The radiation dose, on the other hand, is about 26 nC/kg at the input of the image intensifier tube (Sklebitz and Haendle, 1983). This is less than the dose in conventional tomographic imaging.

Finally, tomoscopy is still in its infant stages and has not found widespread applications in radiology. Research and development, and more importantly clinical results (which appear to be promising so far), will indicate whether the technique will become commonplace.

RESEARCH STUDIES

Image Quality

STUDY 1. Evaluation of Image Quality in Tomographic Imaging. Wolf, M., Stargardt, A., and Angerstein, W.. Physics in Medicine Biology, 22 (5), 1977.

Having presented a discussion of various methods of measuring tomographic MTFs (modulation transfer function) — a function which describes the ability of a system to reproduce detail — and other related factors (for example, influence of MTFs of focal spots and screen-film combinations), the authors discuss the results of their experiments in terms of mathematics and a series of graphs.

Some findings of this study indicate the following:

(a) "That the calculated MTFs of linear, circular and elliptical motion are almost identical with those measured with a line test pattern."

(b) The MTF for hypocycloidal motion was higher using another method (slit method) than that observed when using the line test pattern.

(c) "It can be seen that the MTFs of tomographic blurring, unlike those which occur in other imaging processes, oscillate with appreciable amplitude up to very high spatial frequencis. . . . An oscillating MTF therefore means that the blurring does not always increase when the structures become fine but changes according to the MTF of the type of motion employed. These fine structures of blurred images may be confused with details from the layer to be imaged or do at least make their recognition difficult (spurious signal artifacts)."

STUDY 2. Choice of image recording system in mammography, tomography and cerebral angiography, in terms of system speed, resolution and noise. Haus, A.G. Journal of Applied Photographic Engineering, 4 (2), Spring, 1978.

In this study, the author first discusses the recording systems currently used in the clinical setting for mammography, tomography and cerebral angiography. Only the findings for tomography will be presented here. These are:

(a) For tomography of the middle and inner ear structures, the use of a higher speed screen-film combination is possible rather than the use of regular screens of par-speed and medium-speed film combination "without loss of image quality."

(b) Radiation dose to the patient (in tomography of middle and inner ear) is significantly less when screens with thicker phosphors (lightning plus screens) are used, again "withoug loss of image quality."

Table 8-4

THE EFFECT OF FILTRATION ON DOSE DURING HYPOCYCLOIDAL
TOMOGRAPHY FOR THE MIDDLE EAR, LUNG AND KIDNEY
TOMOGRAMS

(From Krohmer J.S.: Patient dose distributions during hypocycloidal tomography.
Radiology 103:447-450, 1972.)

Technique	Anatomical Location	Measured Dose in Rads	
		No Added Filter*	2 mm Al Added
Middle ear	Center of field	6.61	1.79
77 kVp (no filter)	Right eye	4.44	2.69
80 kVp (2 mm Al)	Left eye	1.25	1.13
50 mA-6 sec	Middle ear (at cut)	0.88	0.90
30 mm diaphragm	Nasopharynx	1.09	0.89
Centered under right eye 3 exposures	Thyroid	0.74	0.75
Lung 60 kVp (no filter) 63 kVp (2 mm Al)	Center of field on skin	0.92	0.46
15 mA-6 sec 30 mm diaphragm	Mid-lung (at cut)	0.37	0.28
Centered over lesion 1 exposure			
Kidney 72 kVp (no filter) 75 kVp (2 mm Al)	Center of field on skin	2.50	1.06
50 mA-6 sec 35 x 45 mm diaphram	Kidney (at cut)	0.28	0.23
Centered over kidney 1 exposure			

*Inherent filter [3] 1.5 mm Al.

(c) With the use of lightning plus screens, "patient exposure and tube current are reduced by more than a factor of 2 compared to the previously
used medium-speed screens."

Radiation Dose Considerations

Radiation exposures in geometric tomography have been documented by a
number of workers for various procedures. A complete discussion cannot be
given here for obvious reasons, however, some selected aspects will be presented.

STUDY 1. Patient dose distributions during hypocycloidal tomography. Krohmer, J.S. Radiology, 103: 447-450, 1972.

The basic objective of Krohmer's study was "to determine patient dose distributions in usual hypocycloidal tomographic techniques and then to investigate two means of reducing this dose." Table 8:4 shows exposure factors for three typical tomographic studies (middle ear, lung and kidney) with the patient in the supine position. The table also gives the anatomical location and the measured absorbed dose in rads on the skin and act "cut". The results indicate that there is a significant decrease in patient dose with added filtration. "Doses at the depth of cut and beyond are modified very little because the decrease with filtration is compensated for by the increase in kilovoltage."

Krohmer also investigated the reduction of eye exposures in middle ear tomography by using 2 mm lead eye shields. The results indicate a reduction in the eye exposure by a factor of 3 and 6 for the contralateral and ipsilateral eyes, respectively. With respect to gonadal shielding during tomography of the kidneys, Krohmer also found that the doses to the female and male gonads were reduced by about 40 percent and about 30 percent (of the unshielded doses), respectively.

STUDY 2. Radiation dose to critical organs during petrous tomography. Chin, F.K., Anderson, W.B., and Gilbertson, J.D. Radiology, 94:623-627, 1970.

This study was performed using hypocycloidal motion, since the motion requires the use of relatively long exposure times. The investigators found that the cornea received the highest dose (more than 10R) and that a single lead shield positioned over the cornea reduced this dose to about 1.0R. They also reported that the lead shields did not interfere with film quality and that positioning of the shields can easily be accomplished by the technologist without causing any inconvenience to the patient.

STUDY 3. Radiation dosimetry in full-chest tomography. Buchignan, J.S., Wagner, W.M., and Howley, J.R. Radiology, 99:175-176, 1971.

In this study, the researchers measured exposure doses to various critical organs during "full-chest" tomography. The results indicate that doses are high and can be reduced for the eyes and thyroid if the examination is performed with the patient in the prone position instead of supine.

SUMMARY

1. Body-section radiography or geometric tomography is a technique whereby layers of the body can be x-rayed using geometric principles.

2. The technique includes longitudinal and transverse axial tomography. In the former, longitudinal body sections are examined by simultaneously moving the x-ray tube and film at a constant speed and in opposite directions.

3. In transverse axial tomography, cross sections can be imaged with the aid of a specialized apparatus designed to rotate the patient and film 360° in the same direction.

4. In tomography, the x-ray tube movement gives rise to an angle, the tomographic angle, which is used to describe the thickness of the layer to be imaged.

5. The layer imaged in tomography is in "focus" on the film and it corresponds to the fulcrum or point at which the x-ray tube and film pivots. The fulcrum lies in the objective plane.

6. Movements of the x-ray tube and film in geometric tomography fall into two broad classes: linear and multidirectional (pluridirectional).

7. In linear tomography, the x-ray tube and film move in a straight line or sometimes the movement can describe an arc.

8. In multidirectional tomography, the tomographic angle is increased (over linear tomographic angles), thus allowing thinner sections to be imaged. The movements involve circular, elliptical and hypocycloidal.

9. In cases where a relatively thick section is required, the principle of zonography is used. The tomographic angles used here range from 0° to 10°.

10. Conventional x-ray equipment can be adapted for linear tomography by using accessory devices which are attached in a specific fashion. Because of several limitations imposed by such a system, specialized tomographic units have become available in radiology departments. One such unit is describes.

11. Multisection tomography is a technique where a number of layers can be imaged with one exposure through the use of a multisection cassette.

12. Other methods of tomography are discussed. These include techniques which are derived from tomosynthesis — the manipulation of the tomographic image by electronic means.

13. The techniques are televised electronic tomography, flashing tomosynthesis, tomoscopy and cinetomosynthesis. Since the image quality is not within acceptable standards, cinetomosynthesis is not described any further.

14. In televised electronic tomography, the cassette is replaced by an image intensifier tube. In a tomographic cycle, the television camera tube produces several images which are recorded n tape. These images are played back and are superimposed on one another in a

storage tube to produce a tomogram.

15. In flashing tomosynthesis, about 24 stationary anode x-ray tubes are used and are all energized at the same time. The image produced is coded in a subsequent processing step. By proper choice of layer orientation, an undistorted focussed image is obtained. The technique does not involve motion of the tube and film.

16. Tomoscopy provides real-time tomographic fluoroscopy using several grid-controlled x-ray tubes, magnetic fields and other control units to provide tomographic images.

17. Finally, some research findings are presented with respect to image quality and radiation dose considerations in geometric tomography.

CHAPTER 9

PORTABLE AND DENTAL X-RAY UNITS

PORTABLE UNITS

PORTABLE x-ray units are used to obtain radiographs of patients who are usually confined to their hospital beds (Figure 9:1) as a result of severe trauma, pathology and other related causes. Within the framework of radiology, the terms portable and mobile are often used interchangeably, al-

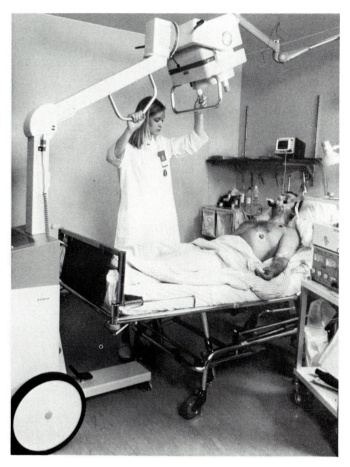

Figure 9:1. Portable radiography. The patient is too ill to be transported to the main x-ray department, hence the radiograph must be taken with a portable (mobile) x-ray unit which is brought to his room. (courtesy of the Siemens Corporation.)

though their literary meanings are quite different. In this chapter, the term portable shall be used to imply that the x-ray unit can be transported to any desired location in the hospital without much difficulty, in contrast to fixed x-ray equipment which is permanently installed in the main department, for example.

A description of portable x-ray equipment typically lends itself to a discussion of:

(a) electrical power requirements.
(b) radiographic output.
(c) the x-ray tubehead and support system.

Electrical Power Requirements

Power sources for operation of portable units in a hospital are usually:

(a) the standard 120-volt (120 V) power outlet (single phase) with a current of about 15 amperes (amps).

(b) special high current (about 30 amps) outlets, usually single-phase 240 volts (240 V).

One portable x-ray unit which uses the power requirements given in (a) above is shown in Figure 9:2. The unit is lightweight, self-contained, easy to operate and consists of a solid-state electronic timer, a collimator, and a variety of portable stands. The tubehead and controls are shown in Figure 9:3. Such a unit could perhaps be used best in radiography of extremities and other small parts, especially in rooms with limited space to work and particularly in cases where patients are in a myriad of traction devices.

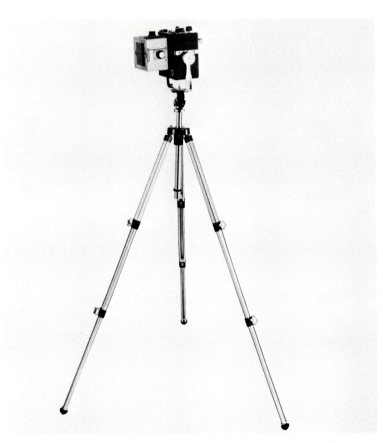

Figure 9:2. A portable lightweight x-ray unit. The output is about 63-65 kVp ad 10-15 mA and the power source is the single-phase, 60 cycle AC 110-130 volt or portable gasoline generator. The timer range is about 0.1 seconds to 5 seconds and the focal spot size is 0.8 mm × 0.8 mm with a total filtration of about 2 mm Aluminum equivalent. The total weight of the generator and stand is 25 pounds. (courtesy of Min X-Ray, Inc., Illinois.)

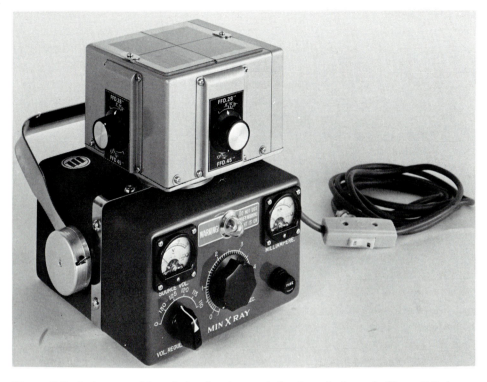

Figure 9:3. A close-up of the tubehead and controls for the unit shown in Figure 9:2. (courtesy of Min X-Ray, Inc., Illinois.)

While standard 120-V power outlets can be found almost in any location in the hospital, high current outlets are built only in certain areas; hence, units operating on these outlets are commonly supplied with a 30-amp plug. In this regard, the units can be used only in these specified areas. Today, this shortcoming has been overcome by the development and introduction of two other kinds of portable x-ray units:

    (a) the capacitor discharge portable unit, and
    (b) the battery-powered ("cordless") portable unit.

The essential features of these two units will be discussed later.

Radiographic Output

"The radiographic output of a portable unit is determined by the current it can take from the mains supply" (Hill, 1977). The output will be high for high-current receptacles and low for low-current receptacles. Portable units are usually classified into three types based on their radiographic output. The typical maximum exposure output for *low-powered, medium-powered* and *high-powered* x-ray units usually ranges from about 10-15 mA at 90 kVp, 40-150 mA at 90-120 kVp and 300 mA at 120 kVp, respectively (Chesneys, 1977).

Rectification

The purpose of rectification is to provide efficient operation of the x-ray tube. Portable units can be:

(a) Self-rectifying, in which case the x-ray tube acts as its own rectifier; hence there are no rectifiers in the high tension circuit. The x-ray tube is connected across the secondary of the high tension transformer.
(b) Half-wave rectified.
(c) Full-wave rectified. These units provide higher exposure outputs and shorter exposure times compared to self-rectified and half-wave rectified units.

X-ray Tubes and Supports

A portable unit consists of a wheel-mounted base onto which is affixed a central column. The x-ray tube is attached to a supporting crossarm which is counterbalanced for vertical adjustments of the tube. A control unit with a number of selectors and indicators is also mounted on the base. Some control units generally house the high tension apparatus.

The tube support system should always provide a wide range of tube motion. Mechanical and electromagnetic locking devices, together with a braking system, are provided for extra safety when using the equipment.

The type of x-ray tube used on a portable unit depends on the maximum exposure output and may be either of the following:

(a) Stationary anode tubes with single focus. These are typical of low-powered sets.
(b) Rotating anode tubes with dual focus. These are typical of high-powered sets.

The tubes are oil immersed and are encased in a lead-lined housing to which suitable beam restrictors (cones, collimators) are affixed. A variety of focal spot sizes are also available.

THE BATTERY-POWERED PORTABLE UNIT

The battery-powered portable x-ray unit does not require a high current outlet for its operation. Because of this, the machine has been popularly referred to as the *"cordless" mobile*. It produces a high exposure output from its own power source, usually a nickel-cadmium (Ni-Cd) battery which can be recharged via the ordinary low current mains outlet. Other advantages of the Ni-Cd power source include:

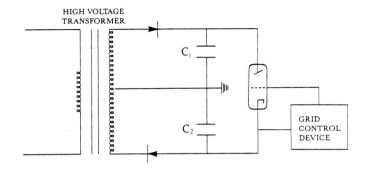

Figure 9:4. Schematic representation of a capacitor-discharge x-ray unit. (From Weaver K.E., Barone G.J. and Fewell T.R.: Selection of technique factors for mobile capacitor energy storage x-ray equipment. *Radiology 128:223-228. July, 1978.)*

(a) longer lifetime (over lead-acid batteries).

(b) no risk of explosion (as is the case with lead-acid batteries).

(c) production of a constant tube voltage.

The battery-powered unit produces direct current (DC) voltage and, therefore, it uses a set of solid-state inverter circuits to:

(a) supply the filament transformer and stator with a 60-Hz AC.

(b) provide the high tension transformer with a 500-Hz AC which is rectified (full wave), via a solid-state bridge circuit, to produce a constant potential (nearly) waveform.

Other features, such as filtration, kVp and mAs settings, will obviously vary for different prototypes. The time taken to recharge the battery from the 120-V supply also varies, but, in general, it takes about 8 hours.

THE CAPACITOR DISCHARGE PORTABLE UNIT

Like battery-powered portable sets, capacitor discharge portable units have found widespread use in radiology. The ultimate goal of a capacitor discharge unit is to produce high exposure outputs (300 mA, 125 kVp) via the standard 120-V power outlets.

In a capacitor discharge unit, the capacitor is used as a storage-discharge device and produces a constant potential. A typical circuit for a capacitor discharge unit is shown in Figure 9:4. The capacitors C_1 and C_2 are positioned between the rectifiers and the x-ray tube. A grid-controlled x-ray tube is used to commence and terminate the tube current. The following events should be noted:

(a) the capacitors are fully charged via the high-voltage transformer.

(b) the x-ray tube will only conduct when the grid bias is removed.

(c) activating the x-ray exposure switch removes the grid bias (brings it to zero) and the capacitors will discharge through the x-ray tube.

(d) the exposure will terminate only when there is a bias (a few kV) on the grid.

The quantity of charge that can be stored on a capacitor is given by the formula:

where Q = CV
       Q = quantity of charge (Coulombs)
       C = capacitance (Farads)
       V = voltage across the capacitor (kV)

For most capacitor discharge units, the capacitance is fixed and is usually one microfarad (1 μF). This would produce a potential of 1 kV per mA stored in the capacitor.

The voltage across the capacitor (V_c) can also be found, if the mAs value is known, from the following relationship:

$$V_c = \frac{mAs}{C}$$

During the discharge phase of operation, when the x-ray tube conducts, the kV decreases by one for every mAs. Hence, if a technologist were to do a chest examination and uses a technique of 80 kV at 10 mAs, the kV will be reduced to 70 kV at the termination of the exposure.

Finally, the following should be considered by the technologist when operating a capacitor discharge unit.

(a) The kV decreases as the exposure occurs (discharge phase).

(b) Higher mAs values will decrease the kV to smaller values by the end of the exposure.

(c) This causes underexposure of the film and delivers more radiation dose to the patient.

(d) The selected mAs should not exceed approximately one-third the selected kV, or the mAs should not be greater than 20 (Weaver et al., 1978).

(e) The grid-controlled x-ray tube decreases the mA to zero; hence "the voltage remaining across the x-ray tube at the end of the exposure is rendered ineffective. . ." (Hendee, Chaney, and Rossi, 1975).

PORTABLE FLUOROSCOPY

Recently, special portable units have become available for fluoroscopy. Such a unit is shown in Figure 9:5. The basic elements of this kind of equipment are:

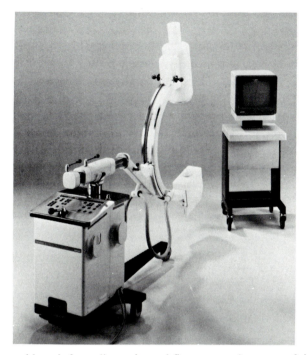

Figure 9:5. A portable unit for radiography and fluoroscopy. (courtesy of the Siemens Corporation.)

(a) the tubehead which houses the x-ray tube and high tension generator. The foci will vary from prototype to prototype; however, effective foci as small as 1.4 mm × 1.4 mm and 0.6 mm × 0.6 mm are available for both radiography and fluoroscopy, respectively. Some units are self-rectified, while others are full-wave rectified using four rectifiers.

(b) An image intensifier tube, the size of which will vary for different prototypes. Recently, a 17-cm intensifier tube has become available.

(c) A C-arm. This is a support which couples the x-ray tube and image intensifier, so that the beam is always directed to the center of the image intensifier tube. Today, greater flexibility of the unit is possible because of extended vertical excursion of the C-arm system from 340 mm to 500 mm and a swivel range of 115° (the customary rotation was 90°).

(d) Closed-circuit television chain. This implies that the components through which current flow form a closed path. These components include a television camera tube coupled to the intensifier tube, coaxial cables, a television control device and a television monitor for viewing purposes. In the past, monocular viewing was common in which case an articulated optical device was used.

(e) A control console which features separate controls for radiography

(70-90 kVp, and up to 30 mA) and fluoroscopy (70-90 kVp and 0.3 to 5 mA), and an electronic timer (0.1 secs to 5 secs). Other controls available on the console include a cumulative fluoroscopic timer that provides a warning signal after 5 minutes, push-button switches for control of the movements of the C-arm, and so on.

More modern portable fluoroscopic units feature *automatic dose rate regulation* (ADR) to ensure that the fluoroscopic mA and kV are adjusted simultaneously to the thickness of the object being examined, so that uniform picture brightness is possible.

These units are commonly used in the operating room, for examinations requiring fluoroscopic control such as cholangiography, hip pinnings, and discograms.

DENTAL X-RAY EQUIPMENT

Dental x-ray units have undergone a complete change from relatively simple equipment to more sophisticated apparatus capable of providing panoramic views of the teeth and other information that can be used in orthodontic studies.

In a simple dental unit, the x-ray tube, high tension transformer and filament transformers are all encased in what is commonly referred to as the *tubehead*. Another characteristic feature is that they are self-rectified. This places a limitation on the maximum exposure output, which, in general, ranges from 7-12 mA at 50-55 kVp. Although clockwork exposure timers are common to older, simple dental sets, electronic timers are now incorporated in modern equipment.

Restriction of the useful beam in dental radiography is accomplished by the use of cones and diaphragms. In this regard, the cone design and dimensions are especially important to:

(a) "assist the operator in accurately aligning the beam with the object and the film" (NCRP Report, No. 35).

(b) "limit the source-to-surface distance to not less than seven inches with apparatus operating above 50 kVp and not less than four inches with apparatus operating at 50 kVp or below" (NCRP Report, No. 35).

Two types of dental cones include *open-ended* cones and those with *plastic ends*. The NCRP points out that open-ended cones are favoured over those with plastic ends, since the latter produce scattered radiation.

Filtration in dental radiography is mandatory, and the minimum total filtration may vary from 0.5 mm to 2.5 mm Al depending on the kVp (NCRP Report, No. 35).

SPECIALIZED DENTAL X-RAY UNITS

Panoramic Units

Panoramic units are designed to provide a special view (panoramic view) of the teeth and mandible, including both temporomandibular joints, on a single film. Two classes of panoramic units are available today: the intra-oral unit and the dental tomograph.

Intra-oral Panoramic Units

The most essential element of an intra-oral unit is that the x-ray tube is positioned inside the patient's mouth. The film is placed outside the mouth and is held by the patient.

Electrical hazards to the patient are negligible since the anode is earthed and is maintained at zero potential. The cathode is cylindrical in shape and is surrounded by a filament, while the anode is long and hollow. The whole unit consists of the x-ray generator (constant potential), the tube support system and the control panel, which displays kV (about 40 to 80), mA (0.25, 0.5 or 1), time 0.06 to 2 seconds) and so on.

Intra-oral radiography offers several advantages, including reduced radiation doses to the skin of the face, time savings in producing radiographs, and comfort for the patient (no gagging, as is the case with single-film dental radiography).

The Dental Tomograph

The dental tomograph is based on a special form of tomography, referred to as *panoramic tomography* or *orthopantomography*. The term implies that a curved layer (the dental arch) can be imaged successfully. The principle of panoramic tomography is shown in Figure 9:6. In the actual equipment:

(a) The x-ray tube is coupled to a curved cassette-holder. This ensures projection of the axis of the object onto the axis of the cassette.

(b) When the cassette is in position, the distance from the axis of the cassette-holder to any point on the cassette is constant.

(c) The tube and cassette-holder are made to rotate at the same speed and in the same direction during the exposure, while the patient remains fixed.

(d) The slit diaphragm plays a role in image sharpness. If the slit is large, then the structures will appear unsharp on the film.

(e) Since the blurring angle is less than 8°, a layer thickness greater than 0.5 cm is always obtained.

(f) Exposure factors will vary depending on the prototype. An exposure time of 15 seconds is not uncommon.

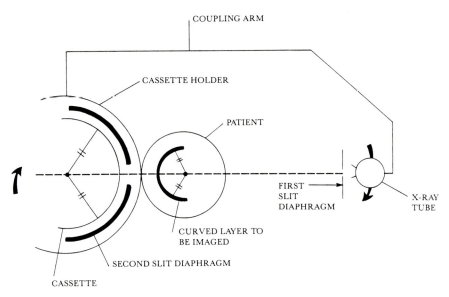

Figure 9:6. The principle of panoramic tomography. See text for further explanation.

(g) Since a narrow slit beam of radiation is used, scatter radiation production is minimal and there is no need for the use of a grid.

(h) In positioning the patient, the desired layer to be imaged is chosen by
adjusting the patient's head backward or forward. This is accomplished by moving the chin holder. Other pointers on the equipment
ensure accurate positioning.

(i) Various studies have shown that the radiation dose to the patient in
panoramic tomography is less for the skin and selected organs when
compared to that received by conventional methods.

(j) The motion used in panoramic tomography is said to be linear (based
on the principles).

(k) The setup procedures and other details will obviously become apparent during clinical training.

A dental tomograph is shown in Figure 9:7, while Figure 9:8 shows an image obtained with the unit.

The Cephalostat

The cephalostat or craniostat is a special kind of dental x-ray unit which
provides, in general, a lateral radiograph of the mandible (including the teeth),
facial bones, and soft tissues of the face, with minimal distortion and magnification. The design of the unit enables the technologist to recreate exactly the
same conditions (positioning of the head, cassette and tube) under which a preliminary series of radiographs were taken. Radiographs of this kind are especially important in orthodontic follow-up studies.

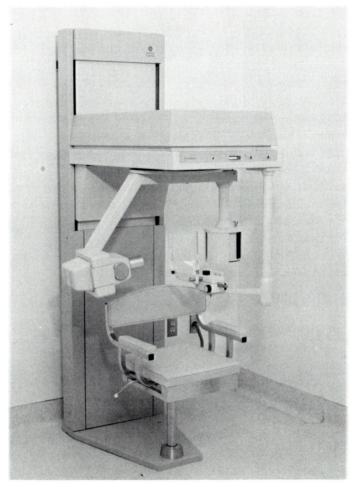

Figure 9:7. A dental tomograph — The Orthopantomograph.

The type of x-ray tube and exposure factors used will depend on the proto-type, however, some units may operate up to 150 mA and up to 125 kVp if long source-to-image receptor distances are used.

The cephalostat consists of numerous components which play a role in accurate positioning of the head. Some of these include an orbital indicator, ear locators, a nasal positioner and a cassette holder.

A cephalostat is shown in Figure 9:9 and the resultant image is demonstrated in Figure 9:10.

Panoramic Zonography

Another dental tomograph is shown in Figure 9:11. This unit is designed for panoramic and tomographic views of the head and neck areas. It provides variable image depth and layer thickness. The tube travels along a preselected

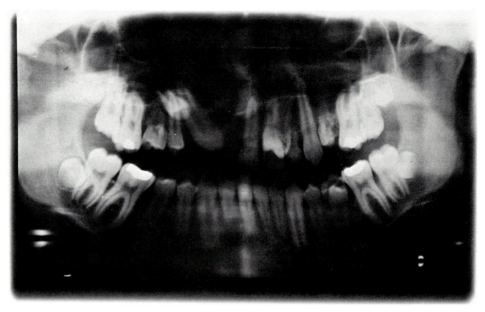

Figure 9:8. An image produced by the orthopantomographic unit shown in the previous figure.

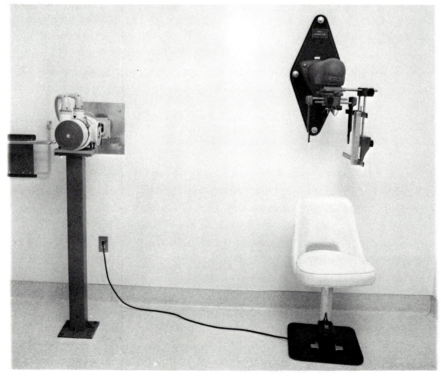

Figure 9:9. The Cephalostat.

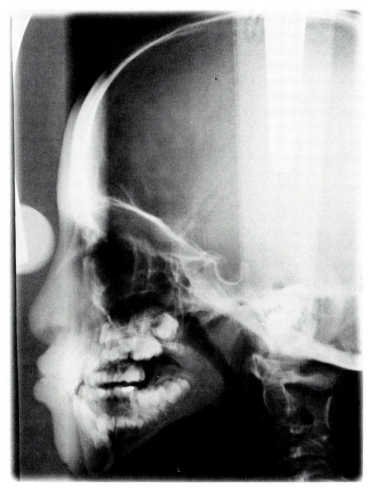

Figure 9:10. An image produced by the Cephalostat.

track matched to the curved structures of the head and neck. The film is always perpendicular to the beam, and the tube motion is synchronized with that of the film.

The unit produces images similar to that shown in Figure 9:8 and is designed to examine the patient in the recumbent position.

RADIATION PROTECTION CONSIDERATIONS

Radiation protection during mobile radiography is of concern to the technologist, since examinations are usually done in rooms not designed for x-ray work.

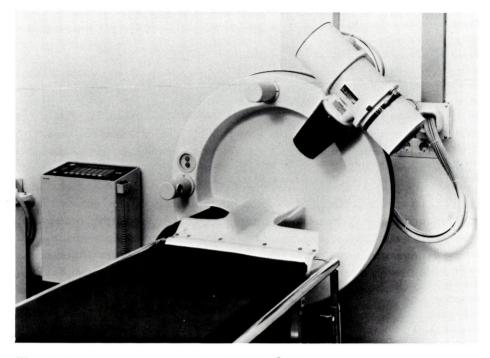

Figure 9:11. A dental tomograph — The ZONARC®. This is a craniofacial zonographic unit which provides up to 9 programs for panoramic tomography views of head and neck areas. Microprocessor control makes program selection easy. Also shown here is a dedicated stretcher for ease of patient handling. Light beam indicators make retakes easy and assist in positioning. (courtesy of the Siemens Corporation.)

The technologist is faced with two problems: leakage radiation from the tubehead and scattered radiation from the patient. Good radiation protection practices are, therefore, of vital importance. Protection can be effective if the three principles of radiation protection are observed. These three principles relate to time, shielding, and distance.

Perhaps the best protection scheme for the technologist during portable radiography is to observe the inverse square law. The law states that the intensity of the radiation is inversely proportional to the square of the distance. This means that the further the technologist is away from the source of radiation (tube and patient), the less radiation she/he is likely to receive. A protection requirement for all mobile units ensures that the exposure cord is long enough (usually 2 m) to allow the technologist to make use of the inverse square law.

Another method of protection is shielding. The technologist must wear lead aprons provided by the department for portable work. Gonadal shielding (patient) must always be used appropriately.

If the time of the exposure is kept as short as possible, then the dose the patient receives is less than with longer exposure times. The use of fast screen/

film combinations ensures very short exposure times in portable radiography.

One final note which deserves mention here relates to radiation exposure of the patient during portable radiography. It is recommended that just prior to making the exposure, the technologist announces this, so that personnel (staff nurses, orderlies) are given the opportunity to make use of the inverse square law.

In orthopantomography, the patient (childbearing age) must be given shielding in the form of a whole-body lead apron. The apron ensures shielding from the neck to the gonads.

OPINION

The Bedside Radiograph

The following is an opinion expressed by Howard J. Barnhard, M.D., (1978) relating to portable radiography. It is included here for the following reasons:

(a) it presents a brief analysis of some of the problems encountered during portable radiography.
(b) it offers a solution to the problems by suggesting a "new technology."
(c) it presents to technologists and other related groups some ideas for research studies.

The Bedside Examination: A Time for Analysis and Appropriate Action. Barnhard, H.J. Radiology, 29:539-540. November, 1978.

"The percentage of mobile-unit/beside examinations continues to grow year by year. Unquestionably some of these patients could have been brought to the Radiology Department for conventional study. Everyone knows anecdotes about the patient found lounging in the solarium after the technologists have brought the unwieldy machine to his room. Certainly such abuses should be corrected. But that does not negate recognition of the clear-cut needs of very ill patients in areas such as surgical and medical intensive care units. We need to take a closer look at the problems and potential solutions rather than continue to be simply frustrated by the increasing number of poor radiographs from this source.

"There are many problems associated with the bedside examination. Technologist time is expensive, including transit of equipment and film to and from the main department. Examinations frequently have to be repeated because of poor quality, further increasing costs. One reason for the poor quality is difficulty in positioning the patient and inadequately corrected variations in tube-to-film distance; moreover, exposures are often too heavy, probably as insurance against the image being too light to be readable. Machines of relatively low milliamperage necessitate long exposures and result in patient motion. Views which might be of great value, such as the lateral projection of the chest, are generally unavailable. All of these problems can only result in lower quality care. In addition, exposure to both patient and technologist is increased by repeated examinations and "overly dark" images. Sometimes it seems that too many studies are being requested, though this is difficult for us to evaluate since we are not standing in the clinician's shoes.

"The solution to these problems can only come from a multifaceted approach. Certainly there is a need for cooperation between radiologists and referring clinicians to reduce unnecessary examinations done outside the department. A significant surcharge for such examinations would be realistic, as it would more adequately reflect their cost; yet, in this day of third-party payers, cost frequently does not seem to greatly influence the decision-making process. Cost analysis may indicate that it is cheaper to have mobile units and film processors scattered throughout the hospital than to waste technologist time in transit, particularly where distances are great, elevator service poor, or both. However, a more productive solution would involve an entirely new technology, including a new technical specialist whose work is considered as critical and prestigious as that of technologists in the special procedures laboratory. Permanent high-powered equipment should be installed in areas of high usage, such as the operating room and intensive care unit. Specially designed beds would accommodate film cassettes. The bed should tilt to a vertical position while supporting the patient and allowing the tubes and other paraphernalia to remain attached. Such a bed would allow lateral views to be made, as well as improved anteroposterior or postero-anterior porojections. An x-ray tube carriage and central generator could service four or more beds. Considering the overall cost that goes into the basic operating room and intensive care unit, this would be a small price to pay for appropriate patient care.

"Although x-ray machines on wheels will still have to remain in use in many areas, they can certainly be made a lot better. Many of the errors made in exposure factors with these units are due to inaccurate "guestimation" of the inverse square law as it applies to distances. Each machine could be equipped with an inexpensive analog computer to accurately adjust these factors. By means of automation, merely extending the measuring tape could be enough to initiate the calculation. At an even more sophisticated level, the distance may be determined automatically by laser or sonar devices. Newly designed mobile machines are moving in this direction, and other innovations are already within our technical grasp if we decide they are worth pursuing.

"Increasing emphasis is being placed on the cost of medical care. Ambulatory care is cheaper and will be used more. Thus, the proportion of truly sick patients in the hospital will increase, leading to further escalation of the percentage of patients requiring examinations away from the department. We cannot sit idly by allowing the obvious to remain unheralded. More esoteric areas such as CT scanning and special procedures rooms have their cadre of advocates in and out of the Radiology Department who also make their needs felt. Bedside examinations lack such advocates. The problem of providing appropriate studies away from the Radiology Department must be responded to in a forthright and imaginative manner."

RESEARCH STUDIES

Dental Orthopantomography

Study 1. Dental Orthopantomography: Survey of Patient Dose. Bartolotta, A, Calenda, E, Calicchia, A, and Indovina, P.L. Radiology, 146:821-823, March, 1983.

In this study, the researchers carried out a dosimetric survey at specific points of the head and neck "in order to estimate the resultant somatic risk. . . ."

Using various commercial x-ray units they made measurements on a Rando "standard man" phantom and TLD-100 LiF dosimeters.

The researchers found that:

(a) in the parotid gland area, absorbed doses were highest.
(b) "absorbed dose rarely exceeds 0.2 mGy (200 mrad) in the anatomical regions studied. . . ."
(c) "that the cummulative maximum absorbed dose the lens in a person undergoing up to 50 orthopantomographic examinations during his lifetime is about 7 mSv (700 mrem), which is neglible when compared with the threshold for onset of opacification that would impair eyesight (15 Sv)."

SUMMARY

1. Portable and mobile x-ray units are classified according to their radiographic output and include low-, medium- and high-powered units.
2. Other important characteristics include power requirements, rectification, and the type of x-ray tube and support system.
3. In general, the standard 120-V power outlet is used, and, in some cases, high current outlets are necessary.
4. Portable units may be self-rectified, half-wave rectified, or full-wave rectified.
5. X-ray tubes for portable radiography can be stationary or rotating anodes. The tube type will depend on the class of portable unit.

6. The battery-powered or "cordless" mobile unit produces a high exposure output from its own power source. It is necessary to recharge the battery pack after using the unit.

7. The advantage of a capacitor-discharge unit is to produce a high exposure output using the standard 120-V outlet. In this unit, the capacitor is used as a storage-discharge device.

8. Several important practical considerations when using the capacitor discharge unit are given. For example, the selected mAs should not exceed approximately one-third the selected kVp or the mAs should not be greater than 20.

9. Portable fluoroscopy implies the use of a unit which includes an x-ray tube, coupled by means of a C-arm to an image intensifier tube. This method of fluoroscopy has become a common practice in operating room radiography.

10. Dental units range from relatively simple machines to sophisticated apparatus. In a simple dental unit, the x-ray tube, high tension and filament transformers are all encased in what is called a tubehead. These units usually utilize a stationary anode tube and operate on self-rectification.

11. Specialized dental units include the dental tomograph and the cephalostat.

12. The dental tomograph is based on the principle of tomography or, more specifically, panoramic tomography.

13. There are several requirements for orthopantomography and these are discussed in the chapter.

14. Radiation protection in mobile radiography involves careful consideration of the fundamental principles of protection which relate to time, shielding, and distance.

15. The chapter concludes with an opinion on portable radiography, expressed by H.J. Barnhard, M.D., and published in *Radiology*. Several reasons for its inclusion in the chapter are given.

16. Finally, the findings of a research study on dose in orthopantomography are presented.

CHAPTER 10

OTHER TECHNIQUES —
PRINCIPLES AND EQUIPMENT

MAMMOGRAPHY

*M*AMMOGRAPHY is a technique for imaging the breast. Initially, the technique was received with much enthusiasm and was therefore used for mass screening. As mammography moved through its developmental stages, it was viewed as a benefit as well as a danger. Controversial reports indicated that the technique increases the risk of breast cancer in asymptomatic women below the age of fifty years. Within this controversial framework, another group of individuals contends that the benefits of mammography are significant and, therefore, contribute to the welfare of the patient.

The controversy gave rise to a further improvement of the technique with emphasis placed on reducing radiation doses while maintaining optimum diagnostic image quality.

Imaging Requirements

Since the human breast is soft tissue, mammography has also been referred to as *soft-tissue radiography* and, therefore, the imaging requirements are somewhat different than conventional imaging.

In mammography, subject contrast is of vital importance, particularly since

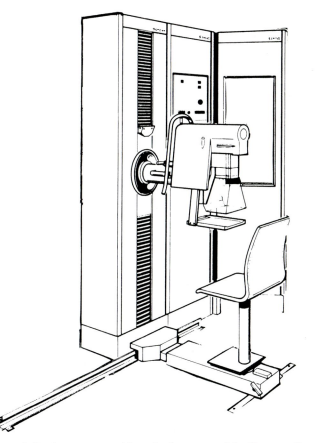

Figure 10:1. A specialized mammographic unit. (courtesy of the Siemens Corporation.)

there are very small differences in density between healthy and unhealthy soft tissues, and especially when microcalcifications are the foci of attention.

The imaging requirements will be discussed with respect to the x-ray source (tube), filtration, and image receptor considerations.

X-ray Source and Filtration

The most important requirement which represents the basis for mammography is the use of low kilovoltages in the range of 25 to 40 kVp. This requirement places special demands on the x-ray tube and filtration.

Until recently, conventional x-ray tubes with tungsten (W) targets were used for mammography. However, in 1969, tubes with molybdenum (Mo) targets were introduced.

Prior to the introduction of specialized mammographic units (Figure 10:1), conventional equipment had to be adapted for imaging the breast. In this case, several modifications had to be made to the equipment, such as modification of the transformer circuitry to facilitate operation in the 25 to 40 kVp range and

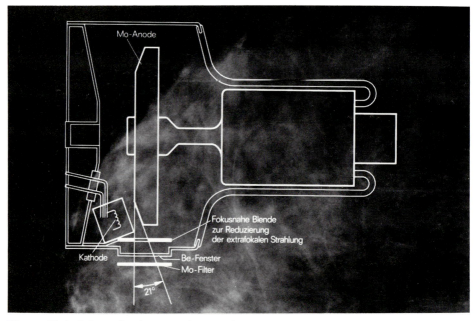

Figure 10:2. Schematic diagram of a molybdenum (Mo) target x-ray tube for mammography, showing the closer spacing of the anode and cathode structures compared to conventional x-ray tubes. The filter absorbs low-energy rays which do not contribute to the production of the image and thus reduces the radiation dose to the patient. (courtesy of the Siemens Corporation.)

removal of the conventional aluminum (Al) filter.

An important feature of the x-ray tube for breast imaging is its emission spectra which is dependent on the target material and the type and amount of filtration. The earlier tubes were made of W-targets with beryllium (Be) windows and aluminum (Al) filtration. The *Breast Exposure: Nationwide Trends* (BENT) study indicated that the higher Al filtration and the W-target tubes result in poor quality when screen/film mammographic image receptor is used. Other tubes such as W-Mo-target, with Al or Mo filtration, can be used to match the spectra to the screen/film combination used to produce better results.

The introduction of Mo-target tubes with a 0.03 mm Mo-filter give a more desirable spectra (soft x-rays) and are capable of producing better image quality than conventional W-target tubes. Another interesting feature of the Mo-target tubes is the closer spacing of the anode and cathode structures as illustrated in Figure 10:2. This arrangement increases the mA for the same temperature of the filament.

Image Receptors

There have been some concerns and uncertainties as to the type of film and screen/film combination for use in mammography to show structural details of the breast to the best advantage. In the past, non-screen, medical and industrial films (direct exposure) were used. These films provided high definition, low noise and high contrast but with high radiation doses. With this concern in mind, other films (higher speed) and screen/film combination became available for use in breast imaging.

In using screen/film combination, a number of points must be considered if high definition is to be maintained. A variety of screen/film combinations are available and a few are listed in Table 10:1. One such combination is the DuPont Lo Dose® Vacuum-Cassette screen/film combination, which consists of a single emulsion film with a thin intensifying screen packed in a vacuum-cassette to ensure good screen/film contact.

Table 10-1

FOUR SCREEN/FILM COMBINATIONS FOR BREAST IMAGING

Screen/Film Combination	Phosphor
1. Kodak Min-R screen with Kodak Min-R film	Gadolinium oxysulfide
2. DuPont Lo-Dose II screen with DuPont Mammography film	Calcium tungstate
3. US Radium Rarex-B (Medium Speed) with DuPont Mammography film	Yttrium oxysulfide
4. 3M Alpha 4 Screen	Gadolinium and lanthanum oxysulfide

Screen/film combination results in reduced radiation doses and the use of shorter exposure times; thus, image blurring due to motion is minimized. The load on the x-ray tube is also reduced and the film can now be processed in a 90-second automatic processor compared to direct-exposure films.

Another type of image receptor for use in breast imging is a charged photo conductive selenium plate. This plate is a requirement for the *xeroradiographic imaging* process (to be discussed subsequently).

Image Quality

The factors influencing image quality in breast imaging relate to compression, image blurring, and scattered radiation.

Scattered Radiation

Barnes (1972) has shown that scattered radiation decreases subject contrast (the effect is more pronounced for thick breasts) and limits visualization of small structures. These limitations, therefore, indicate that the use of a grid to improve contrast is worthwhile.

Conventional grids are not suitable for use in breast imaging because low-energy photons are attenuated by the dense interspace material. The use of grids also results in higher exposure doses to the patient. In view of this, grids are utilized best in film/screen breast imaging when the dose may be offset through the use of higher kVp, increased filtration and a faster image receptor.

Recently, the use of a *carbon fibre/resin* plate (Figure 10:3) has become available for breast imaging. The plate has a high primary transmission and has proven useful in improving subject contrast and visibility of small detail, particularly with low kVp techniques.

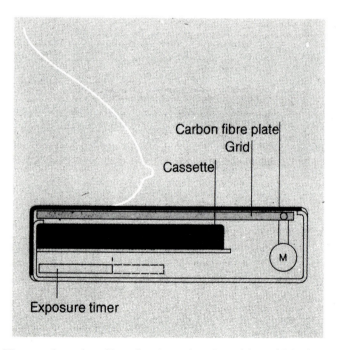

Figure 10:3. The use of a carbon fibre plate in conjunction with a grid for improving subject contrast and visibility of fine detail at low kVp techniques used in mammography. (courtesy of the Siemens Corporation.)

The air gap technique (Chapter 6) is also another means of improving contrast, since the air gap between the breast and the image receptor acts as a grid. Since scattered rays are more oblique than primary radiation, they tend to "fall out" of the air gap and do not reach the film.

Finally, Barnes (1979) has described another method, the *scanning slit technique* (Chapter 6), to provide better results than grids; however, it needs to be developed further for use in breast imaging.

Compression

This is another method to improve subject contrast by reducing the amount of scattered radiation reaching the film. Effective compression also ensures good contact between the breast and image receptor, thus reducing motion blurring problems.

The use of compression and grids in combination will also improve image quality significantly.

Image Blurring

A blurred image is generally not diagnostic. In breast imaging, blurring can be attributed to the geometry of the system (geometric blurring) and to motion.

Motion blurring can be eliminated by immobilization through effective compression.

Geometric blurring is attributed to the size of the focal spot, focal-object and object-image distances. Large focal spot sizes, short focal-object distances, and large object-image receptor distances have a pronounced effect on penumbra formation, and as a result images appear less sharp.

Focal spot sizes for breast imaging may range from 0.6 mm to 2 mm and a focal-image receptor distance of 45 cm is typical. With this distance, a 0.6 mm × 0.6 mm focus is ideal and results in low geometric blurring.

Finally, Figure 10:4 shows the skin exposure dose and image quality obtained with different factors (filter, target, focal spot size, technical factors, developer temperature and so on) for several mammographic systems.

Radiation Dose Considerations

Several workers (Bailar, 1976; Hammerstein et al., 1979; Shrivastava, 1981; Rothenberg et al., 1975) have conducted radiation dose studies in mammography and have reported different values based on the methodology used. The values will not be given here, however, the important consideration for dose studies in mammography are:

(a) the measurement technique.
(b) factors influencing the dose.

Measurement Technique

Recording dose measurements in breast imaging has been carried out using both thermoluminescent dosimeters and ionization chambers. Haus (1982) indicates that the ionization-chamber method is a better technique (in terms of accuracy) and that the chamber be positioned at the surface of the breast where the radiation enters the patient (the bottom of the cone).

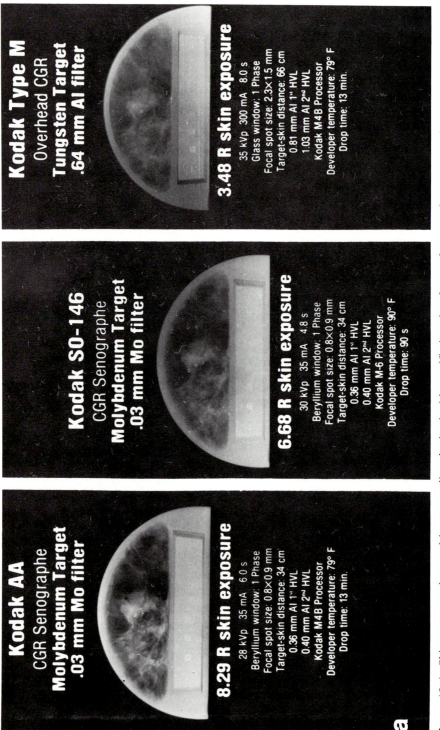

Figure 10:4. Skin exposure dose and image quality obtained with specific imaging factors for several mammography systems. (courtesy of Xonics X-ray Systems.)

DuPont Lo-Dose I

CGR Senographe
Molybdenum Target
.03 mm Mo filter

GE MMX
Tungsten-Molybdenum Target
.03 mm Mo filter

1.58 R skin exposure

28 kVp   30 mA   0.8 s
Beryllium window. 1 Phase
Focal spot size: 0.8×0.9 mm
Target-skin distance 28 cm
0.36 mm Al 1ˢᵗ HVL
0.40 mm Al 2ⁿᵈ HVL
Kodak M-6 Processor
Developer temperature: 90° F
Drop time: 90 s

1.35 R skin exposure

31 kVp   200 mA   0.4 s
Beryllium window: 1 Phase
Focal spot size: 3.2×2.7 mm
Target-skin distance: 57 cm
0.30 mm Al 1ˢᵗ HVL
0.38 mm Al 2ⁿᵈ HVL
Kodak M-6 Processor
Developer temperature: 89° F
Drop time: 90 s

Agfa Gevaert Osray M 3

CGR Senographe
Molybdenum Target
.03 mm Mo filter

1.56 R skin exposure

25 kVp   30 mA   5.0 s
Beryllium window: 1 Phase
Focal spot size: 0.8×0.9 mm
Target-skin distance: 34 cm
0.37 mm Al 1ˢᵗ HVL
0.39 mm Al 2ⁿᵈ HVL
Kodak Processor
Developer temperature: 80° F
Drop time: 7 min.

b

GE MMX
Tungsten-Molybdenum Target
.03 mm Mo filter

0.95 R skin exposure

30 kVp   200 mA   0.3 s
Beryllium window: 1 Phase
Focal spot size: 3.2×2.7 mm
Target-skin distance: 57 cm
   0.29 mm Al 1ˢᵗ HVL
   0.36 mm Al 2ⁿᵈ HVL
Kodak M-6 Processor
Developer temperature: 89° F
   Drop time: 90 s

DuPont Lo-Dose II
CGR Senographe
Molybdenum Target
.03 mm Mo filter

0.84 R skin exposure

28 kVp   30 mA   0.45 s
Beryllium window: 1 Phase
Focal spot size: 0.8×0.9 mm
Target-skin distance: 28 cm
   0.36 mm Al 1ˢᵗ HVL
   0.40 mm Al 2ⁿᵈ HVL
Kodak M-6 Processor
Developer temperature: 90° F
   Drop time: 90 s

CGR Senographe
Molybdenum Target
.03 mm Mo filter

0.86 R skin exposure

28 kVp   30 mA   3.1 s
Beryllium window: 1 Phase
Focal spot size: 0.8×0.9 mm
Target-skin distance: 66 cm
   0.36 mm Al 1ˢᵗ HVL
   0.40 mm Al 2ⁿᵈ HVL
Kodak M-6 Processor
Developer temperature: 90° F
   Drop time: 90 s

C

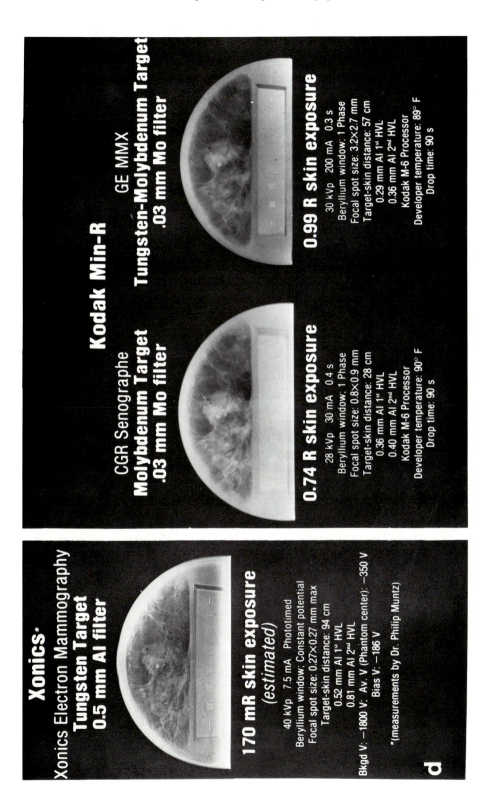

Since risk is an important factor in breast imaging, the absorbed dose rather than the entrance surface dose is "the most appropriate parameter" (when comparing different techniques), simply because the tissue below the surface of the breast "is presumably the tissue at risk for future development of cancer" (Haus, 1982).

Factors Influencing Dose

In breast imaging, several factors affect the dose, and Haus (1982) lists them as follows:

(a) "the ratio of glandular to fatty tissue (which decreases with patient's age),

(b) the quality of the beam,

(c) the area of the breast irradiated (port size), and

(d) the exposure at the entrance surface of the breast."

It is important that these factors be taken into consideration when conducting and reporting radiation dose studies in mammography.

Mammography by Computed Tomography

The techniques of computed tomography are described in Chapter 17. Imaging the breast by computed tomography has been done by Chang et al. (1979) and Gisvold et al. (1979) who used a dedicated computed tomography scanner built by the General Electric Company, Medical Systems Division.

In mammography by computed tomography, the patient is placed prone onto the table and her breast is positioned into a water box through a hole cut through the tabletop. The x-ray tube, which is coupled to a xenon detector array, rotates 360° around the breast to record several x-ray transmission readings. These readings are then fed into a computer which reconstructs an image of the breast.

This method of imaging the breast has been discontinued, since the results (spatial resolution, limitation of the method to certain breast types only, and so on) indicate that the technique is not feasible at this time.

ELECTROSTATIC IMAGING

Electrostatic imaging is a term used to refer to an imaging method whereby x-ray photons are converted into a latent charged image. The image is rendered visible by a special development process.

In this section, two classes of electrostatic imaging will be discussed. These include:

(a) Electron radiography (ionography).

(b) Xeroradiography.

Electron Radiography

Electron radiography (ionography) is a gas-discharge electrostatic imaging method developed by Xonics, Inc. (a science-based company in Van Nuys, California) together with scientists at the University of Southern California.

The two important elements in the imaging scheme are the imaging chamber and the development and fixing processes.

The imaging chamber, shown in Figure 10:5, is an ionization chamber filled with a high atomic number gas, such as xenon or krypton, to a pressure of about 10 atmospheres. The gas is contained within two electrodes which are maintained at a potential of about 10,000 volts.

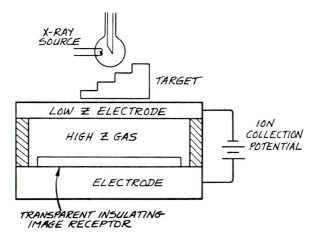

Figure 10:5. The imaging chamber used in electron radiography. See text for further explanation. (courtesy of Xonics X-ray Systems.)

The image receptor is usually a transparent or opaque polyester sheet, the position of which is indicated in Figure 10:6.

Principles of Operation

When x-rays pass through the patient, they enter the imaging chamber and are absorbed to produce multiple electron-ion pairs in the xenon gas. The electrons are attracted to the positive electrode and are deposited on the image receptor to form a latent image. This process is illustrated in Figure 10:6.

The charge deposited at any point is directly proportional to the x-ray flux (number of photons per unit area) at that point.

At the termination of the x-ray exposure, the image receptor is removed from the chamber for processing. The latent image is rendered visible using the so-called *liquid-toner electrophoretic development* process shown in Figure 10:7. In this process the latent electrostatic image is exposed to black toner particles which are positively charged. This action leads to neutralization of the latent

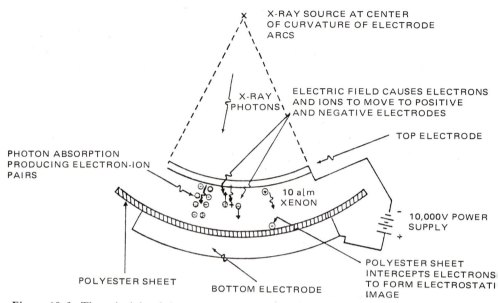

Figure 10:6. The principle of electron radiography. See text for further explanation. (courtesy of Xonics X-ray Systems.)

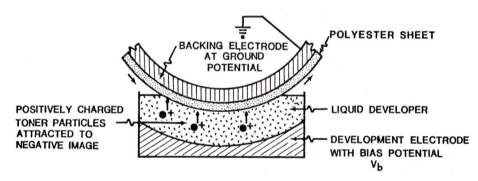

Figure 10:7. Cross-section of the image developer for electron radiography. See text for further explanation. (courtesy of Xonics X-ray Systems.)

charged image. The neutralization is usually proportional to the charge density on the image receptor. After development, the image is fixed chemically to provide a permanent image.

Imaging Characteristics — A Summary

The speed or sensitivity of an electron radiographic system is about twice the speed of conventional screen/film methods, although higher sensitivity is possible.

The resolution of the imaging chamber in electron radiography is higher than that of conventional screen/film systems. In considering other factors, the total resolution of the electron radiographic system is about 10 to 12 line pairs per millimeter (lp/mm) compared to screen/film systems which may be less than 6 lp/mm.

Electron radiography is versatile, in that it can be applied to examinations ranging from extremities to mammographic studies. A more detailed account of the application of electron radiography to mammography is given by Muntz et al. (1977).

Figure 10:8 shows a visual comparison between an electron radiography and a conventional radiograph of the hip and proximal femur and of the kidney.

Xeroradiography

Xeroradiography is a dry non-silver electrostatic imaging method that has been applied to other examinations other than mammography.

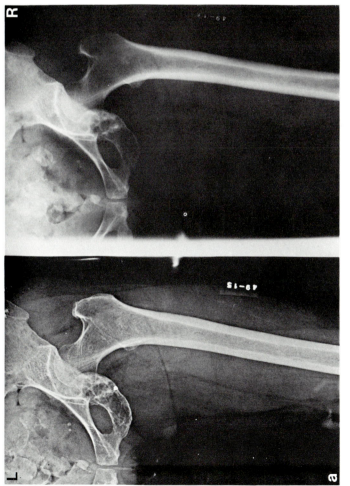

Figure 10:8. Image comparison between electron radiography and conventional x-ray imaging.

(a) Hip and proximal femur. The electron radiographic image on the left gives better fine detail of the metastases in terms of bony destruction and repair than the conventional x-ray image shown on the right, taken under the same identical conditions.

(b) Electron radiography image on the right provides sharper image of the kidney than the conventional x-ray image shown on the left, taken under identical conditions. (courtesy of Xonics X-ray Systems.)

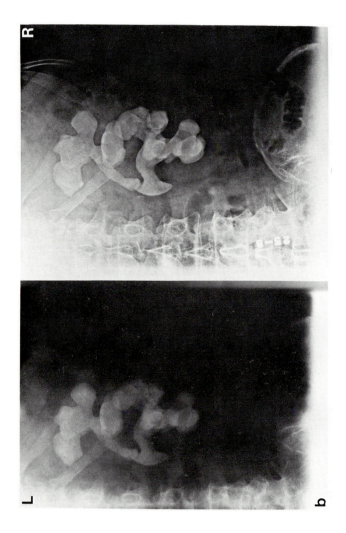

Principles

The method is based on utilization of a photoconductive material, usually selenium, which is deposited on an aluminum base. Together, the base and selenium form the *xeroradiographic plate*, which measures about 24 cm × 36 cm. A plastic coating is applied to the surface of the selenium to protect it from mechanical abrasions that can occur when the plate is being cleaned.

The principles and components of the xeroradiographic process are illustrated in Figure 10:9. The xeroradiographic plate undergoes a charging process whereby positive electrostatic charges are put on the photoconductive surface by the emission of ions from a thin wire. Following this, the plate is then placed in an opaque, lighttight cassette to maintain its charged state. All this takes place in the *conditioner* (Figure 10:9), which also serves to remove any residual latent image that might still be present on a previously used plate. This process is referred to as *relaxation.*

The charged plate is now ready for use. When it is exposed to an x-ray beam, the plate discharges at a rate that is dependent upon the intensity or radiation reaching each point. Areas on the plate which have not received any x-rays will not be discharged. Thus, the exposure of the plate produces a latent electrostatic image which must now be processed to render it visible.

The purpose of the xeroradiographic processor is threefold. First, it develops the latent electrostatic image. Secondly, it transfers and fuses the image onto a sheet of paper, and thirdly, it cleans the xeroradiographic plate so that it can be used again for another examination.

When it is in the processor, the xeroradiographic plate is removed from the cassette to be developed in a closed chamber. While in the chamber, the plate is sprayed with charged powder particles (toner). Those areas on the plate with fewer positive charges will attract less negatively charged powder particles. Those areas with more positive charges will attract more negatively charged powder particles. The latent electrostatic image then becomes visible as a powder image. At this point the powder image is transferred onto a sheet of paper by placing the plate carefully onto the paper and applying some pressure. The powder particles stick to the paper, which must now be fixed to ensure a permanent record.

Fixing the image is accomplished by heating the sheet of paper, which has a characteristic plastic layer. As the plastic is softened by the heat, the powder particles are "deposited" within the plastic layer. The final product is a dry xeroradiograph. After the fixing process is completed, powder particles which may still be present on the plate are removed by a rotating brush as the plate moves into its storage area.

The Xeroradiographic Image

The xeroradiographic image usually varies in shades of blue, since the powder particles used are essentially blue. Thick portions of the anatomy appear

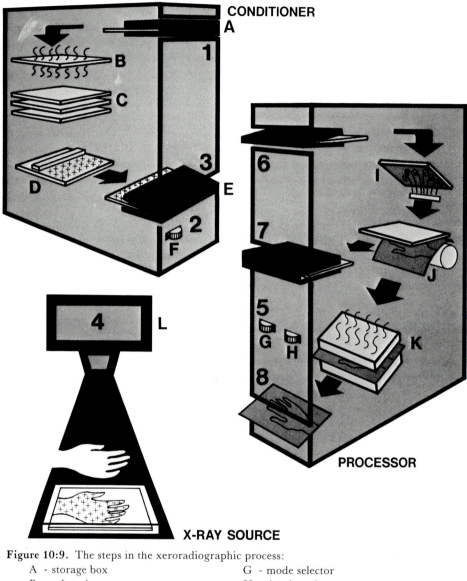

Figure 10:9. The steps in the xeroradiographic process:

A - storage box	G - mode selector
B - relaxation oven	H - density selector
C - storage elevator	I - development chamber
D - plate charging	J - image transfer
E - cassette	K - image fusion
F - contrast selector	L - x-ray tube

(courtesy of Xerox Corporation.)

deep blue compared to thin areas which appear less blue.

In discussing *contrast* in xeroradiography, the term *edge enhancement* is often used. This term describes the sharp demarcation between two different thicknesses of anatomy. For example, more powder will be attracted to the edge region, a region which marks the point where thick and thin parts meet.

In mammography, contrast is small, but in xeromammography contrast may be highlighted by edge enhancement.

X-RAY IMAGING BY REMOTE CONTROL

Remote control in this context refers to all examinations which are carried out in such a way that operation of the equipment and some aspects of patient positioning are automatically controlled from a distance. This concept is shown in Figure 10:10.

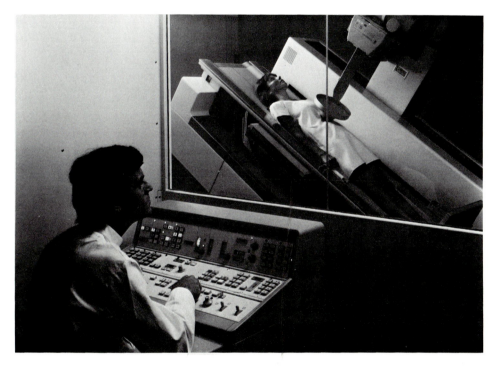

Figure 10:10. The concept of remote controlled radiography and fluoroscopy. The patient is examined from a distance and all personnel are in the control booth. (courtesy of Philips Medical Systems.)

The design considerations for remote-control equipment are important and a common characteristic feature is the ease with which the equipment can be operated. For example, the controls on the panel must be displayed in such a way that there should be no time lost in searching for specific knobs and push buttons. The tabletop should be a floating type to facilitate positioning of the patient. Most remote-control x-ray tables are the 90°/90° tilting type and tilting speeds are usually variable.

The x-ray tube for these units is used for radiography and fluoroscopy and it is usually positioned above the table (overhead fluoroscopy). The image intensifier assembly and recording equipment are thus located under the table. Tube angulation through various degrees and short exporsure times are also characteristic features.

The television monitor is usually positioned at a point along the direction in which the radiologist views the patient. This arrangement enables the radiologist and technologist to study images while observing the patient almost simultaneously.

For some fluoroscopic procedures, automatic and manual brightness control are available. Manual and automatic collimation of the primary beam are possible, in addition to automatic compression devices (Figure 10:10), which are designed for smooth and careful application without causing discomfort to the patient.

In the remote-control radiography, *fluoroscopically controlled patient positioning* is usually a common practice, and in this regard the technologist should:

(a) Place the patient on the table and select all necessary equipment (cassettes) and exposure factors prior to positioning.

(b) Position the patient by conventional means (use manual collimation, centering points and so on).

(c) Lock in automatic collimation if used.

(d) Perform intermittent fluoroscopy and observe the image on the television monitor until the best possible image is obtained.

(e) Make the exposure.

Since this procedure entails some fluoroscopy before radiography, the technologist must make every effort to protect the patient through the use of gonadal shielding, collimation and intermittent fluoroscopy.

The technique of remote-controlled examinations has been a controversial subject. Some people believe that there is a loss of patient contact during the examination since all personnel are in the control booth. They also believe that the patient "feels insecure" because the staff is not close by as is the case with conventional fluoroscopy (spotfilm device). On the other hand, those workers who have used the technique extensively have reported a different viewpoint, as well as their patients. For example, Feddema (1969) has reported that patients who were examined in the conventional manner and who were re-examined with the remote-control technique actually preferred the latter.

The advantages of remote-control radiography and fluoroscopy are increased work load, since examinations can be carried out with greater speed and with more ease, and protection from scattered radiation since all personnel are in the control booth. In this regard, there is no need for protective lead apparel.

HIGH-VOLTAGE X-RAY IMAGING

High-voltage radiography refers to x-ray examinations which are done at voltages higher than 100 kVp.

The fundamental goal of this technique is to produce an image in which the range of tissue densities is increased, thus enhancing the diagnostic impressions of the radiologist.

High-voltage radiography is possible with two-pulse, six-pulse as well as twelve-pulse x-ray generators in conjunction with:

(a) *Appropriate filtraiton.* The filtration should be about 4mm Al, or a 0.1 mm Cu and 1 mm Al filter (added filtration) will also suffice with units operating above 100 kVp.

(b) *Grids* with high "cleanup" efficiencies should be used, becaue at higher kVp values the amount of radiation scattered at small angles increases.

The *air gap* technique can also be used to remove scattered radiation.

(c) *Effective Collimation.* This is mandatory to control the amount of scattered radiation.

Increasing the kilovoltage to the levels used in this technique results in the following advantages:

(a) Shorter exposure times. This is extremely useful in dynamic studies.

(b) The use of lower mAs values than conventional methods.

(c) Improved definition, since smaller focal spots can be used in conjunction with high-definition (slow) intensifying screens.

(d) Increased x-ray output with reduced heating of the x-ray tube. This is useful in examinations which involve rapid sequence exposures.

(e) Reduction in patient dose. Radiation dose is related to kilovoltage and decreases as the kilovoltage increases. This advantage should allow the technologist to use high kVp techniques when doing examinations on young people.

The problems associated with high-voltage radiography are both clinical and technical in nature: for example, increased scattered radiation, loss of contrast and detail in soft tissues are only a few. The technique, however, has found applications in examinations of the chest, spinal column, the obstetric pelvis, hysterosalpingography, gastrointestinal and other barium-related studies.

FIELD EMISSION MEDICAL IMAGING

In conventional radiography, electrons are "boiled off" a filament by the process of thermionic emission. The emitted electrons are accelerated to strike a target by means of a high potential (kV) applied between the cathode and anode of an x-ray tube.

In *field emission* radiography, electrons are "pulled out" of a metal by applying a high voltage between two electrodes: a cathode (emitter of electrons) and an anode. The electrons are emitted in the presence of a strong electric field at the surface of the emitter.

Field emission was discovered in 1897 by R.W. Wood of Johns Hopkins University, and it was some years later before its full potential in imaging was realized.

Basic Principles and Equipment

In field emission radiography, no heat is required to cause electron emission and, therefore, a heating circuit is not necessary. An x-ray generator and a cold-cathode x-ray tube are mandatory pieces of equipment.

The generator has a capacitive storage and operates on 110, 120 volts AC (50/60 Hz, 30A). It is designed to provide very short intense x-ray pulses to facilitate the use of short exposure times. The peak kilovoltage is fixed either at 300 or 350, while the average tube current is 40 mA. This voltage value provides optimum visibility of structures as well as good resolution in chest radiography. The time of the exposure can be controlled manually or automatically to provide optimum density for patients of varying thicknesses.

A field emission x-ray tube is shown in Figure 10:11. The anode is usually made of tungsten, fashioned in the shape of a cone, while the cathode has a hemispherical tip that is extremely small (10^{-4} to 10^{-6} cm). There are four comb-shaped cathode structures from which electrons are emitted. These electrons strike the conical anode to produce x-rays. The conical shape makes it possible to use higher currents (the current density is about 100 million amperes per square cm of the emitter) so that short exposure times (for example, 0.05 microsecond) can be obtained.

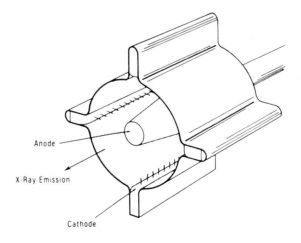

Figure 10:11. The field emission x-ray tube (cold-cathode) showing conical anode and needle-shaped cathodes. (courtesy of Hewlett-Packard.)

The main purpose of developing field emission for medical-imaging lies in the net gain in visibility of certain structures as the kilovoltage increases beyond conventional values. The physical explanations for improved visualization are outlined by Proto and Lane (1978) and only a few are presented here as a summary:

(a) *Absorption coefficients of bone and soft tissue.* The ratio of the attenuation coefficients of bone and soft tissue is significantly reduced. Dyke, Barbour and Charbonnier (1975) have shown that the ratio of attenuation coefficients of bone and soft tissue is 4.5/1 and 1.5/1 at 90 kVp and 350 kVp, respectively. This fact provides the improved visibility of soft tissues which are superimposed by bone.

(b) *X-ray spectrum.* The variation in radiation energy helps to provide a better visualization of chest structures.

(c) *Visual responses.* Bright and dark areas of a 350 kVp radiograph can be viewed at the same time, since the intensity of light to which the eye can respond is more within the acceptable limits.

Dose in Field Emission Imaging

The exposure dose in field emission imaging is substantially less than in conventional x-ray imaging. At high kilovoltages, the entrance dose to the patient decreases. For example, Adran and Crooks (1974) have shown that for a 350 kVp PA chest examination, the entrance dose is 8 mR (2064 nC/kg). The dose for the same examination at 90 kVp is about 24 mR (6192 nC/kg).

Advantages

Field emission medical imaging utilizes a high kVp technique in conjunction with conventional films, screens and scattered radiation grids to provide the following advantages over conventional x-ray imaging:

(a) Lower radiation doses

(b) Greater penetration which provides better visualization of chest structures, especially the mediastinum

(c) Contrast-enhancement at air-tissue boundaries (e.g. thorax and bronchus)

(d) Increased latitude

(e) The use of shorter exposure times which reduces motion unsharpness

(f) Consistent radiographic exposures

PHOTOFLUOROGRAPHY

Photofluorgraphy is the photographic recording of a fluoroscopic image.

In its most basic form, a photofluorographic unit consists of a fluorescent screen (35 cm × 43 cm), which is coupled to a photographic camera by means of a lighttight hood positioned between the screen and the camera.

The patient is positioned in front of the screen which fluoresces when struck by x-rays. The camera then records the fluorescent image, usually on 35-mm, 70-mm or 100-mm high-speed film.

In the past, photofluorography has been used extensively for mass chest surveys. However, because it was necessary (in some instances) to record these examinations on large format films (35 cm × 43 cm), the technique has become obsolete in the practice of radiology. Another limitation imposed by these units is that of high exposure doses. This limitation has led to the development of more efficient photofluorographic units.

Image Intensifier Indirect Exposure Technique

A modern photofluorographic unit is shown in Figure 10:12. It consists of an x-ray image intensifier tube coupled to a high-resolution spotfilm camera. The camera records the image from the output phosphor (screen) of the image intensifier. Presently, these units have not found widespread use in radiology departments.

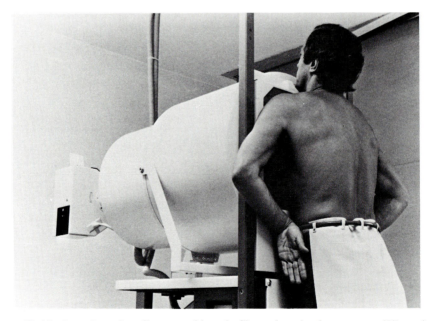

Figure 10:12. A modern photofluorographic unit. Shown here is a large-screen (57 cm. input diameter) x-ray image intensifier tube coupled to a spot film camera (100 mm.) which records the image from the output screen by means of a tandem lens system. (courtesy of the Siemens Corporation.)

The initial experience with this type of unit was published by Raithel, Stahnke, Strum and Valentin (1983), who reported that

> The information yield of the first large-screen x-ray image intensifier tube suitable for chest exposures is investigated and compared with the high kVp technique and the technique of photofluorography for a comparative assessment. It is shown that with respect to the image quality required for the diagnosis of pulmonary fibrosis, the large-screen x-ray image intensifier provides results that are practically identical with those obtained with the high kVp technique, and is thus excellently suited for the surveillance or examination of persons exposed to asbestos or silica dust. In comparison with the photofluorographic procedure, it proves unequivocally superior.

> A major advantage of the new technique is the significant reduction in radiation dose by about a factor of 4 vis-a-vis the high kVp technique and about 14-fold as compared with photofluorography. In addition, it has clear advantages over the high-kV technique with respect to operating costs.

CASSETTELESS RADIOGRAPHY

Cassetteless radiography is an x-ray imaging method which involves the use of special units designed to image the patient without cassettes. A unit consists of a set of supply magazines to hold different sizes of films. In this regard, the method has also been referred to as the *magazine technique* (Siemens Medical Engineering).

Cassetteless x-ray units have been developed to reduce the number of steps required to take a radiograph. This is clearly illustrated in Figure 10:13. They also offer a number of other advantages such as less physical strain and reduced movement of the technologist, smooth working sequence, higher patient throughput because of shorter examination times and so on.

Imaging Properties

A typical cassetteless system consists of a radiographic unit (table and x-ray tube) coupled to an automatic film processor (Figure 10:14). Two such systems are illustrated in Figure 10:15.

The common imaging characteristics are:

(a) an exposure field. This is an area which is in a fixed position on the table. The patient must therefore be positioned over this area which consists of intensifying screens and a scattered radiation grid (moving type). Some units are equipped with two different types of intensifying screens to facilitate selection of the optimum screen type to meet the needs of the department.

(b) a large source-to-image distance (for example, 115 cm), short tabletop-to-film distance (about 4 cm), and uniform film/screen contact.

(c) automatic exposure timing. This can be controlled by push-button selectors.

(d) automatic collimation. This ensures that the x-ray beam is collimated to the selected film size. Manual collimation allows the technologist to collimate smaller than the film size.

(e) a floating tabletop.

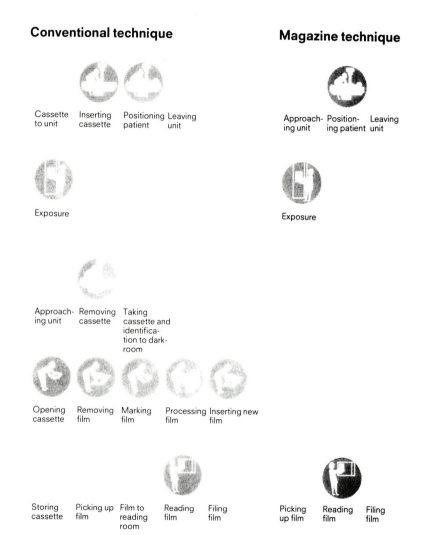

Figure 10:13. A comparison of the workflow for conventional and magazine techniques. (courtesy of the Siemens Corporation.)

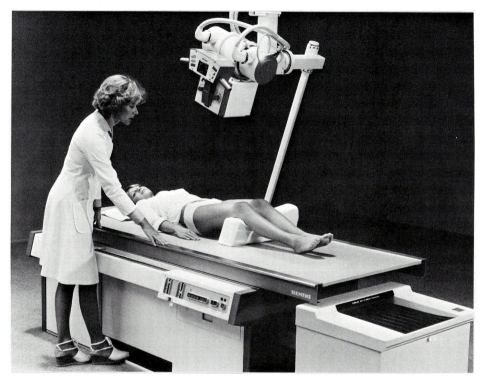

Figure 10:14. A cassetteless radiography unit. (courtesy of the Siemens Corporation.)

Operational Aspects

At the beginning of the day, the supply magazines are loaded in the darkroom. The patient's identification (name, age, sex) is written on a card, which is inserted into an appropriate slot for automatic film identification.

The technologist then sets up all technical factors, including exposure factors, screen type, film size, collimation, left or right side marker selection and all positioning aids to be used in the examination. The patient is then positioned over the exposure field and the correct tube angulation is chosen.

The next step in the sequence of events is to advance the film into the exposure field. This is done by the appropriate push button. When the exposure is terminated, the film is then automatically transported to the processor, where it is developed and ready for viewing within a short period of time.

In its early stages, cassetteless x-ray imaging equipment was restricted to examination of the patient in the recumbent position, however, more recent systems facilitate examinations in the upright position.

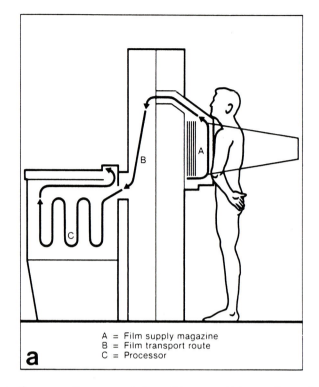

A = Film supply magazine
B = Film transport route
C = Processor

a

Figure 10:15. A diagrammatic representation of two cassetteless radiography units. (courtesy of the Siemens Corporation.)

Fully automatic Bucky set-up with magazine technique

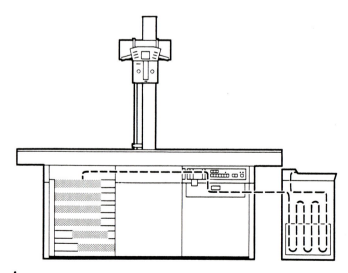

b

FILTRATION IN DIAGNOSTIC IMAGING

The primary beam emerging from the x-ray tube in diagnostic imaging is *heterogeneous* or *polychromatic*. This means that the x-ray beam consists of photons of different energies — that is, the beam consists of long- and short-wavelength x-rays.

The short-wavelength x-rays have high energies and, therefore, penetrate the patient and strike the film to produce an image. The long-wavelength x-rays, on the other hand, are low-energy waves and are absorbed by the patient (in general), thereby increasing the radiation dose. These rays do not play a role in image formation. Since one of the objectives in x-ray imaging is to keep the radiation dose to the patient to a minimum, filters are incorporated into x-ray beams for this purpose.

Definition of a Filter

A *filter* is any material which is placed in the direct path of the primary x-ray beam (useful beam) to absorb, preferentially, low-energy waves which have very little penetrating power. The process by which this is accomplished is called *filtration*.

Types of Filtration

There are three types of filtration that are of consequence to diagnostic x-ray imaging. These are: inherent filtration, added filtration, and patient filtration. Only the first two will be discussed in this section.

Inherent Filtration

Inherent filtration is filtration due to the glass envelope of the x-ray tube, the insulating oil surrounding the glass envelope and the "window" of the tube housing. Any of these materials, therefore, is referred to as an inherent filter. Such filters are always permanent to an x-ray filtration scheme. Since the atomic number of glass is greater than that of oil, it (glass) reduces the intensity (attenuates) of the beam more than oil which provides very little attenuation.

Modern x-ray tube windows are usually made of aluminum (about 0.5 mm), although bakelite has been used in older tubes. Some x-ray tubes have a beryllium window that, in the absence of added filtration, provides low-energy x-rays (soft radiation), which are useful for soft-tissue imaging — for example, mammography.

Added Filtration

An *added filter* is any material placed outside the x-ray tube, in close proximity to the window, for the purpose of selectively removing low-energy x-rays.

The type and thickness of the added filter is partially determined by the kilovoltage at which the tube is operated. As the kilovoltage increases, the thickness of the filter increases.

In diagnostic x-ray imaging, two types of materials commonly used as added filters are aluminum (Al) and copper (Cu). Aluminum is used as a *primary* filter, in contrast to a *compound* filter which is made up of two or more materials, and is generally used at voltages ranging from 50 kVp to 150 kVp at thicknesses between 1 mm to 3 mm. Compound filters are usually used in high-voltage x-ray imaging (above 100 kVp) and a typical filter is made of Al (at least 1-2 mm thick) and Cu (at least 0.1-0.25 mm thick), with the Cu placed closer to the target. The reason for this arrangement is based on the fact that Cu is a more effective absorber of low-energy x-rays. At high voltages, Cu emits soft characteristic x-rays (radiation resulting from high-speed electrons interacting with electrons) which are absorbed by the Al filter directly below it. The same phenomenon occurs with a primary Al filter, however, the characteristic low-energy rays are absorbed by the air gap between the x-ray tube and the patient.

Through this attenuation process, the mean energy of the x-ray beam increases — that is, the beam becomes more penetrating. This process is referred to as *beam hardening*.

Total Filtration

The total filtration for an x-ray imaging system is given by the following relationship:

$$F_T \; = \; F_I \; + \; F_A$$

where F_T = total filtration
F_I = inherent filtration
F_A = added filtration

Heavy Metal Filter Materials

Another common filter in diagnostic imaging is molybdenum (Mo) which is used in mammography equipment. Others include the *heavy elements* gadolinium (Gd), iron (Fe), samarium (Sm), holmium (Ho), tungsten (W) and ytterbium (Yb). Of these, Gd has received more attention in the area of research.

Gadolinium is a *rare-earth* (Group III elements in the periodic table) metal which was suggested by Atkins, Fairchild and Robertson (1975) for use in diagnostic imaging with the introduction of new intensifying screens. In their study, they found that because of the marked attenuation provided by the Gd filter (227 μm thick), there is a twofold reduction of patient skin dose, however, the mAs has to be increased. Another study by Oosterkamp (1961) indicated that Gd filters reduce patient dose in iodine contrast examinations. Yet another study done by Burgess (1981) indicates that at a specified kVp, a Gd filter (250 μm thick), provides better contrast than a 2-mm Al filter, that the same contrast effects can be attained with an increase in 8-10 kVp beyond the kVp used for the Al filter (this leads to a further decrease in patient dose), and that the filter is best suited for imaging thin patients. Finally, Burgess (1981) found "that there is little difference in the relative contrast, tube loading, and the entrance exposure results for a rare-earth screen (Alpha-8) and a calcium tungstate screen (Hi-Plus)."

In a study conducted by Kuhn (1982), Fe was used as a prefilter in reducing patient dose. Kuhn found that the Fe filter (0.15 mm) significantly reduced patient dose compared to the Al (3 mm) and Cu (0.1 mm) filters. He also recommends that the Fe filter be considered for use in cerebral and abdominal angiography, urography and pediatric radiography but not in cardioangiography because of "kinetic unsharpness."

In 1970, Richards, Barbour and Bader et al. published their findings on the use of a Sm (0.2 mm thick) filter in conjunction with dental film. Their results suggest a reduction in skin exposure by 33 percent.

Finally, Villagran, Hobbs and Taylor (1978) studied several heavy elements, including Sm, Gd, Ho, Yb and W, for use as filters in diagnostic imaging. Their results indicated that the reduction in skin dose is attributed to several factors such as the tube kilovoltage, the phosphor of the intensifying screen, the filter material, the thickness of the filter and the thickness of the patient.

Effects of Filters

There are three radiographic factors that are influenced by filtration. These are image contrast, patient dose and the x-ray tube loading (mAs).

The foregoing discussion identified the effects of filters on these parameters, namely, reduced patient dose and increased image contrast.

The tube loading increases in general with filtration. For example, Atkins et al. (1975) and Villagran, Hobbs and Taylor (1978) demonstrated that there is a significant increase in tube loading when gadolinium filters are used. This, of course, will depend on the image receptor phosphor used. Burgess (1981) has shown that with a rare-earth screen (Alpha-8), "a considerable reduction in the tube loading (mAs) can be obtained using the constant contrast approach to technique conversion."

COMPENSATING FILTERS

A *compensating filter* is used to provide an even distribution (uniform) of film density when the part being x-rayed is of uneven thickness, for example, the foot and femur.

A *wedge* of suitable material (Al) may be used as a compensating filter by arranging it so that the thick portion of the wedge is placed over the thin part of the patient and the thin portion (wedge) under the thick part of the patient. Other materials which have also been used as compensating filters include barium plastic compounds, cardboard and corn meal.

Compensating filters have been used very successfully in such examinations as placental localization, the shoulder girdle, the femur and the vertebral column.

Primary X-ray Dodging

Dodging or, more specifically, *image dose dodging* was developed by Edholm and Jacobson, who presented the technique at a meeting of the Swedish Radiological Society in 1970.

The technique uses a series of compensating filters carefully arranged not only to produce uniform film density but also to enhance image quality and reduce radiation dose to the patient.

Several dodging systems have been developed and the results are striking. In this section, only one type of dodging system will be described here. The system has been called the Dodger-T® and it consists of a series of smoothly formed adjustable aluminum wedges (Figure 10:16a). The entire assembly can be attached to the collimator diaphragm as shown in Figure 10:16b. The

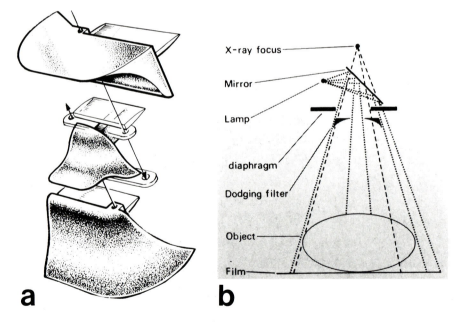

a　　　　　　　　　　**b**

Figure 10:16. A system of compensating filters.
    (a) The Dodger-T®, consists of a series of smoothly-formed, adjustable aluminum wedges which can be adjusted to conform to the patient's anatomy.
    (b) The entire unit can be attached to the diaphragm of the collimator.
(courtesy of Saab-Scania, Medical Division — Sweden.)

wedges can easily be manipulated, and, with the help of a light beam (projected on the patient), the desired arrangement can be obtained. The dodging unit can be applied to all parts of the body except the head. Another system, the Dodger-S® has been designed specifically for radiography of the skull.

It is well known in conventional x-ray imaging that the periphery of structures are sometimes "burnt" out (not visualized) due to the positioning of the patient and/or technical exposure factors used and, in particular, the diffusion of scattered rays from the table, cassette, and screens. Figure 10:17a-b illustrate the *"exposure profile"* and explain why the Dodger-S system, for example, eliminates the "blackening-out" effect, thereby providing uniform film density — that is, all details of the image fall within the exposure range.

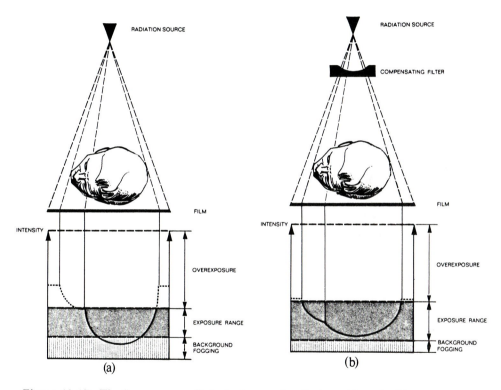

Figure 10:17. The "exposure profile" of a beam of radiation with and without a compensating filter. In (a) some details of the image fall above the exposure range while others fall below. The background fogging produced by scattered radiation destroys image contrast. In (b) all parts of the image are included in the exposure range which is wider than that of (a). Also the background fogging in (b) is smaller. (courtesy of Saab-Scania, Medical Division — Sweden.)

Today, more and more departments are using some form of compensating filtration to provide images of more uniform density.

IMMOBILIZATION EQUIPMENT

The Need For Patient Immobilization

The problem of patient motion in x-ray imaging is an important one. Voluntary and involuntary motion during an examination produces image blurring. A blurred image is of no diagnostic value and, therefore, serves no useful purpose.

In general, the technologist has no direct control over involuntary motion, however, she/he is able to control voluntary motion by careful immobilization of the patient through the use of appropriate immobilization devices. The overall objective in immobilization is to produce sharp images by eliminating patient movement.

Immobilization devices are used to:

(a) provide a direct method of eliminating any unsharpness of images due to motion, thus providing high-quality radiographs.

(b) provide patient safety and comfort.

(c) assist the patient in maintaining a desired position in order to facilitate more efficient and precise positioning.

(d) reduce the number of repeat examinations due to patient motion.

(e) provide adequate radiation protection.

Type of Immobilizing Devices

Immobilizing devices can be put into three classes, namely: general, mechanical and specialized. Since most of these vary in design from manufacturer to manufacturer, a detailed description will not be given here, however, a few characteristic features will be discussed. An important point to remember is that any immobilizing device which is placed in the direct path of the primary beam *must* be radiolucent.

General Immobilizers

These include simple forms such as *sandbags, masking tape, balsa wood, sheets, Polyfoam*® (Leslies Limited, England) pads and blocks and so on.

Sandbags are usually made of durable leatherette and canvas filled with sand. Their gross weight varies from one-half to several kilograms and they are used ina variety of ways. Sandbags are not radiolucent.

Polyfoam is a synthetic foam which is resilient, though and radiolucent. Polyfoam is chemically stable and is unaffected by chemicals which are harmful to natural rubber. It is unaffected by heat at 120°C and may be sterilized. It also has a long life, will not deteriorate if exposed to strong light, and it may be dry-cleaned and even boiled.

Polyfoam blocks and pads come in standard sizes and shapes, and specific dimensions may be obtained from manufacturers to suit individual needs. Shapes may be triangular, circular, wedge, cylindrical (bolsterlike), rectangular, and square.

Polyfoam is very common in departments and has found applications in a number of examinations such as the skull, chest, abdomen, pelvis, upper and lower extremities.

Balsa wood is a special kind of wood that has a characteristic softness. It is radiolucent and can be pressed and shaped (carved) into different shapes for use in patient immobilization. Its capabilities are like those of Polyfoam, but its relatively high cost precludes its use in radiology departments.

Masking tape is a sticky tape which is radiolucent. It can be useful in a variety of ways to assist in patient immobilization. It is recommended that only small parts be immobilized with sticky tape, since large body parts tend to require too much tape for effective immobilization.

Cloth sheets are very practical in immobilization of infants and children. They can be used to wrap the patient securely, thus providing some form of immobilization.

Mechanical Immobilizers

This class of immobilizers are usually of a mechanized nature. They are built with specific features, including locking mechanisms to hold them securely in place for proper immobilization.

Mechanical immobilizers include *head clamps, shoulder pads, hand grips, compression bands, foot support* and so on.

The head clamp is made to fit onto the x-ray table. It consists of two rotating arms which are fitted with pads for safety in immobilizing the patient. By positively engaging these arms, the device can be used to hold the patient's head in any desired position (posterior-anterior or lateral).

Shoulder pads, handgrips and the foot support are other immobilizers which fit onto the table by locking mechanisms. They are very useful in a myelogram examination.

The compression band is usually a plastic or cloth band about 23 cm in width, which can extend across the table. It is used extensively in compression of the ureters during x-ray examinations of the kidneys (intravenous pyelogram). It is also used to improve image quality by compressing and displacing fatty tissue, thus reducing the amount of scattered radiation reaching the film. The band can also be used very effectively in safe immobilization of the agitated patient.

Specialized Immobilizers

These devices generally have a specialized design. Most of them are used in pediatric radiography since immobilization in this respect is a definite challenge, as shown in Figure 10:18.

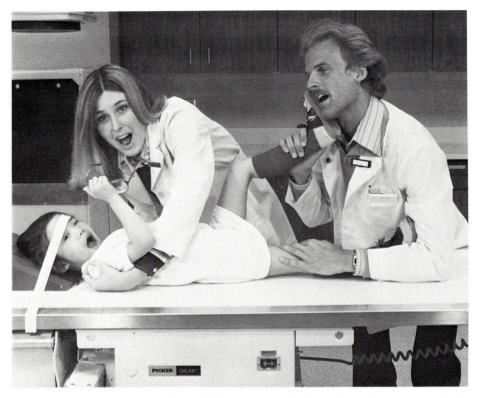

Figure 10:18. The problem of immobilization in pediatric radiography.(courtesy of the Edwin Corporation, Illinois.)

Several types of specialized immobilizers are available commercially and include the following prototypes:

- (a) Tame-em
- (b) The Pigg-O-Stat
- (c) The Baby Chair
- (d) The Mold and Hold positioner and immobilizer
- (e) The Wrigglelator
- (f) E-C-Chair
- (g) The Hugger

A description of these prototypes will not be given in this chapter, since the photographs included here "are worth a thousand words."

Care of Immobilization Devices

Immobilizers should be cleaned as often as possible to protect and increase their life span.

In general, they can be cleaned with isopropyl 70 percent dressing alcohol or with soap and warm water. Periodic checks for the presence of radio-opaque materials, such as barium sulfate, other contrast media, metal clips and pins, glass and so on, are an essential practice of the technologist and the department. These materials can be projected onto the film, thus causing severe artifacts and diagnostic problems.

It is recommended that a special corner of the x-ray room be made available for the storage of immobilizing apparatus. This makes them easily accessible to the technologist.

Applications — A Photographic Atlas

As stated earlier in the chapter, immobilizers have endless use in patient positioning. It is not within the scope of this chapter to describe their applications in radiography. The following photographic atlas (Figure 10:19) serves to orient the technologist, initially, to the domain of radiographic immobilization.

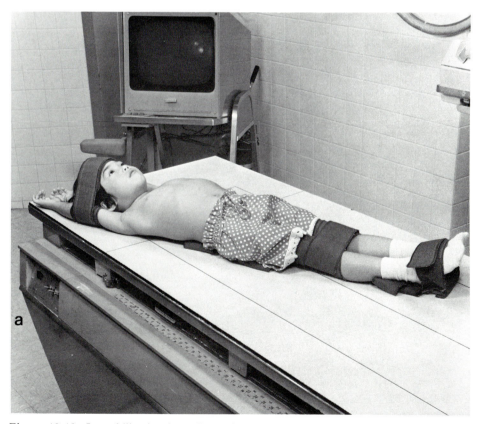

Figure 10:19. Immobilization in radiography — A photographic atlas. (A-E, courtesy of Edwin Corporation, Illinois. F-R, courtesy of Contour Fabricators, Inc., Michigan.)

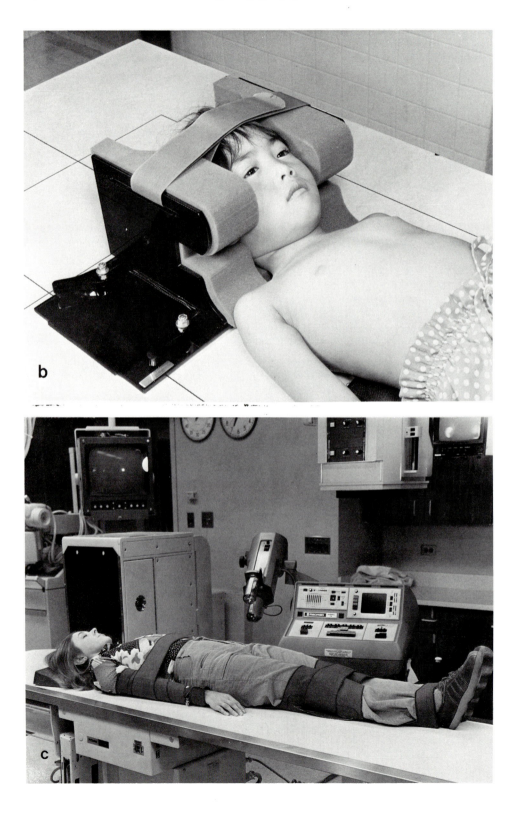

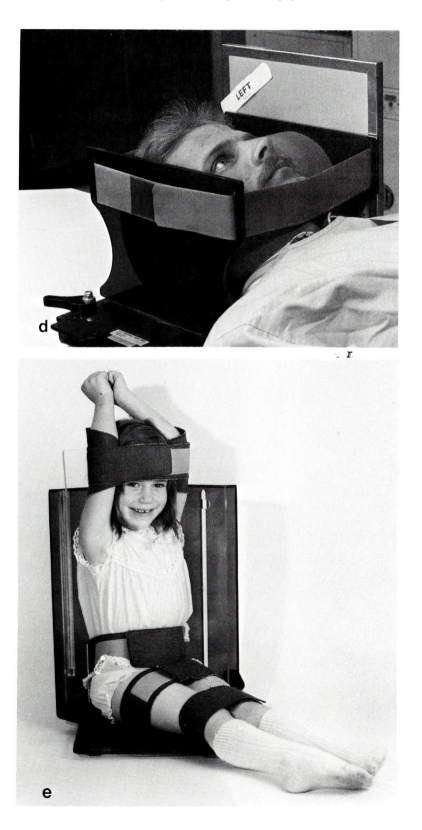

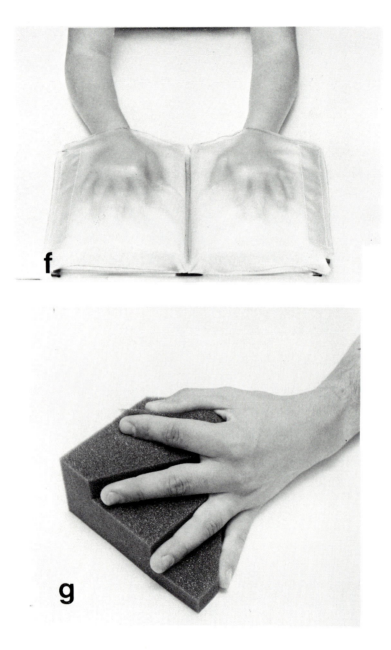

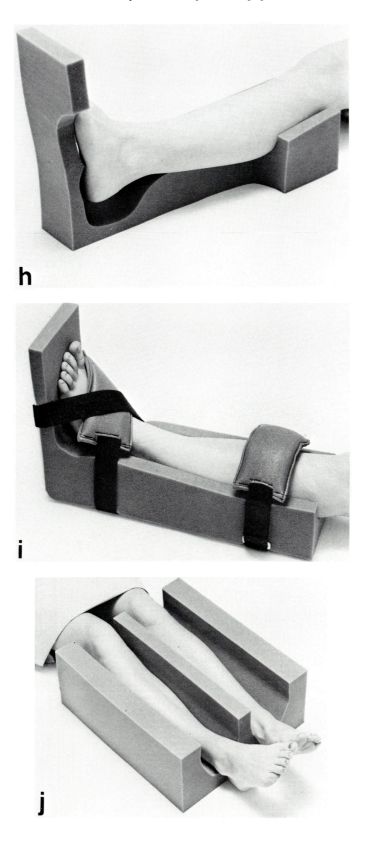

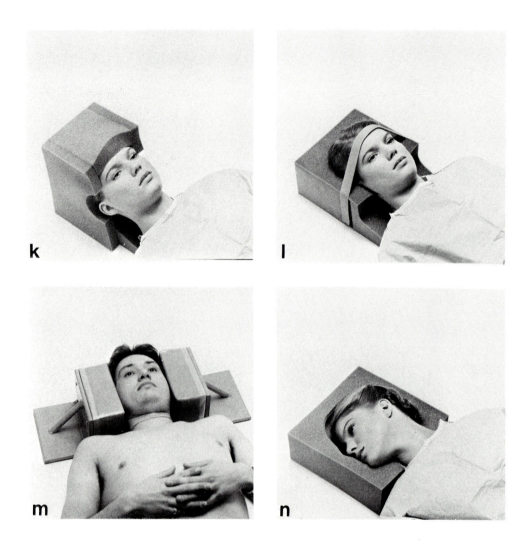

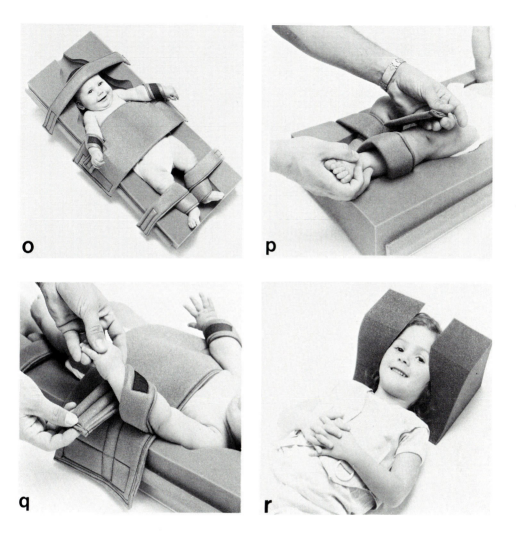

RESEARCH STUDIES

Fluoroscopically Controlled Patient Positioning vs Conventional Positioning

STUDY 1. A comparison of fluoroscopically controlled patient positioning, and conventional positioning, including comparative dosimetry. Leeming, B.W.A., Hames, O.S. Gould, R.H., and Locke, E. Radiology, 124, July, 1977.

The purpose of this study was to investigate the radiation dose to patients who were positioned by technologist-controlled fluoroscopy and by conventional means using the appropriate anatomical landmarks. The researchers used the following formula to calculate exposures in an excretory urography examination specifically selected for this study:

$$R_p = R_r \left[\frac{FSD_r}{FSD_p}\right]^2 (BSF) (mAs)$$

Where R_p = patient exposure per film
R_r = reference exposure rate (mR mAs^{-1})
FSD_r = reference focal-skin distance for R_r
FDS_p = patient focal-film distance
BSF = backscatter factor
mAs = selected mAs

The results of this experiment indicate the following:

(a) Fluoroscopically controlled patient positioning by the technologist is well-founded, because there is no significant increase in the average exposure compared to conventional positioning techniques.

(b) The quality of the examination done by fluoroscopically controlled patient positioning is much better than in conventional imaging because of the tighter collimation allowable by these machines.

(c) The average time of the examination was reduced from 44.6 minutes to 39.5 minutes, allowing more patients to be examined in an 8-hour period.

Automatic Exposure Timing in Xeromammography

STUDY 2. Xeromammographic automatic exposure termination. Zeeman, G.H., Osterman Jr., F.A., Rao, G., Kirk, B.G., and James, A.E. Radiology, 126, January, 1978.

In this study, the authors' main concern was to establish the use of automatic exposure termination (AET) instruments in routine xeromammography. They used a Siemens Iontomat (AET instrument) which consists essentially of an ionization chamber. Having determined several influencing factors, they compared the rate of repeat exposures for both manual and automatic timing. The authors found that:

(a) The AET device produces significant results in xeromammography and that the "uncertainty involved in proper selection of xeroradiography technique factors has been virtually eliminated, however, chamber positioning in the appropriate location is necessary."

(b) "Manual exposure procedures have been proved to be less than ideal (in our experience) due to the number of repeat examinations required."

SUMMARY

1. Mammography is a technique for imaging the breast. It is a soft tissue imaging technique.

2. Imaging requirements for mammography are discussed with respect to x-ray tube and image receptor considerations and filtration.

3. X-ray tubes with molybdenum targets are used, since they provide a more desirable x-ray spectra and better image quality compared to conventional tungsten target tubes.

4. Image receptors include non-screen medical and industrial (direct exposure) films and, more recently, screen/film combinations.

5. The factors influencing image quality, such as compression, image blurring and scattered radiation, are discussed.

6. Dose studies in mammography should take into consideration the measurement technique and factors influencing the dose. Ionization chambers appear to be the best method for measuring dose. The factors affecting dose (such as the quality of the beam) are listed.

7. Mammography by CT is not a practial technique.

8. Electrostatic imaging is a process whereby x-rays are converted into a latent charged image. Two types are discussed: electron radiography and xeroradiography.

9. Electron radiography (ionography) is a gas-discharge electrostatic imaging technique in which multiple electron-ion pairs are produced in xenon gas. The image is rendered visible by a liquid-toner electrophoretic development. The speed of this method is about twice the speed of conventional screen/film imaging.

10. Xeroradiography is a dry, non-silver elctrostatic imaging method which uses a special photoconductive plate. First, the plate is charged, then it is exposed to x-rays which discharge the plate to produce a latent electrostatic image. Second, the image is rendered visible by a special processing method.

11. Remote control x-ray imaging is a method of imaging, whereby the operation of the equipment is carried out automatically from a distance. The basic considerations are described.

12. High-voltage radiography refers to imaging at voltages higher than 100 kVp, in which the objective is to demonstrate an increase in the range of tissue densities. The technique must be used in conjunction with appropriate filtration, grids or the air gap technique and collimation.

13. The advantages of high-voltage imaging are listed.

14. Field emission imaging is a process in which electrons are emitted in the presence of a strong electric field at the surface of the emitter. The purpose of field emission x-ray imaging lies in the net gain in visibility of certain structures as the kilovoltage increases beyond conventional values.

15. The dose in field emission imaging is smaller than in conventional imaging. The advantages are listed.

16. Photofluorography is discussed as a historical note. It is the photographic recording of a fluoroscopic image which has been used in the past for mass chest surveys. A modern photofluoroscopic unit using an x-ray image intensifier is described.

17. Cassetteless radiography involves imaging without cassettes. Films are loaded into special magazines and are brought into an exposure field which features intensifying screens and a grid. Once the film is exposed, it is automatically transported to a processor.

18. Filtration is essential in x-ray imaging. Filters remove the low-energy waves which have very little penetrating power. Filtration can be inherent (due to the glass envelope of the x-ray tube and window of the housing, for example) or added. An added filter is a piece of metal (usually aluminum) placed outside the tube in close proximity to the tube window. The total filtration is the sum of inherent and added filtration. Heavy metal filters such as gadolinium, iron, samarium, holmium, tungsten and so on are the focus of research studies in filtration in x-ray imaging.

19. Image contrast, patient dose and x-ray tube loading are all influenced by filtration. These influences are described briefly.

20. A compensating filter is used to provide a uniform film density when the part to be x-rayed varies in thickness.

21. Patient immobilization is mandatory to produce sharp images. Immobilizers fall into three classes: general, mechanical, and specific.

22. General immobilizers include devices such as sandbags, masking tape, balsa wood, sheets, pads and blocks of Polyfoam.

23. Mechanical devices include head clamps, shoulder pads, handgrips, compression bands and foot supports.

24. Specialized immobilizers are primarily used in pediatric imaging. These include a number of prototypes.

25. A photographic atlas illustrates a few applications of immobilizing devices.

Section B
FLUOROSCOPIC AND X-RAY
TELEVISION EQUIPMENT

CHAPTER 11

PRINCIPLES OF FLUOROSCOPY

THE process of radiography involves observation and recording of *static* (stationary) images on x-ray film. The previous chapters so far have focussed mainly on a description of the production of static images.

Fluoroscopy, on the other hand, is a process by which x-rays are used to study both structure and function, through observation of *dynamic* (moving) images on a *fluorescent screen*.

Fluoroscopy dates back to 1896 when Thomas Edison developed the *fluoroscope*. The theory and mechanics of fluoroscopy were described further in 1935 by Percy Brown and again in 1942 by Edward Chamberlain. At that time, fluoroscopy was referred to as *Roentgenoscopy*.

Two classes of fluoroscopy have been identified in radiology departments, namely: conventional fluoroscopy and intensified fluoroscopy.

CONVENTIONAL FLUOROSCOPY

Conventional fluoroscopy will not be described here in any detail, since the development and introduction of intensified fluoroscopy has rendered the technique virtually obsolete. However, a few essentials are important in order for

251

the student to understand and appreciate the concepts and value of intensified fluoroscopy.

Conventional fluoroscopy is a technique which permits a direct observation of images on a fluorescent screen. A typical arrangement of the imaging components is shown in Figure 11:1. One component that stands out is the fluorescent screen. The screen is also referred to as a *fluoroscopic* screen, and this term will be used throughout the remainder of this chapter.

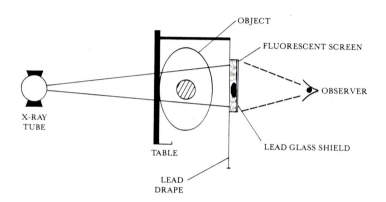

Figure 11:1. The imaging components in conventional fluoroscopy.

Screen Characteristics

Conventional fluoroscopic screens are made of *phosphors* which have the property of converting x-rays to light. In the past, screens were made of silver-activated *zinc cadmium sulfide* (ZnS:CdS:Ag), since it is extremely responsive to x-rays. The reason for the choice of this specific phosphor relates to its light emission. When struck by x-rays cadmium sulfide fluoresces orange, whereas zinc sulfide fluoresces blue. The combination of blue and orange fluorescence produces a yellow-green light emission. This is desirable in conventional fluoroscopy, since the ability to recognize detail is greatest with yellow-green light.

The screen is made of a cardboard base that is coated with *titanium dioxide* to prevent light absorption by the cardboard. The phosphor layer is spread over the titanium dioxide and is coated with a thin layer of *cellulose acetate* to protect the phosphor. Finally, a sheet of lead glass is placed over the cellulose acetate to protect the observer from radiation.

Image Quality

Conventional fluoroscopic screens are highly inefficient, in that their *quantum yield* (ratio of the number of light photons emitted by the screen to the number of x-ray photons striking the screen) is only about 10-15 percent and they exhibit *image lag* or *afterglow* (image persistance after x-rays have been turned off).

Image quality is poor with respect to brightness, contrast and resolution compared to radiographic images and intensified fluoroscopic images.

The *brightness* or *luminance* is extremely low because of the low mA values (low exposure rates) normally used in fluoroscopy, compared to that used in radiography. The brightness can be improved by increasing the thickness of the screen and increasing the mA values, but these lead to problems such as a loss in light transmission, production of scattered rays (for thick screens) and increase in radiation dose for higher mA values. For a significant increase in brightness, the mA value would have to approach 1400-1600 mA, which is not practical for fluoroscopy.

Contrast refers to the difference in brightness (optical density) between adjacent regions in the image. For conventional fluoroscopy, the contrast is generally poor because of the higher kVp values used. In radiography, contrast is improved through the use of lower kVp, but in fluoroscopy this is not the case. If the working kVp is decreased, the intensity of x-rays will decrease and hence image brightness will decrease.

Scattered rays produced by the patient and the screen together produce *fog* which also destroys image contrast.

Resolution refers to the sharpness with which structures can be imaged. In conventional fluoroscopy, sharpness is limited by geometric (focal spot size, object-screen distance and source-image distance) and intrinsic (size of phosphors and thickness of the phosphor layer) factors. The degree of sharpness that can be perceived by the observer is also limited by the low brightness levels.

Viewing Conditions

In the past, conventional fluoroscopy was done in the dark (for maximum viewing conditions) and it was necessary for the radiologist to adapt his eyes to the dark (*dark adaptation*) by wearing red goggles. The process of dark adaptation means that the eye must change from photopic to scotopic vision.

Photopic vision refers to vision caused by chemical changes in the *cones* of the retina of the eye as a result of light stimulation. With photopic vision, the observer can perceive fine detail and discriminate small differences in brightness (intensity discrimination). In conventional fluoroscopy, the cones do not receive enough light for proper image perception, since the brightness level of the screen is low (dim), and image perception therefore becomes a function of the *rods* (another group of light receptors on the retina).

Scotopic vision, on the other hand, refers to vision resulting from light stimulation of the rods. The rods are sensitive to light and do not play a significant role in perception of fine detail.

Sufficient dark adaptation is therefore necessary in conventional fluoroscopy, since sensitivity of the eye is related to dark adaptation time. For example, sensitivity is increased tenfold after 10 minutes of dark adaptation, a hundredfold after 18 minutes and a thousandfold after 50 minutes. In order to maintain the lowest possible exposure rate to the patient during conventional fluoroscopy, the dark adaptation time should be at least 10 minutes.

In summary, the conventional fluoroscopic image lacks detail, brightness and contrast. The ability to perceive detail is restricted by geometric principles, rod vision and the low levels of illumination characteristic of the screen.

If the brightness levels of the image can be increased in some practical way without increasing the dose to the patient, then the observer can use cone vision to see fine details in the image.

INTENSIFIED FLUOROSCOPY

The theory which states that *visual acuity* (ability to perceive fine detail) increases with increasing illunimation has lead to the development and introduction of intensified fluoroscopy.

In simple terms, intensified fluoroscopy is the brightening of the conventional fluoroscopic image through the use of a special electronic device called an *image intensifier tube.* Today, the term *image intensification* is used to refer to intensified fluoroscopy, and, therefore, this term will be used throughout the remainder of this text.

In x-ray image intensification, the image is acquired with less radiation dose and is displayed on a television monitor or other viewing system. Since the image is brighter than the conventional fluoroscopic image, the observer uses cone vision rather than rod vision for image perception. Image intensification has gained popularity throughout the radiologic community, and, therefore, the principles will be discussed in some detail in the next chapter.

EQUIPMENT FOR FLUOROSCOPY

Instrumentation for fluoroscopy includes the following common elements:

(a) A fluoroscopic table.
(b) An x-ray tube for fluoroscopy.
(c) Control for fluoroscopy.
(d) Image intensifier tube.
(e) Image monitoring and recording systems.

The features of the fluoroscopic (RF) table are described in Chapter 3. In review, the table is of the tilting type with moving or floating tabletop.

It consists of a spotfilm device (serial changer) which allows the radiologist to record fluoroscopic images. Present day RF tables make use of an image intensifier tube (which replaces the conventional fluoroscopic screen) coupled to the spotfilm device. Manual and automatic collimation, the use of grid and/ or non-grid techniques and cassette programming are also characteristic features.

The x-ray tube for fluoroscopy has no special features compared to the tubes described in Chapter 5, except for the grid-controlled x-ray tube used in cine-fluorography. The tube is usually the undercouch tube which uses low tube currents (mA) for fluoroscopy, since the x-ray tube is energized for longer periods compared to radiography. However, during radiographic recording of the fluoroscopic image, the tube current must be switched to higher mA values.

Controls for fluoroscopy are several and vary from machine to machine. When a technologist prepares a room for a fluoroscopic examination, she selects both radiographic and fluoroscopic factors suitable for the examination. For fluoroscopy, these factors include kVp, mA, and exposure time.

The fluoroscopic exposure factors are normally high kVp (120 or more depending on the examination) and low mA (0.5 mA to 5 mA). The *automatic exposure timer* is also set up for use during the procedure. The *cumulative fluoroscopic timer* (not an exposure timer) is activated by the fluoroscopic exposure switch and records the duration of time that the patient is irradiated. The timer ranges from 0 to 5 minutes. When the total time of irradiation has reached 5 minutes, the timer breaks the fluoroscopic circuit and terminates fluoroscopy. At the same time, it provides audible and visual (light) signals that serve to remind the radiologist that the patient has been irradiated for 5 minutes. Fluoroscopy is switched back on when the timer is reset.

The brightness of the fluoroscopic image is increased by increasing kVp and/or mA values (fluoroscopy), depending on the subject contrast desired. In the past, manual control was used, but today most units utilize an *automatic brightness control* system.

The image intensifier tube is a special electronic vacuum tube which provides improved image quality with low radiation doses compared to conventional fluoroscopy. The tube also makes it possible for manipulation of images, such as magnification.

The intensified image is usually displayed on a *television monitor* for viewing, although other monitoring systems (*mirror optical systems*) are used. A *television camera tube* and control circuitry are also essential components for monitoring the image. Recording can be done in several ways, such as the use of *videotape* or *disk recorders* and *film*. For film documentation, the image can be recorded on *cine* (movie) and/or *spotfilms*. These require the use of *cine cameras* and *spotfilm cameras*.

In the remainder of this section of the text, the elements described and mentioned above will be discussed further.

RADIATION PROTECTION IN FLUOROSCOPY

Radiation protection in fluoroscopy is a subject by itself and the concepts are usually covered in courses on radiation protection. In this section, only relevant highlights will be pointed out and, therefore, reference will not be made to protection standards and recommendations established by radiation protection agencies.

Protecting the patient from primary radiation involves several measures such as the use of low tube currents, optimum collimation, appropriate target-skin distance (not less than 30 cm and more than 45 cm), keeping the cumulative fluoroscopic time as short as possible, filtration and gonadal shielding.

Personnel protection refers to other measures intended to protect the technologist, radiologist and other support staff (nurses) from scattered radiation. In fluoroscopy the greatest amount of scattered rays arise from the patient, although there are other sources of scattered rays (tube housing, collimator, tabletop, spotfilm device) in the x-ray room.

Protection from scattered rays is important (due to biological effects of radiation) because:

(a) The energy and intensity of the scattered rays vary with the angle of scatter. The greater the angle, the less the energy of the scattered rays, while those rays which are scattered less than 90° to the primary beam have a greater intensity than those scattered in any other direction.

(b) The concepts discussed in (a) above allow the technologist to optimize protection of other staff (including herself) by allowing them to observe the procedure from a position in the room where there is the least amount of scattered rays (if one has to be out of the control booth to observe).

The energy of the scattered rays is just slightly less than that of the primary beam and, therefore, every precaution must be taken to protect oneself from scattered rays not only during fluoroscopy but also during radiography.

In conventional fluoroscopy there is a lead glass shielding on the fluoroscopic screen to protect the observer from primary radiation. In image intensification, shielding requirements are necessary to protect personnel from both primary and scattered rays.

Other means of protection are provided by the lead curtain (drape) that hangs from the spotfilm device (see RF table in Chapter 3) and protective clothing. The lead apron on the spotfilm device must be of a certain size (45 cm × 45 cm) and have a certain amount of lead. Personnel clothing includes lead aprons and gloves which must comply with specific lead shielding requirements established by radiation protection agencies. In general, aprons and gloves have a lead equivalent of at least 0.25 mm.

In remote-controlled fluoroscopy (Chapter 3), scattered radiation levels are high and therefore all personnel must stand behind a protective control booth.

As stated earlier, these various measures have specific radiation protection requirements. Recommendations and standards must be observed in order to achieve maximum radiation protection of patient and operator.

SUMMARY

1. Fluoroscopy is a process which uses x-rays to study the dynamics of structures.

2. Conventional fluoroscopy involves the direct observation of images on a fluorescent screen.

3. The conventional fluorescent screen is made of a special phosphor and other materials. The phosphor is zinc cadmium sulfide which fluoresces yellow-green when struck by x-rays.

4. Image quality in conventional fluoroscopy is poor with respect to contrast, detail and brightness. Several limiting factors include geometric and intrinsic factors as well as those related to viewing conditions.

5. For conventional fluoroscopy, the observer uses rod vision due to the low levels of screen illumination. This restricts perception of fine detail.

6. In intensified fluoroscopy the brightness levels (conventional fluoroscopy) are increased so that the observer uses cone vision for image perception. This incrases visualization of fine detail.

7. The term image intensification is synonymous with intensified fluoroscopy.

8. Equipment for fluoroscopy includes several items, such as a fluoroscopic table, an x-ray tube and control for fluoroscopy, exposure control for fluoroscopy, an image intensifier tube and image recording and monitoring systesm.

9. The image intensifier tube is a special electronic vacuum tube capable of improving the contrast, detail and brightness of the conventional fluoroscopic image.

10. Radiation protection in fluoroscopy is of vital importance and includes a discussion of patient and operator protection measures. A number of measures are identified.

CHAPTER 12

X-RAY IMAGE INTENSIFICATION

IN the last chapter, the principles of conventional fluoroscopy were described. The limitations imposed by this imaging scheme are several and include the need for a completely darkened room, the long dark adaptation time of the observer and, more importantly, the poor visibility of detail and contrast as a result of low levels of brightness of the fluorescent screen.

PRINCIPLES

The fundamental goal of x-ray image intensification is to increase the brightness level of the conventional fluoroscopic image. Increasing brightness will result in a shift from scotopic vision to photopic vision and, hence, will increase visual acuity.

Experiments have shown that visual acuity varies with illumination in an interesting way. It is known from everyday experience that fine print which is difficult to see in dim light may easily be read under higher illumination. This relationship has been worked out and indicates that as the light intensity increases, visual acuity also increase. The principles of image intensification are based on this relationship. If the light intensity from the conventional fluorescent screen is increased, the observer's visual acuity increases and perception of image detail is better. Contrast sensitivity and the speed of perception of the eye are also improved.

Image intensification, therefore, provides the following advantages:

(a) Better viewing conditions.
(b) No dark adaptation.
(c) Viewing under daylight conditions (there is no need for a darkened x-ray room).
(d) More work accomplished with greater speed.
(e) Low radiation doses, since lower tube currents are used — that is, no increase in exposure factors is necessary to obtain an increase in brightness.
(f) X-ray closed-circuit television is possible.
(g) Cinefluorography is possible.
(h) Automatic dose-rate regulation.
(i) Single radiographs with low radiation doses can be obtained.
(j) Serial radiography with low radiation doses is possible.

The concept of x-ray image intensification is shown in Figure 12:1. It is a complex process and is dependent upon modern electronic technology. Image intensification must not be confused with intensifying screen (cassette) action, a rather simple process in comparison.

X-ray image intensification can be defined as the brightening of the fluoroscopic image. Such brightening is achieved by an *x-ray image intensifier tube* (Figure 12:2). According to the National Bureau of Standards Handbook 89, an x-ray image intensifier is "a device which converts instantaneously an x-ray pattern into a corresponding light of higher energy density."

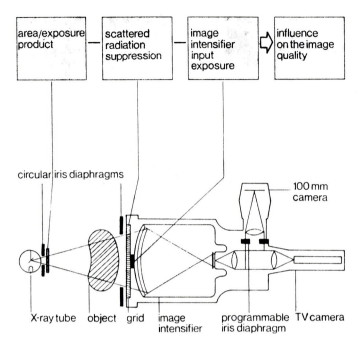

Figure 12:1. The concept of x-ray image intensification. The factors affecting image quality are also shown above the diagram. (From Kollath, Birken and Jötten: Image quality in image intensifier fluorography in relation to patient dose and exposure at the imaging device. *Medica mundi,* Vol. 23, No. 3, 1978.)

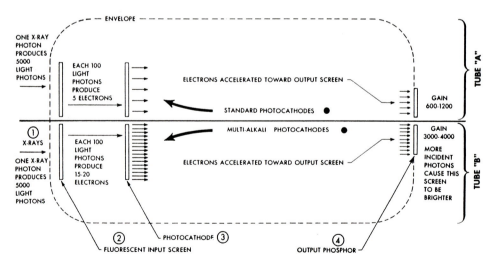

Figure 12:2. The gain in image brightness made possible by an image intensifier tube. Also shown here is a comparison between standard cesium antimony photocathodes (Tube a) and mult-alkali photocathodes (Tube b). (courtesy of Machlett Laboratories, Inc.)

Within the domain of radiology there appears to be four types of x-ray image intensification schemes:

   (a) The x-ray image intensifier tube.
   (b) Solid-state x-ray image intensifiers.
   (c) Reflecting optics image intensifiers.
   (d) Reflecting optics image intensifiers with light amplifier tubes.

The x-ray image intensifier tube has found widespread use in radiology departments throughout the world, and, therefore, it will be described in some detail in this chapter.

The *solid-state x-ray image intensifier* was developed by Kazan who published his report in 1958. His device consisted of a 1-mm thick *photoconductive* (electrical conductivity of a substance when exposed to light or other radiation) layer (cadmium sulfide), an insulator which is opaque to light and an *electroluminescent* (luminescence resulting from a high-frequency discharge from the application of an alternating current to a phosphor such as zinc sulfoselenide) material.

When x-rays strike the photoconductive layer, high-energy electrons are emitted to give rise to a vast number of secondary electrons through a series of collisions. This process increases the electrical conductivity of the photoconductor in the areas which have been struck by x-rays. The image produced is one which varies in conductivity and this causes a variation of the voltage applied to the electroluminescent phosphor.

The electroluminescent phosphor emits a yellow-green light image which corresponds to the x-ray image pattern on the photoconductor. The yellow-green light improves perception of the image. When an alternating voltage is applied between the photocathode and the electroluminescent layer, the light intensity increases significantly.

The solid-state x-ray image intensifier exhibits severe image lag (persistence of the image when the radiation is turned off), and, therefore, it has not been developed for use in radiologic imaging.

The two other methods of image intensification using the *reflecting optics intensifier* and the reflecting optics image intensifier with *light amplifier tube* are almost obsolete in modern imaging trends. Essentially, these two systems consist of a fluorescent screen and mirror optical system to assist in the intensification process. These systems served a useful purpose in the early days of radiology, however, they have been replaced with the x-ray image intensifier tube.

The X-ray Image Intensifier Tube

The most prevalent system of image intensification utilizes the image intensifier tube which provides intensification through a series of conversion events. These include conversion of an x-ray image into a light image, conversion of the light image into an electron image, and finally conversion of the electron image back to a light image of increased brightness than the original light image.

A modern x-ray image intensifier tube is illustrated in Figure 12:3. It is a highly evacuated glass envelope which consists of the following: an input screen, an output screen, a photocathode and an electron lens system. All these components are housed in metal casing which encloses the glass envelope.

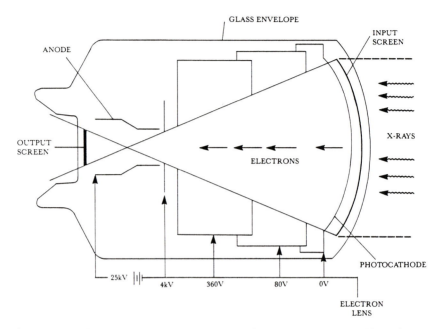

Figure 12:3. The arrangement of components of an x-ray image intensifier tube.

The Input Screen

The screen is made up of a layer of phosphor which is deposited on a thin substrate material such as glass or aluminum. These screens have been referred to as *deposited crystal screens*. Since the crystals are loosely packed, dispersion and reflection of light occur at the surface of the crystals and this lateral spread of light leads to a loss in image resolution.

The phosphor material used in first and second generation input screens is a thick layer of *silver activated zinc cadmium sulfide* (ZnCdS:Ag).

In the mid 1970s, third-generation image intensifiers appeared on the scene. These tubes are designed to eliminate and reduce the problems imposed by first- and second-generation tubes.

Two striking features which make these tubes superior in performance are the phosphor material and the technique used to increase the packing density of the crystals.

The phosphor is sodium-activated *cesium iodide* (CsI:Na) and it has a higher atomic number than zinc cadmium sulfide. The crystals are laid down on the input screen by a *vacuum vapour depositing process*. This process ensures that the crystals are arranged in the direction in which the x-rays travel, therefore causing the light produced to travel along the direction of the crystals. By doing this, lateral dispersion of light is reduced. Figure 12:4a-b shows a comparison of the packing density and crystal structure of both cesium iodide (vacuum vapour process) and zinc cadmium sulfide input screens. In Figure 12:5a-b the lateral dispersion of light is also compared.

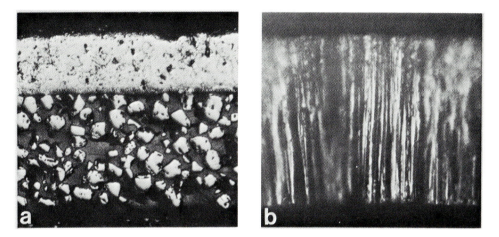

Figure 12:4. A comparison of the packing density and crystal structure of (a) zinc cadmium sulfide and (b) cesium iodide screens of image intensifier tubes. (From Birken and Bejczy: A new generation of x-ray image intensifiers — characteristics and results. *Medica mundi*, Vol. 18, No. 3, 1973.)

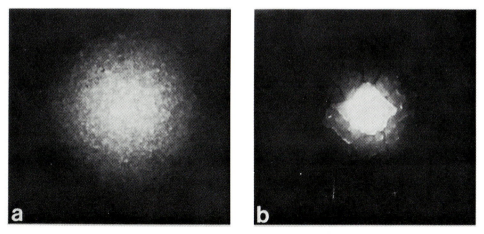

Figure 12:5. The lateral spread of light from (a) zinc cadmium sulfide screen and (b) cesium iodide screen. It is clearly apparent that the lateral spread of light is reduced in b. (From Birken and Bejczy: A new generation of x-ray image intensifiers — characteristics and results. *Medica mundi*, Vol. 18, No. 3, 1973.)

The diameter of input screens usually range from 13 to 30 cm (5 to 12 inches), with 15 cm (6 inches) and 23 cm (9 inches) being the most common ones found in radiology departments. Recently, a 36-cm (14-inch) input screen image intensifier tube has become available to meet the needs of more sophisticated examinations.

Today, the cesium iodide image intensifier tube is widely used and zinc cadmium sulfide tubes are becoming obsolete. The advantages associated with cesium iodide tubes are numerous and include the following:

(a) higher spatial and contrast resolution.
(b) higher conversion factor (to be discussed subsequently).
(c) greater x-ray absorption.
(d) improved quanta detection efficiency resulting in reduced quantum noise.
(e) uniform distribution of resolution over the entire image field.
(f) improved temporal response.

The Photocathode

The photocathode is coated on the concave side of the substrate material on which the input phosphor is deposited. It is a *photoemissive* material, the purpose of which is to convert the light image from the input screen into a corresponding electron image. The photocathode emits electrons in proportion to the intensity of light it receives.

The photocathode is the most inefficient aspect in the chain of conversion events occurring in the entire tube. For example, standard *cesium-antimony* photocathodes will produce 5 electrons for every 100 light photons it receives. The efficiency of electron emission can be increased by using a combination of elements of the alkali metal group. Such photocathodes are known as *multi-alkali photocathodes,* because they consist of a combination of antimony, potassium, sodium and cesium (Sb, K, Na, Ce) and emit three to five times more electrons than conventional photocathodes. This is clearly demonstrated in Figure 12:2. The increase in the number of emitted electrons also produces an increase in brightness at the output screen.

In order to maintain image detail, the substrate material between the input screen and the photocathode is very thin. This material serves to protect the input screen from the alkali metal vapours which are used to activate the photocathode.

The Electron Lens

The *electron lens* consists of a series of concentric cylindrical electrodes (positively charged) which are positioned inside the glass envelope. By applying a high voltage to each of these electrodes (Figure 12:3), the electrons are accelerated across the tube to the output screen at great speeds (increase in energy). Focussing the electrons to the output screen is accomplished by the electric field produced by the electrodes. The image formed at the output screen is now inverted.

The Output Screen

The output screen is much smaller in size than the input screen and, in general, the diameter is about one-tenth the diameter of the input screen. The phosphor (zinc cadmium sulfide) material is deposited on the inside of an optical face plate.

When the high-speed electrons strike the output screen, a light image is formed which is much brighter than the image at the input screen.

In order to maintain good image quality (high definition), the smaller crystals and a thin layer of phosphor coating are used in the construction of the output screen.

Finally, the output screen is plated with a very thin layer of aluminum which faces the photocathode. The purpose of this aluminum plating is to stop the light produced by the output screen from reflecting back into the tube.

The Getters

Image intensifiers contain getters. One is the generally used ion-pump type used to ensure a good vacuum in the tube. The other is the flash getter which acts as a constant absorber of any gases in the tube. The high degree of vacuum brought about by these getters helps to ensure stable and long-lived performance.

The Image Intensifier Tube Housing

The purpose of the tube housing is primarily twofold:

(a) It provides adequate radiation protection by reducing the intensity of x-ray photons which:

(1) pass through the input screen.
(2) are scattered by the input screen.
(3) are produced by electrons striking the output screen.

(b) It serves as a shield against magnetic fields, since these fields can affect the electron beam moving through the tube. The fields may cause decreased resolution, misalignment of the image and even distortion. Magnetic fields are produced, for example, by the electromagnetic locks which hold the tube in a fixed position.

Figure 12:6 shows an image intensifier tube housing. The output screen is seen at the top of the tube.

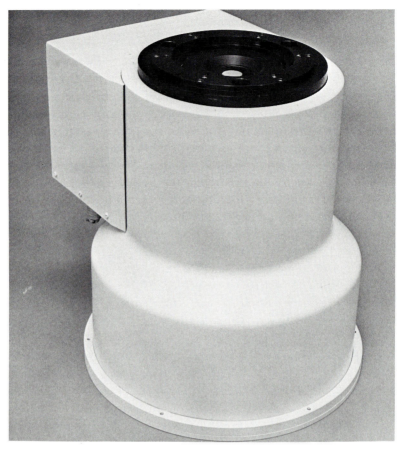

Figure 12:6. The image intensifier tube housing. The output phosphor is at the top of the picture. This image intensifier tube (VXI-600) has been designed with 50% minimum quantum detection efficiency to provide a low quantum noise image to the television camera tube. (courtesy of Varian, Santa Clara, California.)

Operating Principles — A Summary

The basic components of an image intensifier tube have now been described and their fundamental purpose discussed. In review, when x-rays pass through the patient, they fall upon the input screen of the image intensifier tube to produce a light image (one x-ray photon produces about 5000 light photons). The light emitted from the input screen strikes the photocathode to produce electrons. These electrons are then accelerated and focussed toward the output screen by means of an electron lens system. When the electron beam strikes the output screen, light is emitted. The image at the output screen is much brighter than that at the input screen. Since the electrons "cross-over" at the opening in the anode, the image formed at the output screen is inverted.

BRIGHTNESS GAIN AND CONVERSION FACTOR

Brightness gain is defined as the increase in brightness at the output screen of the image intensifier tube. It can be calculated if the brightness level of a conventional fluoroscopic screen (Patterson B-2 screen) is known and only if the same exposure factors are applied to both the conventional fluoroscopic screen and the intensifier tube. Hence,

$$\text{Brightness gain} = \frac{\text{brightness at output screen of image intensifier tube}}{\text{brightness of a Patterson B-2 screen}}$$

Typical brightness gain values range from 1000 to 6000, and as the tube becomes older the value of the brightness gain decreases.

There are two factors which influence brightness gain in image intensifier tubes:

(a) acceleration of the electrons due to the potential difference (voltage) across the tube, and

(b) reduction in size of the output screen. This is sometimes referred to as minification.

The increase in brightness as a result of minification is termed *minification gain,* and this is defined as the ratio of the square of the diameter of the input screen to the square of the diameter of the output screen. On the other hand, the increase in brightness due to acceleration of the electrons is referred to as *flux gain,* which is defined as the ratio of the number of light photons at the output screen to the number of x-ray photons at the input screen.

The following expression gives another relationship for brightness gain and that is:

$$\text{Brightness gain} = \text{minification gain} \times \text{flux gain}$$

There are several drawbacks which one may encounter in trying to determine the brightness gain of an intensifier tube, such as the loss in brightness as the tube becomes older, and therefore there is no way of knowing whether the phosphor or the tube itself has deteriorated. The other drawback is the unavailability of a Patterson B-2 screen in most radiology departments.

The term brightness gain has been superseded by the term *conversion factor,* a more precise and scientific term which enables measurements to be made without much difficulty. The conversion factor is defined as the ratio of the luminance (brightness) of the output screen to the exposure rate at the input screen. The luminance is expressed in candela per square meter (the candela is a unit of luminance such that 1 candela = 0.3 millilamberts) and the exposure rate is expressed in milliroentgens per second.

ELECTRON-OPTICAL MAGNIFICATION

At some point in time during a fluoroscopic examination, particularly when selective functional studies and differentiated diagnosis are important, magnification of the image is desireable.

Magnification is achieved through a technique generally referred to as *electron-optical magnification*. The process is accomplished electronically by changing the voltage on the electron lens system. Figure 12:7 demonstrates this technique. It shows that when electrode two is maintained at a lower voltage than electrode one, a wider divergence of the electron beam results.

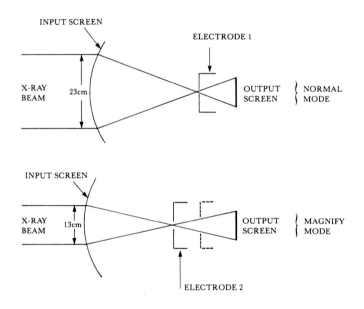

Figure 12:7. Electron optical magnification. When electrode 2 is at a lower voltage than electrode 1, a wider divergence of the beam results. In the magnify mode, the x-ray beam is also collimated to a smaller field size.

Magnification is only possible in a *dual-field* image intensifier tube. A dual-field tube is usually stated as 23 cm/13 cm (9-inch/5-inch), where 23 cm is the diameter of the input screen and is used for panoramic or normal viewing (normal mode). The 13 cm represents the diameter of the central portion of the input screen that will be displayed on the output screen. This simply means that the part of the image which falls in the central 13 cm of the input screen will be magnified (magnify mode). In Figure 12:8, the dual-field principle is illustrated.

When the switch for magnification is activated, the x-ray beam is automatically collimated to fall upon the 13-cm field of the input screen. Other changes which occur simultaneously and automatically include adjustment of the

Large-field technique

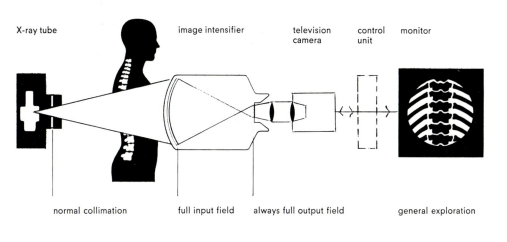

Magnified technique

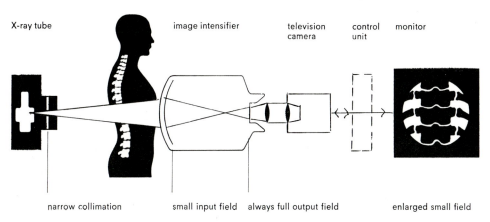

Figure 12:8. The dual-field principle in x-ray image intensification. (courtesy of the Siemens Corporation.)

voltage on the electron lens system and dose-rate control, where the intensity of the primary x-ray beam is increased such that the original brightness level is maintained. It is important to note that when magnification technique is used, the kilovoltage on the control console should be increased by about 15.

With dual-field image intensifiers, it is possible to calculate the *linear amplifi-*

cation factor or the linear enlargement. This is given by the following relationship,

$$\text{Linear enlargement} = \frac{\text{diameter of the input screen}}{\begin{array}{c}\text{diameter of central portion}\\\text{of the input screen that will}\\\text{be magnified}\end{array}}$$

Hence, for a 23 cm/13 cm intensifier tube, the linear enlargement is:

$$\text{linear enlargement} = 23/13$$
$$= 1.8$$

AUTOMATIC DOSE-RATE CONTROL

Image intensification units utilize a concept called *automatic dose-rate control* (ADC) or automatic brightness control as it is sometimes referred to. In order to understand the concept, consider Figure 12:9. As the image intensifier moves from a thick part (upper leg) to a thin part (lower leg), the image brightness at the output screen will change if the exposure factors are not adjusted appropriately. With ADC, image brightness is kept constant by automatic regulation of fluoroscopic voltage and current at the same time. The range of values that can be adjusted varies from about 30 kVp and 0.1 mA to 106 kVp and 6.5 mA for some units. The other important feature of ADC is the reduction in radiation exposure, since the fluoroscopic data (dose rate) are adjusted to the thickness of the object.

There are several methods available to adjust fluoroscopic exposure factors.

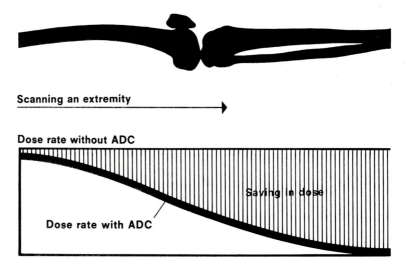

Figure 12:9. Automatic dose rate control. See text for further explanation. (courtesy of the Siemens Corporation.)

The most common method makes use of a sensor to detect the light from the output screen of the image intensifier tube and to send it (light) to a photomultiplier tube which forms part of a control circuit. The signal from the control circuit is then used to alter the x-ray tube voltage or current so that constant image brightness at the output screen is obtained.

Another method utilizes an ionization chamber positioned in front of the input screen. The signal from the chamber is used in the same fashion as the first method just described.

In some units, if the kVp is changed then the mA will not change. If the mA is changed, then the kVp remains fixed. On the other hand, some units alter both kVp and mA. In general, the exposure time is altered when the control circuit changes the kVp, mA or both factors.

IMAGE QUALITY CONSIDERATIONS

Image quality aspects of x-ray image intensifiers have been under study for a number of years. Several factors which influence image quality have been reported in these studies and they include:

(a) Resolution
(b) Contrast
(c) Quantum noise
(d) Distortion

Resolution

Resolution is usually stated in terms of the image intensifier to record line pairs. The concept of line pairs is shown in Figure 12:10. A 23-cm (9-inch) intensifier, for example, has a resolution of about 40-50 line pairs per inch, whereas a 15-cm (6-inch) tube has a resolution of about 45-50 line pairs per inch. Note that the smaller tube has greater resolution. This is because optimizing the electron focussing system is easier to achieve in tubes of smaller diameters. A 15-cm (6-inch) CsI image intensifier can record 4 line pairs/mm compared to a ZnCdS tube which is capable of recording about 2 line pairs/ mm.

Another factor which affects resolution is the composition (thickness and structure) of the input screen. If the screen is very thin with fine crystals, resolution is greater (but there is an associated loss in brightness gain) compared to a thick screen with large crystals (poor resolution but increase in brightness gain). The compact arrangement of cesium iodide crystals increases its packing density by 100 percent and this permits 65 percent x-ray absorption at the input screen, compared to 30 percent x-ray absorption for first-generation image intensifiers with a packing density of 50 percent.

Finally, the image intensifier resolution is influenced by the small focus of

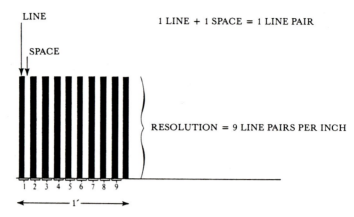

Figure 12:10. The concept of line pairs. One line pair consists of one line and an adjacent space which is equal to the width of the line.

the x-ray tube. From geometric principles, the small focus increases resolution by reducing geometric unsharpness.

Resolution can be measured by a more advanced method using the modulation transfer function (MTF). Students who are interested in the MTF of image intensifiers may refer to the paper by Beekmans (1982).

Contrast

Contrast in an image intensifier tube is defined as "the brightness ratio of the periphery to the center of the output screen" (Christensen, Curry and Dowdey, 1978).

Image intensification does not increase contrast of the fluoroscopic image, but, in fact, there is a loss in contrast. The decrease in contrast is due to the construction of the tube itself along with other factors. One such factor is related to the fact that some primary input x-ray photons pass through the input screen and collide with the output screen. These photons do not play a role in formation of the image but assist in brightening the output screen thus reducing the contrast.

When viewing the intensified image with a television-monitoring system, a fraction of this contrast loss can be regained by proper adjustment of the contrast control on the television monitor.

Quantum Noise

One of the factors which affects resolution of an image is the random quantum fluctuations present in the x-ray beam. These fluctuations can be seen as "the crawling of ants" and this is often referred to as "noise"; hence, the term *quantum noise*. Quantum noise, or scintillation as it is sometimes called, occurs when the number of x-ray quanta (per unit time) falling on the input screen of the image intensifier tube is too low. In order to get rid of quantum noise, the x-ray tube current must be increased, since more photons are needed. Cesium iodide image intensifier tubes exhibit less quantum noise than zinc cadmium sulfide tubes.

Distortion

The input screen of x-ray image intensifiers is a curved surface, and, therefore, the image at the output screen may appear to be curved at the periphery of the field. This type of distortion is referred to as *pincushion distortion* (Figure 12:11). With the cesium iodide image intensifiers there is uniform distribution of resolution over the entire image field.

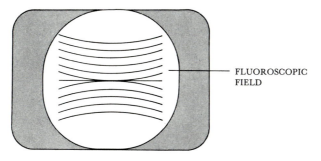

FLUOROSCOPIC FIELD

Figure 12:11. Pincushion distortion of the image due to the curvature of the input screen of the image intensifier tube.

Vignetting

Vignetting occurs to some degree in image intensifier tubes. It is defined as a loss of brightness at the periphery of the image.

LIMITATIONS OF THE IMAGE INTENSIFIER TUBE

In the previous section, several characteristics of image quality were described. It is clear that image intensifiers exhibit performance limitations. These limitations are related to (Wang, Robbins and Bates, 1977):

(a) *Unsharpness.* Image unsharpness is associated with the electron optics and the output screen. The small size of the output screen also contributes to the overall unsharpness of the image.

(b) *Image distortion* due to the curved input screen and electron optics.

(c) *Size and shape of the tube.* These tubes tend to be large and bulky.

(d) *Other problems.* In this regard, Wang, Robbins and Bates (1977) point out that current image intensifiers are "sensitive to voltage drifts, external stray magnetic fields and small dimensional drifts." They would also exhibit space-charge defocussing if the input x-ray pulse exceeds certain dose-rate levels. All these problems are caused by the combination of long electron trajectories, weak cathode field strength, and the small output image size.

OTHER APPROACHES TO X-RAY IMAGE INTENSIFICATION

The limitations imposed by conventional image intensifiers have sparked interest and development of other approaches to x-ray image intensification. Two proximity-type approaches will be described briefly.

Proximity-type Image Intensification

The Panel Electron Tube

The *panel electron tube* is a simple diode proximity-type tube where the input and output screens (essentially the same size) are positioned in close proximity of each other. A schematic of the tube is shown in Figure 12:12. It consists of an input screen, a photocathode, and an output screen which are all enclosed in a metal envelope.

The input screen is made up of an aluminum substrate which is coated with a thin layer of sodium-activated cesium iodide. The photocathode is cesium antimonide. The input screen and photocathode are supported by an aluminum framework and are maintained at a high negative voltage while all other components are placed at ground potential.

The output screen consists of a layer of phosphor deposited on a glass window and an anti-reflective layer deposited on a thin film of aluminum facing the photocathode.

The panel electron tube intensifier system is compact and lightweight, exhibits low image lag, and provides high-quality images with low-dose rates.

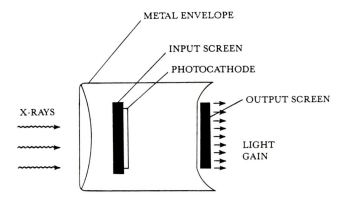

Figure 12:12. A proximity type x-ray image intensifier tube referred to as the Panel Electron Tube ("PET").

Microchannel Plates

A *microchannel plate* is hexagonal in shape and contains a set of hollow glass cylinders which are closely packed together. Each of the cylinders acts as an electron multiplier (Gould, Judy and Bjarngard, 1978).

Conventional image intensifiers use the input screen (phosphor) and photocathode layer to convert x-ray photons to light and electrons, respectively. A microchannel plate provides a direct conversion of x-ray photons to electrons. Figure 12:13 illustrates a microchannel plate x-ray converter which consists of three microchannel plates (A, B and C) stacked together. The first plate, A, converts x-ray photons to electrons, while plates B and C act as electron mulipliers.

The output screen consists of a layer of zinc cadmium sulfide crystals deposited on glass, while the output intensified image is of a large format.

The resolution capabilities of microchannel plates are higher that conventional image intensifiers. For example, Gould, Judy and Bjarngard (1978) have reported a resolution capability of 7 line pairs per millimeter for the mi-

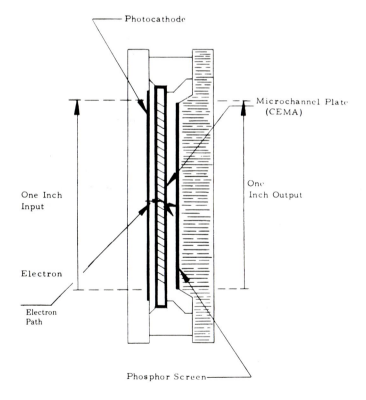

Figure 12:13. Construction of a microchannel plate x-ray image intensifier. (From Balter et al.: A microchannel plate x-ray converter and image intensifier tube. Radiology 110. March, 1974.)

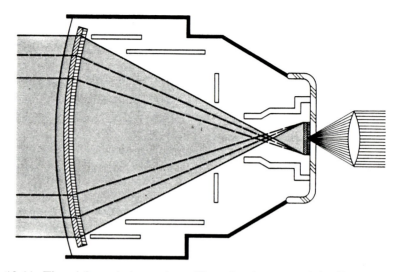

Figure 12:14. The triple-mode image intensifier tube. (courtesy of the Siemens Corporation.)

crochannel plate they studied. In the future, as research continues on microchannel plate x-ray image intensifiers, perhaps they may become commonplace in radiology departments.

LARGE-FORMAT IMAGE INTENSIFIERS

The more common sizes of image intensifiers available in clinical practice are the 15-cm (6-inch) and the 23-cm (9-inch). Recently, large-format image intensifier tubes have become available for diagnostic imaging studies. These tubes feature input screen diameters ranging from 25 cm to 57 cm that can be switched to smaller input fields and highly radiolucent input windows made of aluminum (instead of glass) with thicknesses ranging from 0.8 mm to 1.5 mm. The radiolucency usually ranges from about 92-95 percent. Figure 12:14 illustrates a 57-cm tube with a triple-mode input format (57 cm, 47 cm and 33 cm).

In the next section, features of the 36-cm (14-inch) image intensifier tube are highlighted.

The 36-cm (14-inch) Image Intensifier

The intensifer features an input screen which has a maximum diameter of 36 cm (14 inch) as its most dominant characteristic. This diameter can be switched to a 25-cm (10-inch) field and a 15-cm (6-inch) field, and, therefore, the tube has also been referred to as a *triple-mode* image intensifier.

The new intensifier tube is constructed of non-magnetic metal. Whereas conventional image intensifiers (25-cm and 15-cm) have glass input windows, the 36-cm image intensifier input window is made of a thin layer of *titanium*, thus decreasing the amount of x-rays absorbed (compared to a glass input window).

The performance characteristics of the 36-cm intensifier are good. For example, image resolution is reported to be 34 line pairs per centimeter, 40 line pairs per centimeter and 50 line pairs per centimeter for the 36-cm, 10-cm and 15-cm input fields, respectively. Image contrast is good and the brightness and resolution are uniform throughout the image field.

In switching from the 36-cm field to the 15-cm field the exposure factors must increase accordingly. In this regard also, the conversion factor (hence, the sensitivity) will decrease by a factor of 5 (Hancken, Dietrich and Birken, 1977).

The 36-cm format image intensifier has been applied in imaging the thorax and abdomen quite successfully. Recent studies indicate that the unit can be used also in angiographic work, because it allows for both fluoroscopy and fluorography at the same time. Once contrast medium is injected, the radiologist can follow the flow of contrast and take the appropriate films which are recorded on 100-mm spotfilm by means of a 100-mm fluorographic camera.

It is possible that in the near future, more large-format image intensifiers will become available for use in *digital subtraction angiography*, a new x-ray imaging technique based on digital image processing theory.

SUMMARY

1. The goal of image intensification is to increase the brightness level of the conventional fluoroscopic image, thus increasing human visual acuity by shifting the mechanism of vision from scotopic to photopic vision.

2. As light intensity increases, visual acuity increases. This relationship is the fundamental basis for image intensification.

3. Brightening the imge is made possible by at least four intensification schemes, but only the most common one — the image intensifier tube — is described in some detail.

4. The image intensifier tube is an electronic device which converts x-rays into light of higher intensity. The tube consists of at least four important components: the input screen, the photocathode, the output screen and an electronic lens system.

5. The input screen consists of a phosphor which converts x-rays into light. The light in turn strikes the photocathode (photo-emissive material) which produces electrons. These electrons are accelerated and focussed to strike the output screen (much smaller than the input

screen) which produces a brighter image compared to that at the input screen.

6. The intensifier tube is enclosed in a housing. The housing serves to shield against magnetic fields and provides adequate radiation protection by reducing thc intensity of x-ray photons.

7. The increase in brightness at the output screen is referred to as brightness gain. This term has been replaced by another, the conversion factor, a more precise and scientific term.

8. The conversion factor is the ratio of the luminance of the output screen to the exposure rate at the input screen.

9. The gain in brightness at the output screen is attributed to the acceleration of electrons across the tube (potential difference) and reduction of the output screen diameter (minification).

10. In image intensification, it is possible to magnify images. This is accomplished with a dual-field image intensifier tube, through a technique referred to as electron-optical magnification, in which the voltage values on specific electrodes are changed to cause a wider divergence of the electron beam.

11. Automatic brightness control or automatic dose-rate control (ADC) is a technique in which the brightness of the image is kept constant by regulating the fluoroscopic voltage and current simultaneously.

12. Image quality can be discussed in terms of resolution, contrast, quantum noise and distortion. Each of these is described briefly, especially the factors influencing resolution and contrast.

13. Several limitations of the image intensifier tube are pointed out and these relate to unsharpness, image distortion, the size and shape of the tube, and other problems.

14. Other approaches to image intensification involves the use of the panel electron tube and the microchannel plate. The panel electron tube is a simple diode with input and output screens positioned very close together with a photocathode in between them. The microchannel plate consists of a set of hollow glass cylinders closely packed together. Each of the cylinders acts as an electron multiplier.

15. More recently, large-format image intensifiers have become available for use in x-ray imaging. The main feature is a large input screen with a diameter of 36 cm. Other features include a titanium window (instead of glass) and good performance characteristics with respect to resolution and contrast.

CHAPTER 13

IMAGE MONITORING CONCEPTS

IMAGE TRANSMISSION
HIGH RESOLUTION X-RAY TELEVISION
SUMMARY

THE output image on an image intensifier tube cannot be viewed directly because of its increased brightness and small size. Various approaches are available to transfer the image from the intensifier to subsequent systems for display (television monitor), viewing and recording.

IMAGE TRANSFER MECHANISMS

The methods of image transfer are shown in Figure 13:1 and include lens, mirror, and fibre optics coupled to television monitoring.

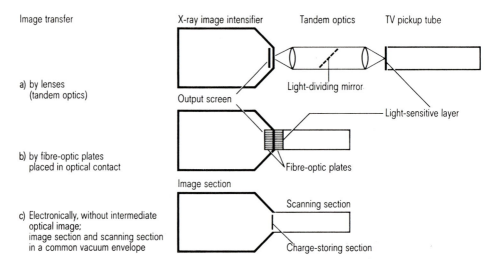

Figure 13:1. The methods of image transfer from the image intensifier tube to the television camera tube. (From Hofmann, F. W.: Image transfer from the x-ray image intensifier to subsequent systems. *Electromedica* 4., 1972.)

Lens and Mirror Optics

These optical systems are based on the use of mirrors and lenses for image transfer and display. Although mirror viewing systems are becoming obsolete in diagnostic imaging, a review of the basic physical concepts is worthwhile since they apply to other components (tandem optics).

A *mirror* is a polished surface capable of reflecting images. Mirrors can be plane, spherical (concave or convex) or parabolic.

A *lens* is a piece of glass with one or both sides curved to allow light rays to diverge or converge to a point. Lenses can be concave or convex as seen in Figure 13:2.

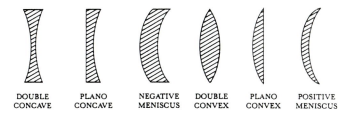

| DOUBLE CONCAVE | PLANO CONCAVE | NEGATIVE MENISCUS | DOUBLE CONVEX | PLANO CONVEX | POSITIVE MENISCUS |

Figure 13:2. Concave and convex lenses.

Lenses and mirrors bring about refraction and reflection of light. In *reflection,* light rays are returned from an illuminated surface which is not itself a luminous source. *Refraction,* on the other hand, is the bending or change in direction of propagation of light when it travels from one medium to another. These two properties are shown in Figure 13:3.

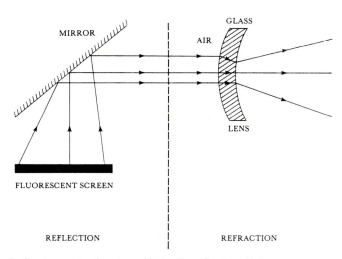

Figure 13:3. Reflection and refraction of light. In reflection, light rays are returned from an illuminated surface (mirror) which itself is not a luminous source. In refraction, light rays change direction (bend) when they travel from one medium (air) to another (glass).

If certain conditions are not met when mirrors and lenses are used independently, rays of light from the outer portions of these devices will not intersect at the same place as those coming from the central portion, as seen in Figure 13:4a and therefore the edges of the image will be blurred. This behavior which

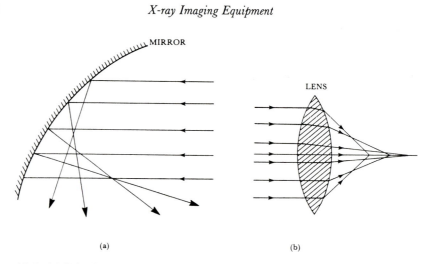

(a)   (b)

Figure 13:4. (a) Spherical aberration. Rays of light from the outer portions of the lenses and mirrors do not intersect at the same point as those arising from the central portion. This behavior arises from the spherical curvatures of lenses and mirrors. (b) The correction of spherical aberration.

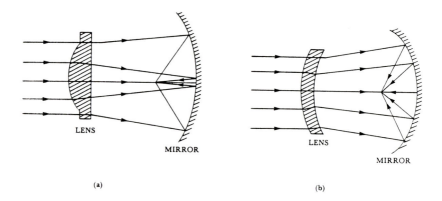

(a)   (b)

results from the spherical curvatures of the lens and mirror is referred to as *spherical aberration.* These aberrations can, however, be corrected by careful arrangement of and use of both lenses and mirrors (catadioptric systems) as shown in Figure 13:4b. One such system is the *tandem optical system* (Figure 13:1), which features a plane mirror to redirect the light, an objective lens, and a field lens. The objective lens is mounted in front of the output screen and collects all the light to form an image of the original object. The field lens focuses and directs the image to the television camera.

Fibre Optics

The limitations imposed by a lens and mirror optical system are several and include a loss of image quality due to a decrease in brightness during image transfer and vignetting. The image also has to be transferred through a long distance from the output screen to the input target of the television camera tube. This has the consequence of a bulky system. These limitations can be removed by a fibre optical system.

Fibre optics utilize light-conducting glass fibres. It was first used in image intensifier tube technology where the output window was a fibre optics glass plate. The principle of light and pattern transmission through a fibre optics plate is illustrated in Figure 13:5a. When the plate is used as the frontal window of the television camera tube, it is possible to couple the image intensifier and the television camera tube directly without using an optical lens system as illustrated in Figure 13:5b.

The advantages of fibre optics coupling for use in diagnostic x-ray imaging are:

(a) compact construction.
(b) no loss in image quality during image transfer.
(c) practically no vignetting.
(d) elimination of contrast loss (due to light scattering in the glass) by isolating the fibres from each other.

The disadvantage are several and include:

(a) Photographic recording must be done off the television monitor, since direct access to the image on the output screen is not possible. This method entails a loss of image quality.
(b) Control of the light intensity between the output screen and the television camera tube is not possible. (This is important for fluoroscopy.)
(c) Image rotation on the television screen is not possible. With lens and mirror optical systems, rotation of the image is possible by rotating the television camera tube about its optical axis.
(d) The appearance of dark spots and blemishes on the viewing field caused by damaged or deformed glass fibres.

Presently, fibre optics coupling is used in mobile fluoroscopic units (operating room). In procedures such as cinefluorography and spotfilm techniques, fibre optics coupling results in a considerable loss of image quality.

Television Monitoring

One of the important advantages of image intensification is that *television fluoroscopy* is possible. This means that the image at the output screen is transferred (via lens or fibre optics) to a television-monitoring system (Figure 13:6).

Essential Elements

One of the first requirements of a television system is that it must be capable of transmission and reception of a *still picture*. A still picture consists of a large number of light and dark areas, where each small area of light or shade is

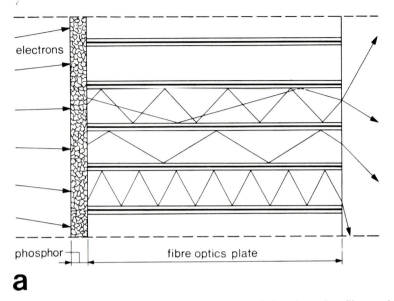

a

Figure 13:5. (a) The principle of light and pattern transmission through a fibre optics glass plate. (b) The coupling of the image intensifier tube and television camera tube with the fibre optics plate. (From Botden P.J.M., Feddema J., and Vijverberg G.P.M.: First results with an experimental integrated image intensifier television system. *Medicamundi* 14. No. 3., 1969.)

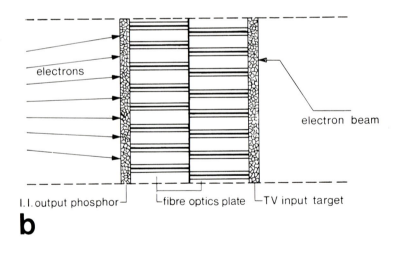

b

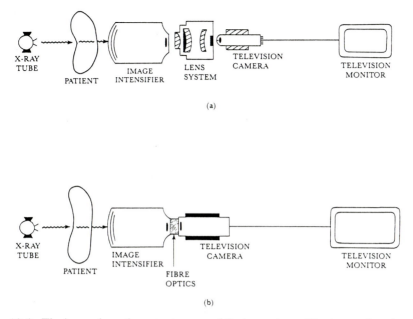

Figure 13:6. The image from the output screen of the image intensifier is transferred to a television camera tube through a lens system (a) or a fibre optical system (b). The television camera tube faces the output screen.

referred to as a *picture element.* The scene to be televised, therefore, is made up of picture elements which are transmitted to reproduce the original scene.

The other essential elements are:

(a) *a television camera tube.* This is a photoelectronic tube capable of converting visual information (a light pattern or the scene to be televised) into electrical information (a varying electrical signal — the signal voltage).

(b) *an image-reproducing tube.* This is the television picture tube or *kinescope.* The tube is capable of converting the varying signal voltage from the television camera tube back into a visual pattern. The screen of the picture tube reproduces the original scene by duplicating its picture elements.

The transmission and reception of still pictures may be achieved by two methods:

(a) a radiolink, as in broadcast television where transmission through the atmosphere is aided by antenna and receivers.

(b) closed-circuit television using special conducting cables.

Closed-circuit television (or *direct-wire* television) has found widespread applications in such areas as education, industry, traffic control, medicine and diagnostic imaging. In closed-circuit television the signal from the television camera tube is connected directly to the television picture tube by a length of cable. Such a cable is referred to as a *coaxial cable*. The conductor is located in the center of the cable which has a protective, grounded metallic sheath around it.

The most basic form of closed-circuit television for diagnostic imaging is shown in Figure 13:7.

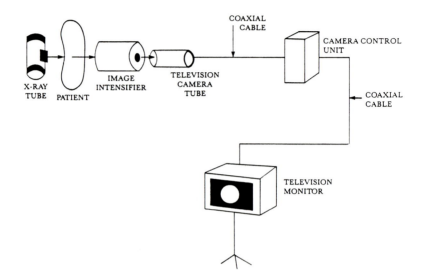

Figure 13:7. The most basic form of closed-circuit television in diagnostic x-ray imaging.

TELEVISION CAMERA TUBES IN DIAGNOSTIC IMAGING

The purpose of a television camera tube is to change visual information (light image) into electrical signals. The light image is first captured by a lens which focusses it onto a photosensitive surface of the camera tube.

There are a number of camera tubes available today such as the image orthicon, the vidicon, the Plumbicon® and the isocon. Although the *image orthicon* has been used in television fluoroscopy, it is mainly used in broadcast television. The image orthicon has been replaced by the *vidicon* and the *Plumbicon* tubes, which are widely used in diagnostic imaging and it is for this reason that they will be described in detail in this section. The *isocon* is the largest of the camera tubes mentioned here and, although it is used mainly in broadcast television, it is part of the imaging scheme of the *dynamic spatial reconstructor (DSR)*. The DSR is a highly specialized computed tomography scanner, and the only one in the world is located at the Mayo Clinic.

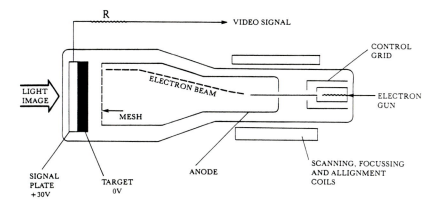

Figure 13:8. Schematic representation of the Vidicon television camera tube. See text for further explanation.

The Vidicon Camera Tube

The vidicon camera tube is an evacuated glass envelope about 16 cm (6.25 inches) long and about 2.5 cm (1 inch) in diameter. The essential components are a photosensitive target plate, an electron gun, and a series of external coils surrounding the glass envelope. The coils and glass envelope are both enclosed in the camera housing. The arrangement of these components is shown in Figure 13:8.

The Target

The target of the vidicon consists of two layers. One is a thin layer of conducting material coated on the inner surface of a glass face plate which acts as a signal-plate electrode for the output signal. The other is a thin layer of photo-semiconductor materials, usually *antimony trisulfide* (Sb_2S_3).

The Electron Gun

The electron gun consists of a cathode which is heated to give off electrons by the process of thermionic emission. The control grid (Figure 13:8) shapes the electron into a beam. The electrons are then accelerated by another grid to enter the scanning section of the tube where they are focussed onto the target. Before the electron beam approaches the target it encounters a wire mesh, which, together with the signal plate, slows down the accelerating electrons from the electron gun and allows them to strike the target at right angles.

External Coils

These coils include focussing, deflecting and alignment coils. They are positioned outside the glass envelope. The electron beam is focussed to a point on the target by the focussing coil, while other coils (vertical deflecting and horizontal deflecting coils) allow the electron beam to move up and down and side to side, respectively, in scanning the target of the camera tube.

Principles

When light from the image intensifer output screen falls on the photocon ductive layer, it emits electrons in proportion to the intensity of light. The target now becomes positively charged in the areas struck by light and, therefore, acts like a charged capacitor. As the electron beam approaches and scans the target, it meets the charge deficiency and fills the target by a deposition of electrons on the surface. This process discharges the capacitor and causes a current to flow through the resistor, R (Figure 13:8). The resultant voltage is called the *video signal*. All video signals coming from the camera tube must be amplified in some way (camera control unit) before they are sent to the television picture tube.

The Plumbicon

The Plumbicon (N.V. Philips Company) is a *lead oxide* (PbO) vidicon, that is, it uses lead oxide as the photoconducting layer rather than antimony trisulfide. The principle of operation is essentially the same as the standard vidicon camera tube.

Advantage and Disadvantage of Camera Tubes

The advantages and disadvantages of three camera tubes are summarized in Table 13:1.

Table 13-1

SOME ADVANTAGES AND DISADVANTAGES OF THREE
TELEVISION CAMERA TUBES

TV Camera Tube	Advantages	Disadvantages
Image orthicon	High sensitivity — can perform at low levels of illumination. Reduced Image Lag. Increased detail preservation.	Expensive. Increased noise in signal. Complex (requires elaborate circuitry). Large size (gives rise to bulky equipment).
Vidicon	Inexpensive. Small size. Simple operation. Reduced Image distortion. Less noise in signal.	Less sensitive than image orthicon. Increased image lag at low levels of brightness. Reduced image contrast.
Plumbicon®	Improved image contrast compared to the vidicon. Reduced image lag compared to the vidicon. Almost no noise in signal.	Decrease in detail visibility. Slightly larger than the vidicon. Expensive.

The image orthicon is very expensive and can transmit at low levels of brightness. It also exhibits practically no image lag. The vidicon, on the other hand, is less expensive but exhibits image lag. This makes it impractical for x-ray examinations such as cardiac and arterial catheterizations but suitable for hip pinnings or any other procedure which involves repair of the anatomy by metal pinning.

The Plumbicon exhibits shorter image lag than the vidicon and, therefore, it is suitable for examining moving structures.

THE TELEVISION MONITOR

The television monitor consists of the *picture tube* and associated electronics. The picture tube is shown schematically in Figure 13:9. It is a cathode ray tube, a funnel-shaped evacuated glass envelope with an electron gun at the narrow end of the tube.

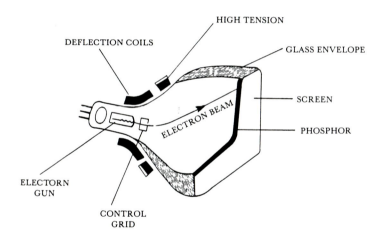

Figure 13:9. Schematic illustration of the television picture tube.

The expanded end of the tube forms the screen, the inner surface of which is coated with a fluorescent material which emits light when struck by electrons. One of the primary constituents of the fluorescent material is zinc sulfide.

The varying output video signal from the camera tube is applied to the control grid of the television monitor. The beam of electrons emitted from the electron gun will also vary in intensity. Since there is a high voltage (10 kV) on the anode at the expanded end of the tube, the electron beam is accelerated at high speeds to strike the fluorescent screen. The brightness at a specific area on the screen depends on the number of electrons striking that area. The more electrons, the brighter the area or region. The image created on the screen will therefore vary in degrees of brightness.

Scanning in the Picture Tube

The area scanned on the target of the camera tube is referred to as a *raster*. The electron beam in the camera tube traces at least 525 lines on the target at a rate of 30 times per second, with each complete scan being referred to as a *television frame*.

The same process occurs in the picture tube. The television picture is therefore made up of lines (Figure 13:10), and the number of lines (525, 625 or 1050) will vary from system to system.

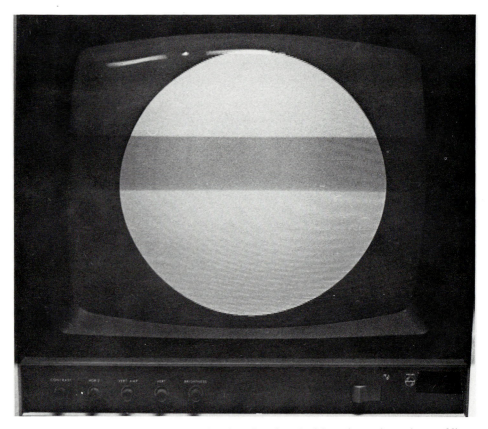

Figure 13:10. The television screen, showing that the television picture is made up of lines. In this photograph the horizontal scan lines are clearly seen. Also, in the absence of vertical synchronization, the picture rolls up and down the screen (the dark band across the screen).

The scanning of the screen may be either progressive or interlaced. In *progressive scanning* the electron beam begins at the top left corner of the screen, then it moves horizontally to the right and then back to the left for a second line, but this time a little lower than the first. As the beam completes the last line at the bottom right corner, it makes a diagonal sweep to the upper left corner to commence a new scanning sequence. This method of scanning is referred to as *horizontal linear scanning*.

One of the drawbacks of sequential scanning is that of flicker in the television picture. This flicker can be eliminated by the *horizontal interlaced scanning* technique. In this method, each picture frame (525 lines) is divided into two fields (odd and even), where each field is made up of 262 ½ lines. An odd field contains odd-numbered lines (1, 3, 5, 7, 9, and so on), whereas an even field contains even-numbered lines (2, 4, 6, 8 and so on). A complete picture frame, therefore, consists of an odd field interlaced with an even field and this effect eliminates flicker. For a 60-Hz field frequency (North America), a frame is completed in one thirtieth second and in one twenty-fifth second for a 50-Hz field frequency (Europe).

Synchronization

Another essential requirement in a television system whether it be broadcast or closed-circuit television is that of *synchronization*. Scanning the target plate of the camera tube must be synchronized with scanning the picture tube screen for a faithful reproduction of the picture or image. This is accomplished by special synchronizing signals or pulses (sync, for short) from the camera tube to the television monitor.

The signals include horizontal sync and vertical sync. In the absence of vertical sync the picture rolls up and down the screen (Figure 13:10). Without horizontal sync, the picture appears as diagonal segments on the screen. Synchronization, therefore, ensures that the picture elements on the target plate of the camera tube have the same relative position as those reproduced on the screen of the picture tube. The horizontal and vertical controls on the television monitor are used to adjust images that are out of synchronization. The mechanisms for synchronization are complex and are not within the scope of this text.

COLOR TELEVISION

Principles

The same principles governing black and white television also apply to color television with a few additional requirements. These requirements include the use of three camera tubes, special signals for transmission and a receiver which is designed to reproduce color information.

Figure 13:11 illustrates the principle of color television. The color light (scene) is first separated into three *primary colors* — namely, red, green and blue — by optical filters. These primary colors are used because they can be combined to produce a wide range of colors. Tube 1 (Figure 13:11) "picks up" the-red parts of scene or picture, tube 2, the green portions and tube 3, the blue portions of the scene. Video signals are therefore obtained for the red, green and blue portions of the scene. The three video signals are then combined to generate two signals for transmission to the color television monitor. The two signals are:

(a) The *luminance signal*, which contains brightness variations of the scene, that is, this signal has black and white information and intended for black and white television monitors.

(b) The *chrominance signal*, which consists of the red, green and blue aspects of the scene is intended for color television monitors.

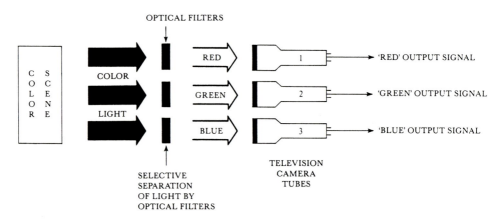

Figure 13:11. The principle of color television. See text for further explanation.

In order to reproduce the color scene on the color monitor, both signals (luminance and chrominance) are combined to produce the original red, green and blue video signals.

The Color Television Monitor

A color television monitor is shown in Figure 13:12. It is an evacuated glass envelope which consists of three electron guns. The phosphor screen contains red, green and blue dots arranged in groups of three. There is also a thin metal sheet called the *shadow mask* which contains numerous tiny holes where each hole is in line with a dot trio. The function of the shadow mask is to ensure that each beam from the three electron guns excites its respective color dots without exciting the other two dots.

Each video color signal is applied to one of the three electron guns to produce a beam that will excite its respective color dot. For example, the red video signal is "fed" to the "red" gun which will produce a beam of electrons to excite the red phosphor dots. The blue signal goes to the "blue" gun to excite the blue

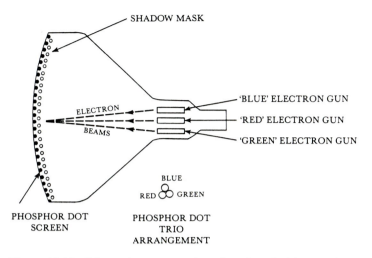

Figure 13:12. Schematic representation of a color television monitor.

phosphor dots and so on. Each beam converges at the proper angle over the entire screen such that the three beams pass through one hole in the shadow mask for each dot trio. This process results in the reproduction of a color picture.

The application of color television principles in diagnostic imaging has not received widespread attention. Although color television has been used in *color subtraction techniques,* much more work remains to be done to reproduce a scheme which is practical for use in clinical fluoroscopy.

Color television can be used to assist in the study of anatomic structure, motion of organs, the flow of contrast media and also provide an increase in density and contrast of the image.

TELEVISION PICTURE QUALITY

The qualities of the television picture that are of importance to the technologist are resolution, contrast, brightness, aspect ratio, image noise and lag.

Resolution

Television resolution depends on the number of picture elements that can be faithfully reproduced and the *bandpass* or *bandwidth* (range of frequencies that can be transmitted by the television system) of the video signal. Picture elements ae made up of lines; resolution, therefore, depends on the number of scanning lines. The greater the number of lines and the higher the bandpass, the better the resolution.

The line rate for conventional television chains is 525 (60-Hz field frequency) and 625 (50-Hz field frequency). Today, high resolution (more than 525 and 625) television chains are available and the essential charcteristics will be discussed subsequently.

Contrast

This quality is related to the intensity difference for the black and white portions of the picture. Contrast relates to brightness, and since brightness is controlled by the video signal voltage, contrast is also related to the video signal. Contrast can be adjusted by the contrast control on the monitor. This adjustment alters the amplitude of the video signal.

Brightness

Brightness is the overall intensity of illumination of the picture and depends on the monitor high voltage and the voltage on the grid-cathode circuit. When the brightness control on the monitor is adjusted, the average level of the video signal changes. This is not the case with the contrast control which changes the video signal only slightly. For the best possible image, it is important to adjust these two controls together.

Aspect Ratio

This quality is of less importance to the technologist. It is the ratio of the width to the height of the picture frame. The standard aspect ratio is 4:3 which makes the picture wider than it is high. If the aspect ratio is not maintained, then the picture will appear too thin or too wide.

Noise

When viewing television images the technologist may notice the "snow" effect. This effect is a result of *electronic noise* and occurs with very weak video signals.

Lag

The problem of lag was mentioned earlier in the discussion of the vidicon tube which exhibits image lag. This lag results in image blurring on the picture tube.

VIEWING DISTANCE FOR TELEVISION IMAGES

The proper viewing distance for television images is given to be four to eight times the picture height. Table 13:2 shows the optimum viewing distance for four common monitor sizes with a 525 line rate. If it is necessary to view the screen at a closer distances, then television systems with higher line rates must be used.

Table 13-2

MONITOR VIEWING DISTANCE FOR A 525-LINE TELEVISION SYSTEM.

(Courtesy of General Electric Company,
Medical Systems Division.)

Monitor Size (diagonal of the Kinescope)	Kinescope Height	No. of Lines Per Inch	Line Separation	Optimum Viewing Distance	Region of Distinct Vision
8	4.8″	102	.010″	33″	11.4″
14	8.4″	58	.017″	58″	20″
17	10.2″	48	.021″	70″	24″
21	12.6″	39	.026″	87″	30″

OTHER TELEVISION APPLICATIONS IN DIAGNOSTIC IMAGING

Apart from television fluoroscopy, the other television applications which deserve mention here are electronic subtraction, electronic harmonization and digital fluoroscopy.

Electronic Subtraction

A method of *photographic subtraction* was described as early as 1935 by Professor Ziedses des Plantes. The method is extremely useful in examinations employing contrast media (for example, angiography) where, in some cases, small vessel detail tends to be obliterated by bony structures.

In photographic subtraction, a *scout film* is first obtained, followed by a *subtraction mask* which is a negative of the scout film. This negative is made by superimposing a subtraction film (for example, Dupont Cronex Subtraction Film) on the scout film and then exposing them to light in a special unit used for copying and subtracting radiographs. The next step is to obtain a film with contrast media. This film is then superimposed on the mask and an unexposed film is then superimposed on both of these. All of these are then exposed to light, and the end result is a film which shows only the contrast-filled vessels (a composite image).

In television fluoroscopy, it is possible to obtain a composite image by means of *electronic subtraction.*

The principle of electronic subtraction is shown in Figure 13:13. Two radiographs (scout film and film with contrast) are placed side by side on a film illuminator. The images are "picked up" by two television cameras which are operating synchronously. Two signals are, therefore, sent to an amplifier which produces a subtraction signal. This signal is conveyed to the television monitor via the television central control unit. The subtraction is such that likebrightness values are cancelled out, and the image (the subtraction image) can be displayed either in the positive or negative mode. With electronic subtraction, the brightness and contrast and the degree of cancellation of like features in the two images can be varied. The image can be recorded photographically or by videotape.

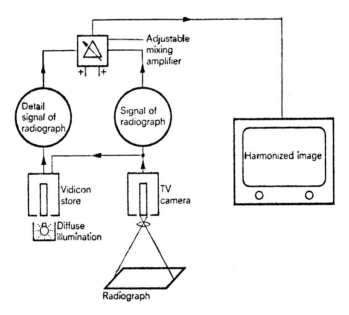

Figure 13:13. The principle of electronic subtraction. See text for further explanation. (courtesy of the Siemens Corporation.)

The electronic subtraction technique is particularly useful in examinations such as angiography, myelography, pyelogrpahy and so on, but it has not become very popular in diagnostic x-ray imaging.

Electronic Harmonization

The purpose of electronic harmonization is to enhance fine details in an image and to reduce the contrast of large area details. The resultant image is said to be harmonized.

In Figure 13:14 the principle of *electronic harmonization* is shown. The radiographs to be harmonized is scanned by one television camera tube. The signal obtained from this tube is referred to as the main signal. In harmonization, the other television camera tube operates as a "vidicon store" which turns the main signal into a detail signal. By mixing the main signal with the detail signal in a mixing amplifier, a mixed signal is obtained, which produces the harmonization picture on the monitor screen.

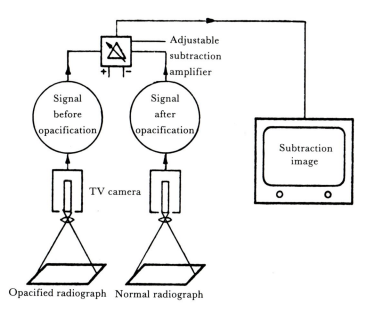

Figure 13:14. The principle of electronic harmonization. See text for explanation. (courtesy of the Siemens Corporation.)

The order of magnitude of fine details can be enhanced in a series of steps by push-button selectors placed on the television monitor of the electronic harmonization unit. The degree of mixing between the main and detail signals is continuously adjustable.

Electronic harmonization is especially useful in mammography where microcalcifications can be seen better than in the original radiographs. It is also useful in skeletal radiography, in which bone structures are clearly demonstrated to show pathological changes, and in examinations involving the use of contrast media. As in the case of electronic subtraction, this technique has not found widespread use in diagnostic imaging.

Digital Fluoroscopy

Digital Fluoroscopy is based on the application of digital image processing techniques (Chapter 18) to television fluoroscopy.

The technique essentially involves conversion of the video signal (analog signal) into digital information through the use of a digital image processor and a control computer.

Digital fluoroscopy has received much enthusiasm and the technique has gained widespread applications. The technique offers several advantages over conventional imaging and forms part of a larger imaging scheme referred to as *digital radiography*. For this reason it will be discussed in a separate chapter.

IMAGE TRANSMISSION

The information obtained from a fluoroscopic examination is instantaneously presented to the radiologist for viewing on a television screen via closed-circuit television. In addition, the fluoroscopic image can also be transmitted to subsequent major departments in the hospital, such as the operating room and emergency department. Such transmission of images not only facilitates communication between radiologists and physicians but it can also be used as a teaching tool. Radiographs can also be viewed in remote areas in the hospital without having to transfer them out of the department.

Images can also be transmitted out of the hospital to clinics and other institutions by means of microwave transmission, however, there is a delay of a few seconds before the image is ready for viewing.

The idea of image transmission to remote areas other than in the hospital has gained popularily within the radiologic community, however, because it is in its developmental stages at this time, it will not be discussed further.

HIGH RESOLUTION X-RAY TELEVISION

The conventional x-ray television chain cannot reproduce faithfully the high-quality images provided by the new generation of x-ray image intensifiers (CsI). Therefore, a high resolution x-ray television (HRXTV) system was designed to eliminate this problem. The characteristic feature of the HRXTV chain is its *improved transmission properties*.

A detailed account of the HRXTV chain is given by Haendle, Horbaschek and Alexandrescu (1977). The following account is a summary of their paper with respect to the HRXTV chain.

The improved transmission properties of the HRXTV chain is shown in Figure 13:15. Improvements have been made to the lens, camera tube, video amplifier and the picture tube.

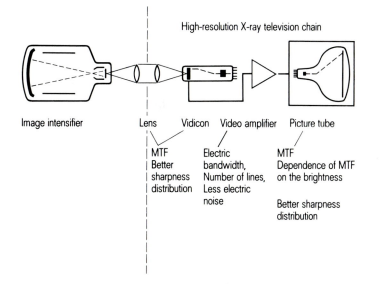

Figure 13:15. The improved transmission properties of high resolution x-ray television. Only the improvements as a whole lead to better image quality. (From Haendle, J. Horbaschek H. and Alexandrescu M.: High-resolution x-ray television and high-resolution video recorder. *Electromedica* 3-4., 1977.)

The lens has been improved to provide better resolution and a more uniform image field. The camera tube has been designed with a much better electro-optical system and an improved magnetic deflection and focussing scheme for the electron beam. The next link in the television chain — the video amplifier — has been designed to facilitate a wider bandpass and also provides a decrease in electronic noise. The change made to the television monitor are with respect to the electron optics, the deflection system and the number of scan lines. Both the electron optics and the deflection system have been improved. Brightness levels are also higher.

The number of lines for the HRXTV has been increased by a factor of two. For the 60 Hz field frequency, the previous 525-line system has been increased to 1050 lines and to 1250 lines for the previous 625-line (50 Hz field frequency). The effect of HRXTV on picture quality compared to the conventional x-ray television chain is clearly demonstrated in Figure 13:16. The authors (Haendle, Horbaschek and Alexandrescu) also gave visual comparison between the 625-line and a 2000-line television system (laboratory model)

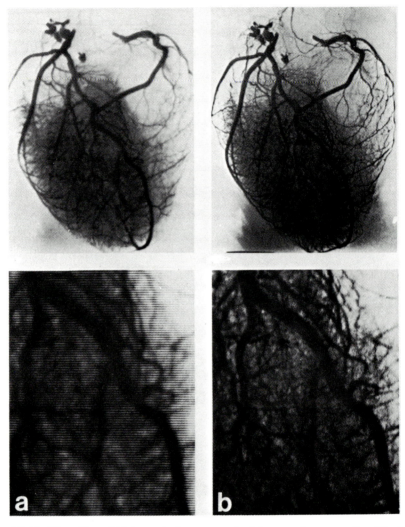

Figure 13:16. The effect of high resolution x-ray television on picture quality. The images shown in (a) (top and bottom) were taken with a conventional x-ray television system while those images (top and bottom) shown in (b) were recorded with a high resolution televison chain. (From Haendle J., Horbaschek H. and Alexandrescu M.: High-resolution x-ray television and high-resolution video recorder. *Electromedica* 3-4., 1977.)

through photographs recorded off the respective television monitors. This comparison is shown in Figure 13:17.

Finally, the HRXTV chain can transmit up to four million bits (binary digit) of information compared to 1.3 million bits for conventional x-ray television systems. This has implications for digital x-ray imaging. The HRXTV chain is particularly useful in digital fluoroscopy where maximum information is needed for digital image processing and reconstruction.

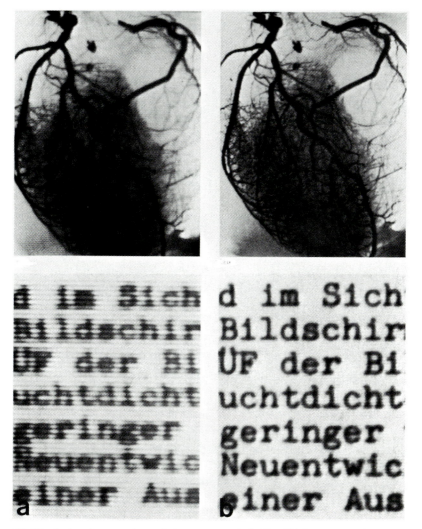

Figure 13:17. A visual comparison of pictures recorded off a 625-line conventional x-ray television monitor (top and bottom) images shown in (a) and a 2000-line laboratory high-resolution x-ray television monitor (b). (From Haendle J., Horbaschek H. and Alexandrescu M.: High-resolution x-ray television and high-resolution video recorder. *Electromedica* 3-4., 1977.)

SUMMARY

1. A number of approaches are used to transfer the image from the output screen of the image intensifier tube to subsequent systems for display, viewing and recording.
2. Since the lens and mirror optical system is one approach, it is described and reviewed with respect to definitions, reflection, refrac-

tion, and spherical aberration.

3. Another approach to image transfer is based on fibre optics. Fibre optics utilize light-conducting glass fibres and offer a number of advantages, such as compact construction, no loss of image quality during image transfer, no contrast loss, and practically no vignetting. Disadvantages are listed.

4. Yet another method is television monitoring which requires the mechanism to transmit and receive a still picture, a television camera tube, and an image-reproducing tube such as a television picture tube.

5. The transmission and reception of still pictures may be accomplished by two methods: a radiolink (as in broadcast television) and closed-circuit television.

6. Since closed-circuit television is widely used in imaging departments, it is dealt with in some detail in the chapter.

7. A television camera tube is a device which converts a light image into electrical signals. Three camera tubes were identified and only two — the vidicon and the Plumbicon — are described, since they are widely used in imaging applications.

8. The vidicon and Plumbicon are based on the principle of photoconductivity but differ in respect to their photoconductors. The vidicon uses antimony trisulfide, whereas the Plumbicon uses lead oxide.

9. The advantages and disadvantages of camera tubes are discussed briefly.

10. The television picture tube is a cathode ray tube. It consists of funnel-shaped glass envelope with an electron gun at the narrow end of the tube. The purpose of the tube is to convert the electrical signals received from the camera tube into visual information.

11. Two approaches to scanning in the picture tube are available. These are sequential (or progressive) and interlaced. Sequential scanning involves a horizontal linear scanning technique in which each line (television) is scanned one after the other (progressive). Interlaced scanning involves a horizontal interlaced scanning technique in which each picture frame (525 lines) is divided into two fields (odd and even), each consisting of $262\frac{1}{2}$ lines. An odd field contains odd-numbered lines and an even field contains even-numbered lines. A complete picture frame then consists of an odd field interlaced with an even field. This method eliminates flicker.

12. In the television principle, synchronization is important — that is, the scanning in the camera tube must be synchronized with the scanning in the picture tube for a faithful reproduction of pictures.

13. Color television principles are discussed briefly. In color television, at least two signals are important: the luminance signal and the chrominance signal. The luminance signal has black and white infor-

mation for use with black and white television monitors. The chrominance signal consists of red, green, and blue signals for use with color television monitors.

14. The color television monitor consists of three electron guns, and the phosphor screen features red, green, and blue dots arranged in groups of three. A thin metal sheet, called the shadow mask, ensures that each beam from the three electron guns excites its respective color dots without exciting the other two.

15. Color television techniques in x-ray imaging have been applied in color subtraction techniques.

16. The qualities of television pictures are the resolution, contrast, brightness, aspect ratio, image noise and lag. A description of each of these is given.

17. The proper viewing distance for television is given to be four to eight times the picture height.

18. Other television applications in diagnostic x-ray imaging include electronic subtraction, electronic harmonization and digital fluoroscopy.

19. Image transmission encompasses communicating images to other remote areas either within the hospital (closed-circuit television) or by microwave transmission to remote areas outside the hospital.

20. The main feature of a high resolution x-ray television system is its improved transmission properties. Such improvement has been made possible by refinements in the lens camera tube, video amplifier and the picture tube. These are described briefly.

CHAPTER 14

IMAGE RECORDING — PRINCIPLES
AND INSTRUMENTATION

A N integral component in any imaging scheme is image recording. The information collected from the patient must not only be displayed in a meaningful form for viewing, but it must also be recorded in some way to provide permanent images.

In x-ray imaging, a variety of methods are available for recording images. The most prevalent method involves recording images on non-screen film (direct exposure) or on a screen/film combination (indirect exposure). In this context, the film is placed on the tabletop or in the Bucky diaphragm. The film is subsequently exposed to radiation passing through the patient and a latent image is formed. The latent image is then rendered visible through chemical processing of the film and a permanent image is obtained.

Other methods of recording images fall into two categories, namely: *static recording* and *dynamic recording*. The method described above is an example of static recording in which case the image is presented as a fixed photographic image.

In dynamic recording, a series of images are obtained in a short time. The time separation between each individual image is extremely short. If these images are projected by suitable means (special projector), the effect of motion results.

Dynamic recording is used primarily to study the physiology of organ systems, although structural details (static recording) can be observed as well.

DYNAMIC RECORDING METHODS

Dynamic recording methods include cineradiography (serial radiography), cinefluorography, spotfilming using serial exposures, videotape and videodisk recording.

Videotape Recording

Videotape recording (VTR) is a magnetic recording process. Recording x-ray images on magnetic material has been under investigation for some time. In 1959, Oosterkamp and Schut pointed out for the first time how x-ray images can be recorded using the television video signal. They used a magnetic memory wheel to record single television images.

Recording moving television images was already developed in television studios, but it was r.ot applied to x-ray imaging at that time, since the equipment was too complex. It was not until 1963 that a simple recorder was developed for application in x-ray imaging. One of the speical features of this device was the capability of recording serial television images.

Today, videotape recording is a popular and widely used technique, and, therefore, it will be described here in some detail.

Essential Characteristics of the Videotape Recorder

VTR is used in conjunction with fluoroscopy (image intensifier and television chain) to record fluoroscopic examinations so that immediate playback is possible. To perform this task efficiently, the recorder must be capable of the following, as pointed out by Barella and Genefaas in their 1969 publication:

(a) *"Optimum" image quality.* Factors related to image quality are sharpness, contrast and noise level of the image. Sharpness or the degree of detail which can be put on the tape is a function of the particle size of the magnetic material on the tape, tape width and the size of the head gap in the recording head. These will be discussed later in the chapter. The contrast of the reproduced image depends on the circuitry which is used to transform the information on the tape into a video signal during playback. Special measures are taken to prevent a loss of image contrast by including demodulator circuits in video recorders. The noise level of the recorded image is affected by the overall frequency range that can be put on the tape via the recorder itself and by the grainy structure of the tape.

(b) *Simple and logical operation.* Since a number of manipulations (record, rewind, playback, etc.) have to made on the recorder during fluoroscopy, it is important that the user understand the operating principles in order to record successfully.

(c) *Reliability.* To ensure maximum recording conditions, the video recorder must be mechanically stable and electronically reliable. The mechanical aspects of the recorder include such elements as the rotating video recording head and tape threading, etc. Electronic reliability is achieved by temperature compensation of the specialized circuitry, while other electronic controls allow for constant tape speed during recording and playback. Interfering signals are not picked up by the recorder during recording, because the grounding of its circuitry is separated from earthing points of other x-ray equipment in the same room.

Barella and Genefaas (1969) have also pointed out other characteristics which have become common to more recent video recorders used in x-ray imaging. These are:

1. *Endless loop:* In various examination techniques it is of importance to record short fluoroscopy phases and to play these back immediately and repeatedly (e.g., recordings of test injections in angiocardiography and simultaneous video recording with the cine run to check what is being filmed). With the normal tape this cannot be done quickly and simply. Winding back and searching for the exact passage on the tape costs time and one's impression of the image becomes vague as a result. For these reasons use is made of an endless tape (loop) which is suitable for some minutes of recording. This form of operation offers, moreover, the possibility of employing intermittent fluoroscopy (dose reduction). It also opens up important vistas especially in surgery (with practically static objects).

2. *Stationary image/slow motion:* The reproduced image can be stopped, for example, for a close study of a specific phase. The recorded images can also be shown in slow motion (⅓ of the normal speed; forwards and backwards). This feature greatly facilitates retrieval of specific phases of an examination, which are required for study.

3. *Sound Dubbing:* In addition to the recording of sound simultaneously with the fluoroscopic image, sound dubbing offers the possibility of adding audio signals after the fluoroscopic image has been recorded. For instance, a commentary on the playback images (diagnosis, patient data, etc.) can be spoken on the tape.

4. *Automatic tape stop:* During the examination, the recorder should claim as little attention as possible from the medical personnel. It is therefore provided with an end-stop, so that one does not have to keep a wary eye on the amount of tape running from one reel to the other. In addition, a buzzer sounds five minutes before the end of tape is reached.

Magnetic Tape and Recording Head

Two essential components of the video recorder used in imaging are the magnetic tape and the recording head.

Magnetic tape (videotape) consists of a plastic base, (mylar) usually acetate or polyester coated with a 1-mm thick emulsion of fine magnetizable particles. These magnetizable particles are usually *iron oxide,* but recently *chromium dioxide* and magnesium dioxide have become available for use on some videotapes.

The tape is about 2.5 cm to 5cm wide which includes tracks along the upper and lower edge for recording sound.

The degree of detail that can be recorded on the tape is influenced by the tape width and the size of the magnetizable particles. In general, the greater the width and the smaller the particle size, the greater the detail that can be recorded.

The *recording head,* or more precisely, the *video head* (because it also functions as a playback device), is a circular or rectangular iron core with a very narrow gap between its poles. This gap is referred to as the *head gap.* The width of the head gap is very narrow (about 0.001 mm), since it plays a role in the degree of detail that can be recorded (usually the smaller the gap, the greater the detail that can be recorded).

Another component of the video recorder is the *head drum,* since it contains the video head which rotates very rapidly in the gap of the drum during recording. In Figure 14:1, the video recording head and head drum are shown.

In some video recorders, recording is affected by means of two video heads which are displaced 180° from each other and which can rotate very rapidly in the gap of the head drum. At the same time, the magnetic tape is lead spirally and must be guided precisely over the head drum, as is illustrated in Figure 14:2.

Recording and Playback Principles

In the recording process, the output video signal (a varying output voltage)

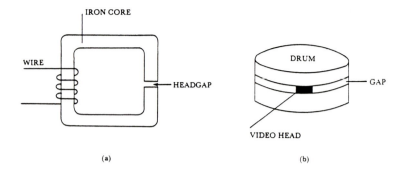

(a)   (b)

Figure 14:1. (a) The video head, showing the head gap and wire wound around an iron core. The wire receives the output video signal from the television camera tube and creates a magnetic field at the gap. The field varies in intensity because of the variation in brightness from the output screen of the image intensifier tube. The video head, positioned in the head gap of the head drum, is shown in (b).

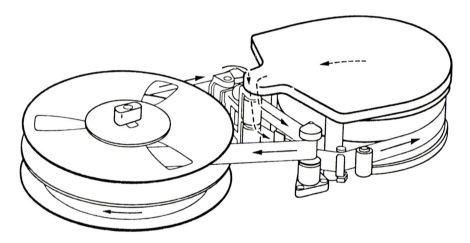

Figure 14:2. The magnetic tape runs past the head drum precisely guided. (courtesy of the Siemens Corporation.)

from the television camera tube is directed through the coil of wire which is wound around the video head (Figure 14:1). This signal produces a varying magnetic field across the gap of the video head. As the tape passes across the gap, various portions of it become magnetized, depending on the strength of the magnetic field at the gap.

In playback (or replay), it is first necessary to rewind the tape. During playback, as the magnetized tape passes the head gap, it induces a magnetic field at the gap. This field in turn induces a varying electric current in the coil of the video head. The current is used to provide a varying output voltage (video signal) which is transmitted to the electron gun of the television monitor.

To record maximum information on the tape, it is wound spirally over the head drum and maintained at a high speed relative to the video head. This is necessary to allow each television frame to be recorded along a sloping track as shown in Figure 14:3 (one recorded track represents one full television frame). Also seen on the tape in Figure 14:3 are synchronization tracks which can be recorded in the middle or on the edge of the tape.

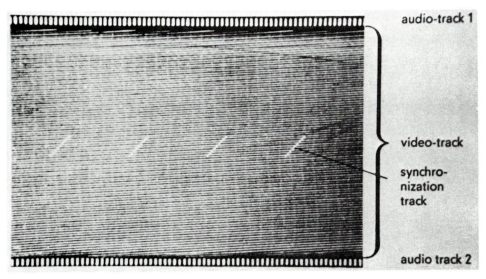

Figure 14:3. Section of videotape showing video, audio and synchronization tracks. The tracks have been made visible with iron powder. (courtesy of the Siemens Corporation.)

Synchronization in videotape recording is accomplished by special synchronization circuitry which is necessary to ensure that:

    (a) only one television field is recorded for one rotation of the video head.
    (b) the same tracks are scanned during recording and playback.

Videotape recorders also feature slow/stop motion. In slow motion, the tape is made to run at a lower speed than that of the recording speed, although other factors are taken into consideration. In stop motion, the video head is positioned on the tape such that it "reads" out continuously one recorded track. In this case, only one single television frame is displayed on the monitor screen.

Advantages of Videotape Recording

The advantages associated with videotape recording are:

    (a) Instantaneous replay of the recorded image.
    (b) The image can be played back repeatedly.
    (c) The capability of stop and slow motions during replay.
    (d) Reuse of the tape after erasures.

(e) Use of the tape as a permanent record.
(f) Easy storage of tape.
(g) Lower radiation doses to patients since lower tube currents (fluoroscopic mA) are used.
(h) By adjusting suitable controls on the television monitor, the contrast and brightness of the recorded image can be increased or decreased.

Later in the chapter, videotape recording will be compared with other methods of recording x-ray images.

Videotape recording can be used in several types of x-ray examinations but is most effective in those which involve the use of contrast material.

A video recorder for use in x-ray imaging is shown in Figure 14:4a, while the dimensions are given in Figure 14:4b.

Storage of Videotape

In the storage of videotapes, the following should be considered:

(a) Tapes must be stored in a dust-free environment. They should be packaged in boxes or plastic bags or appropriate storage containers.
(b) Proper humidity and temperature conditions must be maintained, since changes in these conditions may damage (breakage due to tension) the tape.
(c) The tape should be stored on its edge, since poor climatic conditions (humidity and temperature) may damage its edges if it is stored flat.
(d) Tapes must be shielded from strong magnetic fields. This is particularly important if tapes are stored near a magnetic resonance scanner.

Videodisk Recording

Videodisk radiography is a technique which involves the use of *magnetic videodisks* and *laser videodisks* to record and play back single (static recording) or a series (dynamic recording) of television images. This technique has gained popularity recently and has found applications in Bucky table with television, general x-ray work (for direct storage of spot exposures), and particularly in operating room radiography.

Magnetic Videodisks

A magnetic videodisk is a *video memory device.* It is a magnetic recording process, the principles of which are akin to videotape (a video memory device) recording. The principal advantage of videodisk recording is that of rapid access of the information stored on the disk for instant replay and in slow motion if desired.

A magnetic videodisk is similar to a phonograph record except that it is a more rigid plate which is coated on one or both sides with a thin film of magnetic particles such as iron oxide (a ferrite material). The disk is about 45

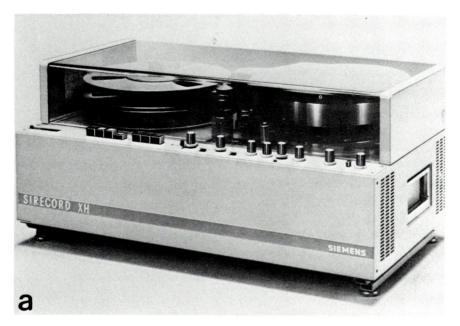

Figure 14:4. (a) A high-resolution video-recorder (SIRECORD XH) for use in diagnostic x-ray imaging. (b) The dimensions of the recorder. (courtesy of the Siemens Corporation.)

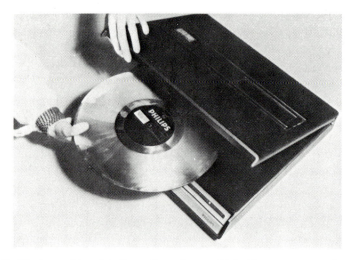

Figure 14:5. The laser video disk (from Oosterkamp, W.J.: New concepts and progress in instrumentation for cine and video radiology. *Medicamundi, Vol. 19, No. 3, 1974).*

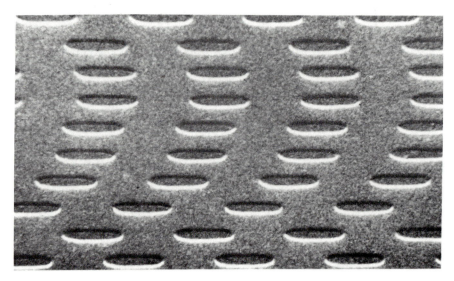

Figure 14:6. Photograph of the surface of a laser videodisk taken by a scanning electron microscope. The video signal is stored in a spiral track in a series of depressions (pits) by varying the distance and elongation of these pits. (From Oosterkamp, W.J.: New concepts and progress in instrumentation for cine and video radiology. *Medicamundi*, Vol. 19, No. 3, 1974.)

cm in diameter and is divided into concentric tracks which are read by a stationary read-write video head. During operation, the disk rotates at a high speed and the head "floats" over it (due to the compressed air created by the high rotation speed) to extract the information.

Laser Videodisks

Laser videodisk recording is a non-magnetic recording technique which is an alternative to magnetic tape and disk recording.

The laser videodisk is similar to a phonograph record (Figure 14:5). The information is stored in a series of microscopic (elliptical) depressions, as shown in Figure 14:6, by altering the basic shape of each depression and the distance of the depressions. The disk is coated with a thin layer of highly reflective material.

During operation, the disk rotates at very high speeds (about 1500-1800 revolutions per minute) and is scanned by a laser light. In Figure 14:7, the laser light (created by a 1 mW helium-neon laser) is directed to the depressions on the disk by means of a beam splitting prism, a movable mirror which follows the tracks and a lens. The light is then reflected back from the disk to strike the photo diode to generate a video signal; audio signals are also possible (Compaan and Kramer, 1973).

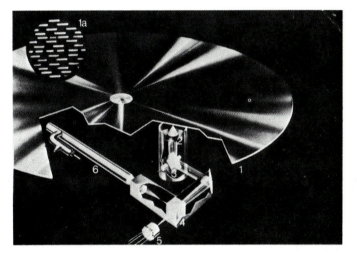

Figure 14:7. Schematic illustration of the operation of a laser video disk. The laser light is directed to the depressions on the disk by means of a beam splitting prism, a movable mirror and a lens. (From Oosterkamp, W.J.: New concepts and progress for cine and video radiology. *Medicamundi,* Vol. 19, No. 3, 1974.)

A 30-cm laser videodisk is capable of recording 45,000 television frames and providing about one-half hour of television display. Information can be retrieved very quickly with identification of single pictures, and slow motion is also a characteristic feature.

Applications

The use of videodisk recording in x-ray imaging is increasing rapidly. Already, magnetic videodisks are used quite extensively in computed tomography.

Videodisk recording may be used in the operating room and in general diagnostic work primarily for reduction in patient dose.

The following description of a study conducted by Birken and Franken (1975) provides the first illustration of the use of the videodisk recorder in imaging.

In their method, they used a single-track videodisk recorder to record spot exposures (by way of the image intensifier) which can be displayed immediately on a television monitor. This technique, referred to as *television storage of spot exposures,* is illustrated in Figure 14:8. In describing the principle of television storage of spot exposures, the authors state:

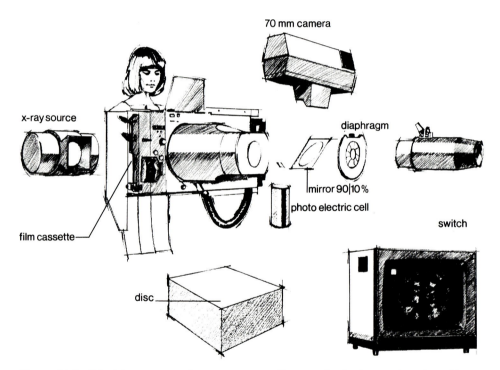

Figure 14:8. Television storage of spot exposures. See text for further explanation. (From Birken, H. and Franken, A.J.: Use of the single-image store in general and pre-operative x-ray diagnostics. *Medicamundi*, Vol. 20, No. 3, 1975.)

The release of a spot exposure initiates the partial closure of an iris diaphragm between the x-ray image intensifier output and the television camera during the preparation time for the exposure. The excessive light which would otherwise fall on the Plumbicon during the exposure is thus reduced to the necessary level for producing the television image signal. At the same time, the scanning electron beam in the television tube is suppressed. An electric charge pattern corresponding to the light image is built upon the Plumbicon target. At the end of the exposure, the charge pattern which carries the information is scanned. The single image signal thus obtained is fed to the television monitor and the disc store. Once the image has been recorded, the store switches to playback without any visible interruption and remains in this state until a new television-stored image of a further exposure appears or until fluoroscopy is started again.

The authors also report that:

A clinical trial in general x-ray diagnostics confirmed the usefulness of immediate evaluation of spot exposures by means of the television storage medium during the examination. It is felt to be particularly advantageous for recording rapid movements in examinations of the esophagus and stomach. The stored television image shows immediately in these cases whether the desired phase has in fact been recorded. Spoilt radiographs due to untimely breathing can be recognized and repeated immediately where necessary. Because of the greater certainty, it has also been posible to reduce the number of exposures per examination and thus lower the radiation dose.

It is important to note that because videodisk recording and videotape recording are primarily used for different purposes, comparisons of the two should not be made. A comparison between videodisk recording and spotfilm recording might be more appropriate.

A second illustration of the use of videodisk recording in x-ray imaging is provided by Zatz, Finston and Jones (1974) of Stanford University School of Medicine and Health Physics Office.

They used a mobile image intensifier television system and integrated it with a videodisk recorder, another television monitor (for viewing the recorded image), and a camera to photograph the image for application in operating room procedures requiring x-ray control. The basic layout of their imaging scheme is shown in Figure 14:9. When the foot switch is activated, fluoroscopy commences for about 0.38 seconds and the image recorded on the disc is immediately replayed on the other monitor. Since the foot switch is spring-loaded, it returns to the videodisk radiography position when released. This factor ensures that the unit cannot be utilized unintentionally in the fluoroscopic mode.

Radiation dose measurements were carried out for hip pinning and transphenoidal hypohysectomy examinations using tissue equivalent phantoms. Values for these measurements shown in Table 14:1 indicate a significant reduction in exposure to patient and staff compared to conventional fluoroscopic imaging.

Spotfilm Recording of Serial Exposures

Spotfilm recording of serial exposures is a dynamic process in that a serial radiographic technique is used. In this technique, up to six frames of film are exposed per second. This means that each individual image is separated only slightly in time and, therefore, the series of images can portary the effect of motion.

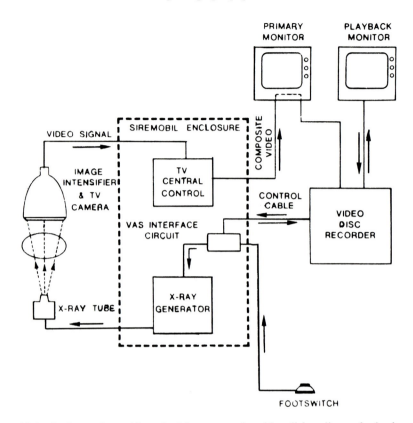

Figure 14:9. An image intensifier television system for video disk radiography in the operating room. (From Zatz, L. et al.: Reduced radiation exposure in the operating room with video disk radiography. Radiology, 110, Feb. 1974.)

Table 14-1

COMPARISON OF RADIATION DOSE BETWEEN VIDEODISK
RADIOGRAPHY AND CONVENTIONAL FLUOROSCOPY IN
THE OPERATING ROOM FOR TWO PROCEDURES
REQUIRING X-RAY CONTROL

(Courtesy of Zatz, L.M., and et. al.: *Radiology* 110:475-477,
February 1974.)

Location	Fluoroscopy (mR/min)		Video Disk Radiography (mR/5 exposures)	
	Small Field	Large Field	Small Field	Large Field
Simulated AP Hip Pinning (85 kVp 0.9 mA)				
Operator's body	0.29	1.15	0.008	0.028
Operator's hands	4.2	17.8	0.10	0.38
Patient's skin	1,170.0	1,270.0	25.0	26.0
Simulated Transphenoidal Hypophysectomy (70 kVp 2 mA)				
Operator's body	0.37	1.33	0.01	0.03
Operator's hands	8.5	39.2	0.20	0.90
Patient's skin	1,300.0	1,350.0	30.0	30.0

Spotfilm recording of serial exposures is accomplished by a *spotfilm camera* — a large-format camera which has become commonplace in fluoroscopic imaging. Figure 14:10 shows a functional diagram of a spotfilm camera. These cameras presently use 70-mm, 90-mm, 100-mm, nd 105-mm roll or cut film (single film), although the 100-mm and 105-mm film formats are more prevalent.

The camera consists of a film magazine, a film transport mechanism and the associated optics for film exposure and identification of patient.

The film from the supply magazine is transported to the exposure position (film stage) by the film transport mechanism which is motor driven. During the exposure, the output image from the intensifier tube is directed through the objective lens-mirror combination onto the film. At the same time, patient data and other film markings (exposure plane and consecutive exposure number) are also recorded onto the film.

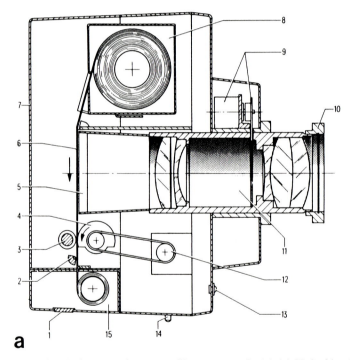

a

Figure 14:10. Functional diagram of two spot film cameras. In (a) (1) Unlocking button, (2) Film cutting knife. (3) Film pad roller. (4) Film transport (motor driven). (5) Film stage. (6) Film. (7) Cover. (8) Supply magazine. (9) Auxillary shutter. (10) Rapid connection flange. (11) Objective. (12) Counter mechanism drive. (13) Pilot lamps. (14) Film transport button. (15) Take-up magazine. (courtesy of the Siemens Corporation.)

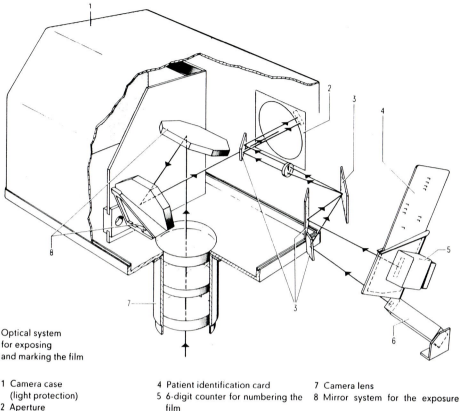

Optical system
for exposing
and marking the film

1 Camera case
  (light protection)
2 Aperture
3 Mirror and lens system for marking the film

4 Patient identification card
5 6-digit counter for numbering the
  film
6 2-digit counter
  (exposures per patient)

7 Camera lens
8 Mirror system for the exposure

b

Image Distribution

The spotfilm camera is optically coupled to the x-ray image intensifier tube by means of an *image distributor*, as is illustrated in Figure 14:11. The image distributor ensures that the camera records the image from the output screen of the intensifier tube. This is done by using a system of lens-mirror combination for splitting the light beam from the intensifier tube. The beam splitter usually transmits about 90 percent of the light to the film camera (either the spotfilm camera or cine camera) and the remaining 10 percent to the television camera. In Figure 14:12, the spotfilm camera is shown coupled to the image intensifier tube.

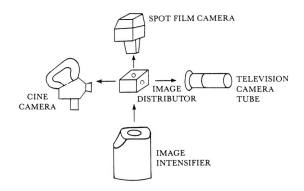

Figure 14:11. The image distributor splits the light from the image intensifier output screen such that the camera used for recording (either the spot film camera or cine camera) receives about 90 percent of the light, with the remaining 10 percent transmitted to the television camera tube.

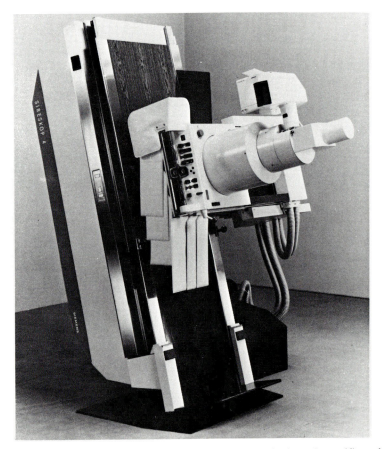

Figure 14:12. The spot film camera (top-right) is coupled to the imge intensifier tube via the image distributor. (courtesy of the Siemens Corporation.)

Advantages

The advantages of spotfilm camera imaging are several and include:

(a) Low radiation doses, since the image is recorded off the intensifier tube (low tube currents are used in intensified fluoroscopy) and there is no switching from fluoroscopic to radiographic exposure factors as is the case with cassette-loaded spotfilm recording (to be discussed subsequently).

(b) The low doses permit the use of small focal spots with short exposure times. This reduces geometric and kinetic blurring and ensures optimum image quality (good detail).

(c) Efficient operation and time savings. Since the camera supply and take-up magazines have a large capacity, there are no errors in changing films (as is the case with cassette-loaded spotfilm recording). Patients can be examined very quickly and the staff are involved in less work.

(d) Correct exposures. Automatic exposure ensures uniform image quality. Consider Figure 14:13 which illustrates the principle of the Sircam spotfilm camera recording method (a Siemens unit). In this unit, the kVp and mA set by the Vidomatic® (automatic dose rate control system) during fluoroscopy are converted automatically by the Sircamatic control system into optimum exposure values for the film. The Iontomat® is an automatic exposure timer which limits the time for the exposure of the film.

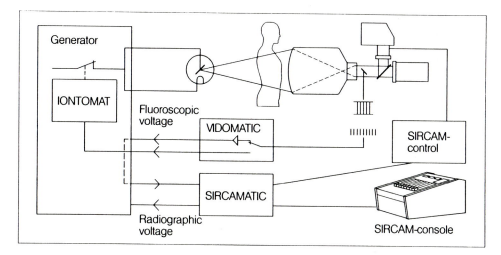

Figure 14:13. The principle of automatic exposure in the spot film technique based on the SIRCAM® (Siemens) spot film camera recording. See text for further explanation. (courtesy of the Siemens Corporation.)

(e) The high exposure rate (up to 6 frames per second) which can be achieved with spotfilm camera recording not only makes the technique suitable for use in gastrointestinal examinations but also in angiocardiography, coronary augiography, urology, pediatric imaging, and in the operating room.

Cinefluorography

Cinefluorography is a method of x-ray cinematography whereby the image from the output screen of the intensifier tube is photographed on 16-mm or 35-mm film (Table 14:2) using a cine camera. The cine camera is optically coupled via the image distributor (Figure 14:11) to the image intensifier tube so that it receives the image from the output screen.

Table 14-2

BASIC FEATURES OF 16 mm AND 35 mm CINEFLUOROGRAPHIC FILM

Film	Width of Frame	Length of Frame	Number of Frames per Foot	Remarks
16 mm	10.5 mm	7.5 mm	40	Less expensive. Easier to project.
35 mm	22 mm	18 mm	16	Greater image quality.

The main elements of a cinefluorographic imaging system are:

(a) A cine camera with suitable film.
(b) Synchronization of film movement with x-ray production.
(c) A cine film projector.

The Camera and Framing Methods

The camera is an integral part of the cinefluorographic system. It is essentially the same as that used for professional or "home" movies. The camera is an optical device which uses a converging lens system to collect the light from the output screen of the image intensifier tube and to focus it onto the film.

A typical cine camera is shown in Figure 14:14. Apart from the lens system, it features a film magazine, a pressure plate and a shutter.

The *speed* of the lens is given by the f-number and refers to the time obtained for an adequate exposure. The *f-number* is defined as the ratio of the focal length of the lens to the diameter of the lens opening. The lens opening is re-

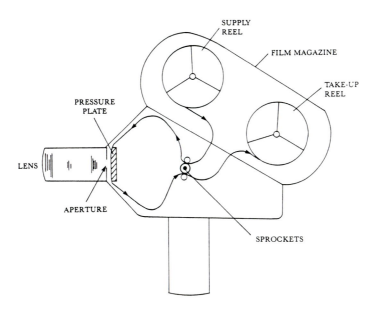

Figure 14:14. Schematic illustration of a typical cine camera. The threaded path of the film is shown and the direction of film movement is indicated by the arrows.

ferred to as the *aperture* and its function is to permit light to enter the camera. An f-number of 2.5 simply means that the aperture of the lens is two-fifths of the focal length. A lens with such a large aperture (smaller f-number) is relatively fast since it allows a great amount of light into the camera. A lens with a smaller aperture (larger f-number) allows less light into the camera.

The *shutter* controls the exposure by rotating in between the aperture and the lens, thus admitting light only for a prescribed time. When the shutter covers the aperture, the film is advanced by means of a *pull-down mechanism* which fits into the perforations on the film. The pull-down mechanism also permits intermittent movement of the film. When the aperture is uncovered by the shutter, the film advances so that other frames may be exposed.

The *pressure plate* holds the film flat and firm in order to avoid image blurring due to motion as the film passes the aperture.

In preparing the camera for use, the magazine must first be loaded. This can be done in the darkroom or in subdued light, depending on the type of film. The pressure plate is then opened and the film is positioned between the aperture and pressure plate, with the pull-down mechanism inserted into one of the perforations on the edge of the film. The film is then threaded in between sprockets (which move it through the camera at a constant rate) to form upper and lower loops (Figure 14:14). These loops are important, since they facilitate intermittent movement of the film through the *film gate* (aperture and pressure plate assembly) so that individual frames can be exposed. Before using the camera, it is recommended that the technologist run the camera to observe that the loops and the threaded path of the film are maintained.

Exposure rates (frames per second or framing frequency) for cine cameras may vary from camera to camera and range from 8 to 64 frames per second (fps). The coverage of a certain area on the film is referred to as *framing*. In general, three types of framing methods are of concern in cinefluorography. The first is *underframing*, in which case the diameter of the circular fluoroscopic image is smaller than the width of the frame. The second is *exact framing*, where the diameter of the fluoroscopic image is exactly the same as the width of frame. In the third method of framing, *overframing*, the diameter of the fluoroscopic image is larger than the width of the frame.

In exact framing, no portion of the image is lost, while in overframing, portions of the image are lost.

Framing considerations are important, since the framing method influences the patient exposure dose and the size of the image. If proper collimation schemes are not maintained, the radiation dose can be high for different framing methods, since the area of the patient exposed may be different than the area exposed on the film. For example, with exact framing no portion of the image is lost, but the field size is about 1.3 times as large as the image intensifier input screen. The patient therefore receives excess radiation not incident on the image intensifier (if a square or rectangular field size is used). For overframing, the area of the patient exposed is about 2.1 times greater than the area exposed on the film (Christensen, Curry and Dowdey, 1978).

The framing method also determines the size of the image on the film which is related to the magnification due to the lens system. In general, image size increases as framing increases and as the image intensifier tube increases (in size), the size of the recorded image decreases.

Cine Film

It is important to use the correct film for cinefluorography to maintain optimum image quality. The film camera records the image from the output screen of the image intensifier tube and, therefore, it is useful to consider the light emission from the screen, since the film must be compatible with the light emission.

The emission is yellow-green, and, hence, the film must be chosen to accommodate the range of wavelengths in this region. In this respect, both *orthochromatic* (sensitive to green, yellow and blue) and *panchromatic* (sensitive to red, orange, yellow, green, blue and violet) films are used.

Cine films must also have a wide exposure latitude and low contrast.

The camera unit and film are important tools in cinefluorography. The camera must be checked regularly to ensure that it is free from dust and other particles and that its components are in perfect working condition.

Synchronization

In cinefluorography, the film is exposed only when the shutter is opened and therefore it seems reasonable to produce x-rays only when the camera shutter is opened and not when it is closed. This can be accomplished by *synchronization,* a concept which is associated with the following:

(a) A method whereby x-rays are produced only when the film is stationary and the camera shutter is opened.

(b) Movement of the film is constant such that each frame receives the same amount of x-rays.

A non-synchronized cinefluorographic unit generates x-rays continuously whether the camera shutter is opened or closed. This method is referred to as *non-pulsed cinefluorography* and it has become obsolete for the following reasons:

(a) Unnecessary exposure of the patient.

(b) Unnecessary loading of the x-ray tube during the time the camera shutter is closed.

(c) Frames of the film may be unequally exposed, especially in full-wave rectified units where short exposure times are used.

In *synchronized* cinefluorographic units, the exposure is synchronized with the opening of the shutter. This method is referred to as *pulsed cinefluorography.*

There are at least three methods of pulsed cinefluorography, but only the most recent one will be described here. Pulsed cinefluorograpy using the grid-controlled x-ray tube is shown in Figure 14:15. The cine camera consists of a synchronizing commutator which controls the cine pulse attachment. When the grid of the x-ray tube is at a negative potential, electron emission is blocked (no elections flow towards the target) and no x-rays can be produced. The apparatus is so arranged that when the shutter is opened, the grid voltage is removed and electrons can flow again to strike the target and to produce x-rays.

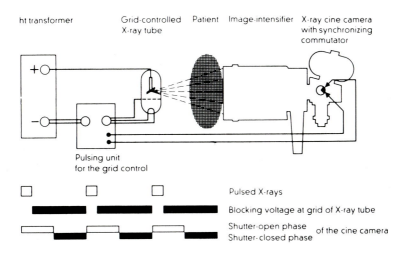

Figure 14:15. The principle of pulsed cinefluorography using a grid-controlled x-ray tube. (courtesy of the Siemens Corporation.)

Pulsed cinefluorography is an extremely useful technique in clinical x-ray imaging since:

  (a) it reduces radiation exposures to the patient by about 50 percent compared to non-pulsed units.
  (b) it reduces the tube loading because the tube is not subject to such loading during the shutter-closed phase of camera operation.
  (c) it increases image sharpness due to the very short exposure times made possible with the grid-controlled x-ray tube.
  (d) the frame speed can be changed during the cine series.

Radiation Dose Considerations

A number of factors influence the dose in cinefluorography and the following formula, which may be used to calculate doses in cinefluorograpy, illustrates this:

$$D = K \frac{I \times T \times V^n}{d^2}$$

where D = dose (r)
  I = tube current (mA)
  T = exposure time (seconds)
  V = potential difference (kV)
  d = distance (from focus to the point where the dose is measured)
  n = 2.

The precise value of n is related to other factors such as filtration (inherent and added), the range of the voltage used, and the type of rectification. Yet, other factors that must be considered include the type of film, filming speed, processing, type of camera, and the speed of the lens.

In general, synchronization, framing frequency and the f-number are considered the more important factors in terms of dose. Synchronization reduces the dose by about 50 percent. As the number of frames per second (framing frequency) increases, the dose increases proportionately. Since the f-number determines the speed of the lens and the amount of light incident on the film, it is recommended that for optimum results the aperture be set at two f-numbers below the maximum aperture setting (Christensen, Curry and Dowdey, 1978).

Summary of Components

A cinefluorographic x-ray unit is complex in design and function. There are numerous components and factors which must be considered when using this method of x-ray imaging. These elements include synchronization, framing, the camera and its components, the film, and radiation dose considerations.

Rapid Serial Radiography

Rapid serial radiography or *cineradiography,* as it is sometimes referred to, are two terms used to descirbe a method of dynamic recording whereby a series of images are acquired at rapid rates in order to study physiologic phenomena. The term cineradiography is used in this context because the effect of motion may be observed if these images are projected by a movie projector. In practice, no such projectors exist, since large-film formats (for example, 35 cm × 35 cm) are used. The observer must therefore view the images and adapt his visual perception to study the motion effect and physiologic phenomena.

The first rapid serial radiographic equipment was described by Howard Ruggles in December 1925. In 1929, H. Jarre designed a similar concept which was used in the study of certain physiologic phenomena such as spasm of the tracheobronchial tree. In Table 14:3, other developments in the history of rapid serial radiographic equipment are summarized.

Table 14-3

SOME DEVELOPMENTS IN THE HISTORY OF RAPID SERIAL
RADIOGRAPHIC EQUIPMENT

PERIOD	INVENTOR	RAPID SERIAL CONCEPT
1934	P. Caldas	Rapid cassette changer.
1934	E. Moniz	Escamoteur (manually-operated cassette changer).
1938	Vande Maele	Rapid film changer using perforated roll film.
1942	Sussman and others	Rotating wheel cassette mechanism.
1943	Sanchez-Perez and Carter	Motor-driven cassette changer with collecting tray.
1949	Gidlund	Roll-film changer.
1953	Rigler and Watson	Roll-film changer.

Principles and Equipment

Two categories of equipment for rapid serial radiography exist and they are:

(a) film changers
(b) cassette changers

A basic scheme common to both types of these imaging devices is shown in Figure 14:16. The scheme consists of an exposure area, a storage area for unexposed films (or cassettes with film), a storage section for exposed films and/or cassettes, and transport mechanism.

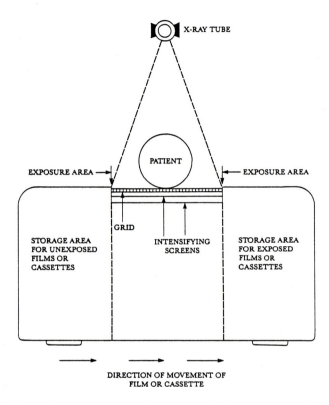

Figure 14:16. Schematic representation of an automatic film or cassette changer for cineradiography.

The fundamental principles of rapid serial radiography involve a critical timing of film movement out of the storage section into the exposure area and out of the area into the receiving magazine (film cycle). Another critical time period involves a signal to the x-ray generator to indicate when the exposure should be made. This signal orginates from the film or cassette changer once the exposure switch is activated.

The *timing cycle* of film changers includes the *zero time* and the *phasing-in time*. When the x-ray generator receives the signal from the changer, there is a short time delay before the exposure. The fraction of this delay time which is constant (characteristic of all serial changers and is due to the time taken to close relays and so on) is referred to as the zero time. The zero time is also referred to as the *anticipation time*, since the actual exposure can be determined beforehand by the exposure switch. In three-phase x-ray units, the zero time is extremely short and is therefore negligible.

The phasing-in time is related to the phasing of the power cycle (AC current) and the time in which the changer sends a signal to the x-ray generator to start the exposure. The phasing-in time is variable and is important in cases where the maximum permissible exposure time has to be calculated by the radiologist or technologist. The maximum permissible exposure time is related to the filming rate (exposure rate — up to 12 per second) of the changer. If the filming rate is increased, then the maximum permissible exposure time will be shorter.

In the past, cassette changers for rapid serial radiography were used, but, because of certain problems imposed by the mechanics of the system, film changers have gained popularity and have become commonplace in angiographic studies.

Several types of film changers are available commercially (the *AOT*, which means "*angio-t*able," is a cut-film changer, the *PUCK* film changer is a cut-film unit, the *ELEMA* roll-film changer, the *Franklin* roll-film changer, and so on).

The Puck film changer is shown in Figure 14:17a and is illustrated in Figure 14:17b. It is a light-weight cut-film changer capable of holding about 20 films (35 cm × 35 cm or 24 cm × 30 cm) with an exposure frequency of 3 exposures per second.

It consists essentailly of a film changer, a loading magazine, a receiving magazine and a program selector. The film changer is controlled by the program selector and a hand switch. The exposure area consists of an upper exposure plate which is made up of a carbon-fibre-reinforced resin (high strength and low x-ray absorption material compared to aluminum), intensifying screens and a pressure table which provides good screen/film contact.

The program selector with punch card operation (Figure 14:18) coordinates the desired exposure sequence to release the injection of contrast media (via the injector) and forward and reverse tabletop motion.

The punch card is used to determine the number of films in a series and the exposure program. It has a maximum range of 20 seconds and is prepared by the operator who selects the programming by pressing out prepared holes using a stylus.

A typical layout of the equipment for rapid serial radiography is shown in Figure 14:19. Although this figure only illustrates the concept of *single-plane operation* (one film changer to image the patient in anterior-posterior or vice-versa position), *bi-plane operation* is commonplace in angiography. In bi-plane angiography, two film changers are used simultaneously to image the patient in both the anterior-posterior and lateral positions. Figure 14:20 shows examples of the use of the film changer in rapid serial radiography.

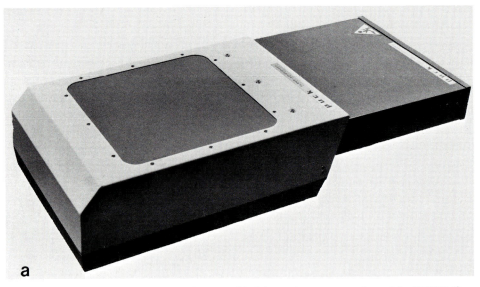

Figure 14:17. (a) The PUCK film changer: (b) Schematic representation of the PUCK film changer. (courtesy of the Siemens Corporation.)

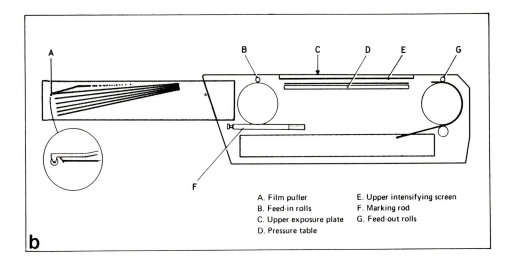

A. Film puller   E. Upper intensifying screen
B. Feed-in rolls   F. Marking rod
C. Upper exposure plate G. Feed-out rolls
D. Pressure table

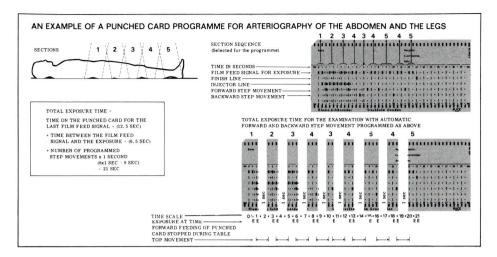

Figure 14:18. The program selector with punch card operation (courtesy of the Siemens Corporation.)

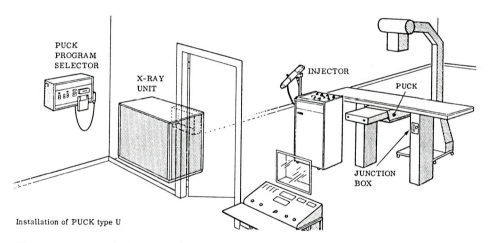

Figure 14:19. Typical layout of equipment for rapid serial radiography. (courtesy of the Siemens Corporation.)

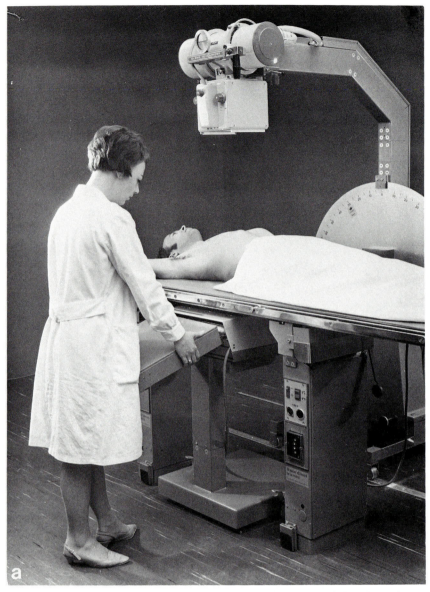

Figure 14:20. The clinical use of the PUCK film changer for rapid serial radiography. (courtesy of the Siemens Corporation.)

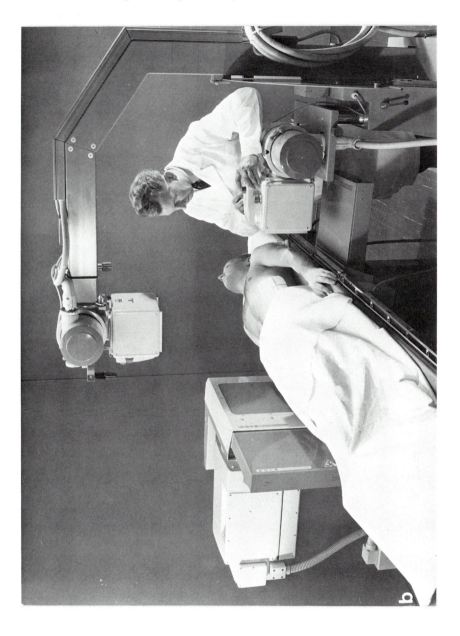

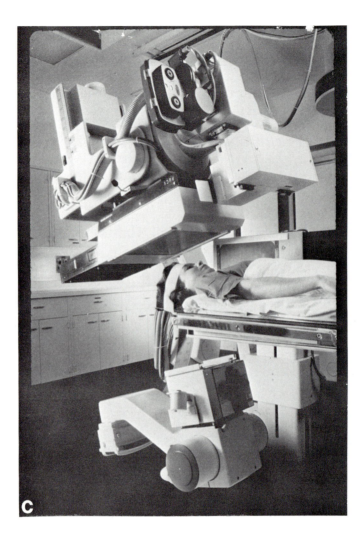

Large-Field Serial Radiography

The size of the exposure field for the method of rapid serial radiography discussed previously is usually 35 cm × 35 cm, since the typical film size is 35 cm × 35 cm.

Large-field serial radiography is a technique which is used to image the femoral-popliteal arterial system. A characteristic feature of large-field serial radiography is an exposure field larger than 35 cm × 35 cm. Such a field provides radiographs which cover an area from the lower abdomen to the lower limbs.

In this technique exposures are made in rapid sequence, and, to maintain optimum results, certain requirements must be met. These are:

1. A long source-to-image distance since this ensures a large exposure field coverage. A minimum of 182 cm is recommended to ensure a

field coverage of 35 cm × 129 cm. To obtain this distance, the x-ray tube is usually mounted onto a fixed ceiling support or to a ceiling flange.

2. Special long cassettes with dimensions such as 35 cm × 129 cm. In cases where this film size is not available, three 35-cm × 43-cm films are loaded into the cassettes.

3. An asymmetrical beam-limiting device to ensure that the primary beam is restricted only to the surface area of the cassette (a rectangular field).

4. Suitable methods to obtain uniform radiographic density and optimum contrast, since the part being imaged varies in thickness (abdomen, thighs, lower limbs). These methods include:

   (a) The anode heel effect. The patient's feet are always placed towards the anode end of the x-ray tube.

   (b) Special film/screen combinations of high and medium speed at the abdominal and thigh regions, respectively.

   (c) A graduated or compensating filter affixed to the asymmetrical beam-limiting device. In most cases a graduated filter made of three wedges of aluminum is used, where the largest wedge is positioned towards the patient's feet.

5. Automatic cassette changers. An example of a rapid serial cassette changer is shown in Figure 14:21. This prototype uses five 35-cm × 129-cm cassettes which are stacked and protected so that both exposed

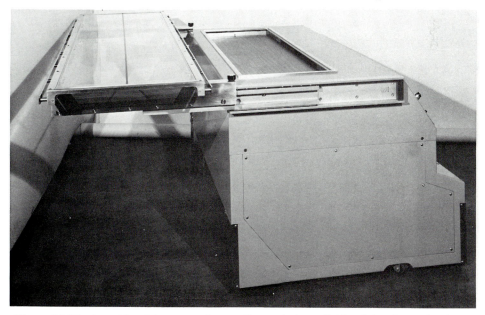

Figure 14:21. A rapid serial cassette changer for use in large field serial radiography. (courtesy of B.C. Medical, Montreal, Canada.)

and unexposed cassettes are not affected by the radiation beam during the examination. In this unit, the cassettes are exposed at the same source-to-image distance. This concept eliminates any magnification effect.

Step-Wise Shifting of the Tabletop in Combined Angiography of the Abdomen and Legs

In modern rapid serial imaging, film changers are the most prevalent method used in angiography. A method referred to as *step-wise shifting of the tabletop* (Figure 14:22) has become common in this practice.

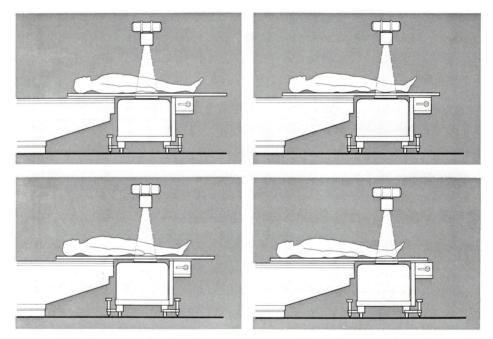

Figure 14:22. The principle of combined angiography of the abdomen and lower limbs with stepwise shifting of the table top. (courtesy of the Siemens Corporation.)

In this method, the tabletop is shifted step-wise by a moter-drive mechanism. The direction of motion of the tabletop is such that it is always in the opposite direction to the flow of contrast media.

The apparatus includes film changer and an exposure number/step selector which allows the technologist to preselect the number of images to be recorded on each body region. An example of a radiographic program of this type is given in Figure 14:23. In this program, two films are taken at 0.8 sec and 1.1 sec after the start of the injection, at Step I. At Step II, two more films are taken at 4.4 sec and 5.8 sec after the start of the injection. At Step III, four

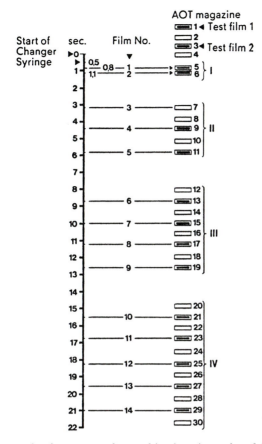

Figure 14:23. An example of a program for combined angiography of the abdomen and legs with step-wise shifting of the tabletop. See text for further explanation. (courtesy of the Siemens Corporation.)

films are taken at 8.8 sec, 10 sec and 12.2 sec after the start of the injection, and so on. At the end of the series, 14 films would have been taken in 21 sec after the start of the injection.

During the procedure, as the patient is shifted, the tube voltage (kVp) is automatically reduced to compensate for the variation in thickness of the body regions.

STATIC RECORDING

The recording of fixed radiographic images on magnetic or non-magnetic (for example, film) material which are not separated by very short time intervals is defined as *static recording*.

The most popular method of static recording is conventional radiograpy in which a film or film/screen combination is used in conjunction with the Bucky mechanism.

Table 14-4

COMPARISON OF FOUR X-RAY IMAGE RECORDING SYSTEMS

(From Rich, J. E., Television in the Radiology Department. The General Electric Company, 1969.)

	DYNAMIC RECORDING		SPOT RECORDING	
	CINE	VTR	SPOT FILM	VDR
Recording Time (1)	108 sec	1 hour	Single exposure	20 sec
Maximum Frame Rate	60-120/sec	30/sec	1/sec	30 sec
X-ray mA (2)	10	3.5	200	3.5
Processing Time	1 hour	Instant	90/sec	Instant
Library Storage	Easy	Possible	Easy	Difficult
Reusability	$22,000 (3)	$23,000	$4,000	$27,000 (4)
Relative Resolution	2	4	1	2

(1) At maximum frame rate.
(2) Normalized for equal kVp and exposure time.
(3) Includes image intensifier.
(4) Includes image intensifier, television camera/monitor.

The other method of spotfilm recording is accomplished with the spotfilm device, typical of some fluoroscopic units (Chapter 3). Such a device uses a large-format film on which one (full spot) or several different (coned spots) spot exposures are recorded by switching from fluoroscopic to radiographic factors. This technique is referred to as *conventional spotfilm recording* or the cassette-loaded spotfilm technique. It provides high-quality images and uses more radiation compared to spotfilm camera recording.

Other methods of static recording include spotfilm camera recording of single exposures and videodisk recording of single images. In the former, the method of recording is the same as previously described, except in this case the camera records only single images which are not obtained by rapid-sequence exposures. In the latter, the principle of recording is the same as previously described except only single images are stored. These images are not obtained by the rapid-sequence exposure concept and therefore the images are not separated by very short time intervals. The effect of motion cannot be perceived if these single images (obtained by static recording) are projected by a suitable projector.

COMPARISON OF IMAGE RECORDING METHODS

Comparing different image recording methods is an extremely difficult task, because there are several factors which must be taken into consideration in order to present a reasonable comparison.

Rich (1969) gives a comparison of cine, videotape, spotfilm and videodisk recording systems in which he examines several significant parameters of each. These are summarized in Table 14:4.

RESEARCH STUDIES

Image Quality Comparison — 105-mm spotfilm and cassette-loaded spotfilm.

STUDY 1. Comparison of Image Quality of 105-mm film with Conventional film. Skucas, J., and Gorski, J.W. Radiology, 118:433-437, February, 1976.

In this study, the researchers compared the quality of the images obtained with a 105-mm spotfilm camera and the cassette-loaded spotfilm technique (fluoroscopy with spotfilm device). They found that:

> The contrast, resolution, geometric and motion unsharpness, mottle and overall impression of 105 mm film were compared to these qualities in conventional spotfilm. It is believed that conventional filming is superior for low contrast objects and cooperative patients whereas with uncooperative, obese patients, the 105 mm filming modality would decrease motion unsharpness.

Radiation Dose — 100-mm spotfilm vs. Full-Scale Radiography

STUDY 2. Radiation Dose in Hysterosalpingography: Modern 100-mm Fluorography vs. Full-Scale Radiography. Seppanen, S., Lehtinen, E., and Holli, H. Radiology, 127:377-380, May, 1978.

In this study, the researchers' overall objective was "to determine comparative radiation doses of modern 100 mm fluorography and full-scale radiography with special reference to hysterosalpingograpy."

The basic equipment for this study involved the use of automatic density control, a CsI image intensifier tube, a 625-line TV system with a 2.5 cm vidicon tube, a 100-mm spotfilm camera with a maximum speed of 3 exposures per second and CRONEX SF2 (Dupont) film for fluorography. On the other hand, the full-scale radiography method utilized Type 2R film (3M) with Ilford fast tungstate intensifying screens.

In their abstract, the authors' state:

Radiation doses of modern 100 mm fluorography and full-scale radiography were compared experimentally and applied to hysterosalipingography. It was determined that 100 mm fluorography reduced the doses by 28-29½ per exposure and 37-47½ per examination compared with full-scale radiography performed with fast tungstate screens in identical conditions (70-80 kV, 400 mA). The dose during one minute of videofluoroscopy was equivalent to the doses produced by one exposure in full-scale filming and three to four exposures in 100 mm filming. Although electronic magnification in 100 mm fluorography increases the doses by two or threefold, these are still less than the doses in full-scale radiography.

SUMMARY

1. Image recording encompasses a variety of methods which range from non-screen film, the use of screen/film combination (static recording) to dynamic recording.
2. Dynamic recording includes techniques such as videotape and videodisk recording, cineradiography (serial exposures), cinefluorography and spotfilm methods using serial exposures.
3. Videotape recording is a magnetic recording process acomplished by a videotape recorder. The characteristic features of the recorder are its ability to provide optimum image qualtiy, reliabiltiy, simple and logical operation, and endless loop, stationary image and slow-motion, sound dubbing and automatic tape stop. A short description of each of these is given.
4. Two essential components of the recorder are the magnetic tape and recording head. The tape consists of magnetizable particles, while the recording head (video head) is a circular or rectangular iron core with a very narrow gap between its poles.
5. In recording information on the tape, the signal from the television camera tube produces a varying magnetic field across the gap of the videohead. As the tape passes the gap, it is magnetized depending on the strength of the magnetic field at the gap.
6. In playback, the magnetized tape passes the gap to induce a magnetic field which in turn induces a varying elecrtrical current in the coil of the videohead.
7. Synchronization is necessary in videotape recording to ensure that only one television field is recorded for one rotation of the videohead and that the same tracks are scanned during recording and playback.
8. The advantages of videotape recording are listed.
9. For storage of videotape, the environment must be dust-free and maintained at the proper temperature and humidity. The tape should also be stored on its edge and be shielded from strong magnetic fields.
10. Videodisk recording can be done using magnetic videodisks and laser videodisks. Magnetic videodisks are video memory devices similar to

a phonograph record. The disk is coated with magnetizable particles which are read by a stationary read/write videohead. The principles of recording are similar to videotape recording.

11. Laser videodisk recording is a non-magnetic recording technique in which information is stored in a series of microscopic depressions cut into a disk similar to a phonograph record. During operation, a laser light reads the depressions on the disk. The light is then reflected back to a photodiode which produces a video signal.

12. Videodisk recording may be used in the operating room and in general radiography to reduce patient doses.

13. Spotfilm recording of serial exposures requires a spotfilm camera. The film camera consists of an optical system which captures the image from an image distribution system.

14. The image distributor ensures that the light from the output screen of the imge intensifier tube is distributed to the television camera tube and the film camera. Usually, 10 percent of the light is directed to the camera tube, while the remainder (90½) goes to the film camera.

15. The advantages of spotfilm recording are listed.

16. Cinefluorography is x-ray cinematography where the image from the output screen of the intensifier tube is recorded by a cine camera which is coupled to the image distributor.

17. The cine camera is an optical device which uses a converging lens system to capture the light from the intensifier tube. The speed of the lens is given by the f-number, while the lens opening is the aperture. The shutter controls the exposure.

18. The coverage of the film is referred to as framing. Three framing methods — under framing, exact framing, and over framing — are discussed.

19. Cine film must be compatible with the light emission from the image intensifier tube, and in this regard both orthochromatic and panchromatic films are used.

20. Synchronization in cinefluorography is important. This method (pulsed cinefluorography) ensures that the exposure and the opening of the camera shutter are synchronized to prevent unnecessary exposure of the patient, unnecessary tube loading and unequal exposure of film frames.

21. Radiation dose in cinefluorography is discussed in terms of synchronization, framing frequency and the f-number.

22. Rapid serial radiography or cineradiography is essentially a dynamic recording process. Two classes of equipment are described: film changers and cassette changers. These changers are based on cirtical timing of film movement during recording. The timing cycle is discussed in terms of the zero time and the phasing-in time.

23. Large-field serial radiography is a technique which utilizes an exposure field larger than 35 cm × 35 cm. This technique requires a long source-to-image receptor distance, special long cassettes, an asymmetrical beam-limiting device and suitable methods to obtain uniform film density and contrast.

24. Static recording refers to a process of recording fixed radiographic images on magnetic or non-magnetic material which are not separated by very short time intervals.

25. The most popular methods of static recording, conventional film or film/screen methods and spotfilm recording of single exposures on large-format film are described. Another method, videodisk recording of single images, is also described.

26. A comparison of the different image recording methods is given in table form.

27. The results of two research studies on image quality comparison (105-mm spotfilm and cassette-loaded spotfilm) and radiation dose (100-mm spotfilm vs. full-sclae radiography) are given.

Part B

DIGITAL IMAGING TECHNOLOGY

Section C

DIGITAL IMAGE PROCESSING
AND COMPUTERS

CHAPTER 15

DIGITAL IMAGE PROCESSING

HISTORY

THE history of processing images by a digital computer (digital image processing) goes back several decades and its developement continues to attract attention in a number of areas.

Digital image processing may be regarded as an interdisciplinary subject since it revolves around physics, mathematics, engineering and computer science. It therefore has a wide spectrum of applications, for example, it has been applied to problems in physics, biology, anatomy and physiology, weather forecasting, electron microscopy, criminology, industrial radiography and space studies.

Digital image processing had significant developments at the Jet Propulsion

Laboratory of the California Institute of Technology where it was used in space studies involving the challenge to put a man on the moon. The images that were sent back from unmanned space craft such as *Ranger, Surveyor* and *Mariner* were all subject to digital image processing techniques. The processing of the poor and degraded images that were sent back not only enhanced them but restored them as well.

In general, the use of digital image processing in the space program has had a significant impact on applications in other fields. More recently, digital image processing has found widespread applications in medicine and particularly diagnostic imaging, where it has been applied successfully in techniques such as computed tomography, digital radiography, magnetic resonance imaging, nuclear medicine and ultrasound.

The increasing interest in digital image processing is primarily attributed to advances in micro-electronic technology and complex mathematics that can be carried out by a digital computer which has become more affordable.

IMAGE REPRESENTATION

Analog Images

To understand digital image processing, it is important to realize that an image can be represented in a number of ways. Images can also be formed in several ways.

In photography, the image of an object is formed by focussing light rays on film. The film is then processed in specific chemical solutions to render the image visible. In radiography, when a beam of x-rays passes through a patient, the transmitted x-rays (the x-ray image) are projected onto x-ray film. The film is then processed in chemical solutions to render it visible.

The two examples just given are images formed by the *photochemical process*. Other examples of *visible images* are pictures such as paintings, drawings and optical images (formed by lenses and lasers). Images can also be formed by *photoelectronic* means. In this process the images can be represented as electrical signals.

Last but not least, images can also be represented as mathematical functions and by non-visible means, such as temperature and pressure.

The images discussed so far are *analog* in form. This means that the information is continuously available in comparison to information which is available in discrete units, such as pulses. The popular sine wave is a classical representation of an analog signal. It varies continuously with time.

Digital Images

Digital image processing makes use of a digital computer so that any data going into the computer must first be converted into *digital form* (numbers).

Therefore, analog information (analog images) must be changed into digital information which the computer can use to process the data (Figure 15:1). This type of conversion is referred to as *analog-to-digital conversion* and it requires the use of an analog-to-digital converter (ADC). This will be discussed subsequently.

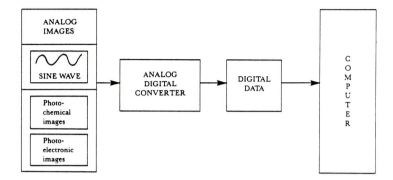

Figure 15:1. Block diagram of the conversion of analog information to digital data for input into a digital computer.

The computer then performs the necessary processing on the digital data and may display the results in digital form (that is, as a digital image) as shown in Figure 15:2.

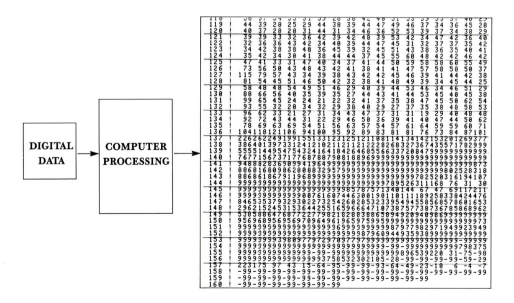

Figure 15:2. Data may be displayed in digital form.

DEFINITION OF DIGITAL IMAGE PROCESSING

From the previous discussion, a formal basic definition of digital image processing can be given. *Digital image processing* is a technique whereby digital information (numerical data) is fed into a computer which performs specific operations (processing) on the data to generate images that may serve a more useful purpose.

By definition then, digital image processing has a number of advantages, since the computer-processed information can be manipulated in a number of ways to provide benefits with respect to image synthesis, image enhancement, storage and display.

STEPS IN DIGITIZING AN IMAGE

Scanning

How can the images formed by photochemical and photoelectronic means be converted into digital data? Consider an image formed by the photochemical process, a transparency (slide), for example. The first step in digitizing the picture involves dividing it up into an array of small regions. This process is known as *scanning* and it is illustrated in Figure 15:3. Each small region in the picture is referred to as a *pixel,* a contraction for *picture element.*

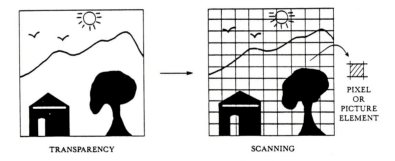

Figure 15:3. The process of scanning in digitizing an image. The transparency (picture) is divided up into a large number of picture elements or pixels.

Sampling

The next step involves a process called *sampling.* In sampling, the brightness of each pixel is measured by using special devices, such as a photomultiplier tube. In an example given by Cannon and Hunt (1981), a small spot of light projected onto a transparency passes through it and is detected by a photomultiplier tube. The transmitted light intensity is converted into electrical impulses by the photomultiplier tube and these impulses are compared with the signal obtained when no slide is in the path of the original light. This process is sampling, where the relative brightness at each pixel is sampled or measured. This is illustrated in Figure 15:4. The process of sampling is done for the entire image.

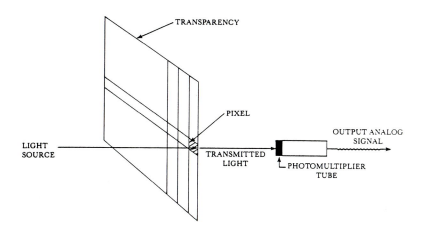

Figure 15:4. The process of image sampling. The brightness at each pixel location is measured with the aid of a photomultiplier tube or other suitable device.

Quantization

The third and final step in digitizing an image is *quantization*. Since the brightness values obtained during sampling are still analog signals, they must be converted into digital information before they can be fed into the computer. Quantization is a process whereby each brightness value is assigned a discrete number (0, a positive or a negative number) called a *gray level*. An image would therefore be made up of a range of numbers or gray levels. The total number of gray levels is called the *gray scale*. Figure 15:5 shows the process of quantization resulting in a four-level gray scale.

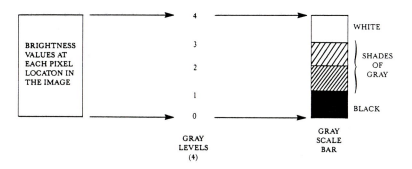

Figure 15:5. The process of quantization. Each measured brightness value is assigned an integer (0, + or - number) called a gray level. The gray levels can be transformed into a gray scale.

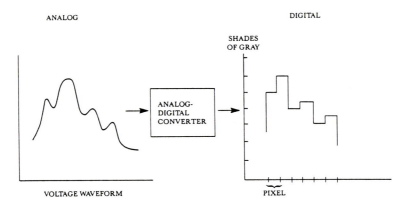

Figure 15:6. Analog-to-digital conversion. The continuous voltage waveform (left) is converted into a discrete or digital representation (right) by the ADC.

An image can have 2, 4, 8, 16, 32, 64, and so on, gray scale levels. In the case of two gray levels, the gray scale would show black and white only. In the case of 64 levels, one end of the gray scale would be black, the opposite end white, and shades of gray represented in the middle.

Analog-to-Digital Conversion

The process of analog-to-digital conversion is shown in Figure 15:6. The continuous analog signal is converted into a discrete digital representation by the analog-to-digital converter (ADC).

The faithful transformation of the analog signal to a digital signal depends on the "depth" of the ADC. This conversion is discussed in more detail in the chapter on digital radiography (Chapter 18).

An ADC with more "depth" will produce a more faithful reproduction of the original signal. The number of gray levels would also be higher. For example, a 2-bit ADC (Chapter 18) will generate $4(2^2)$ gray levels, while a 4-bit ADC will generate $16(2^4)$ gray levels. Most digital image processing systems including those used in medical imaging have at least 8-bit ADCs ($2^8 = 256$ gray levels) and 10-bit ADCs ($2^{10} = 1024$ gray levels.).

IMAGE PROCESSING OPERATIONS

The result of quantization gives an image which is now broken down into digits. These digits are then sent to the computer for processing.

The computer uses suitable programs to process the data to generate a desired result. Image processing operations include such techniques as *manipulation, restoration, enhancement* and *analysis*.

Image manipulation refers to image magnification and windowing (Chap-

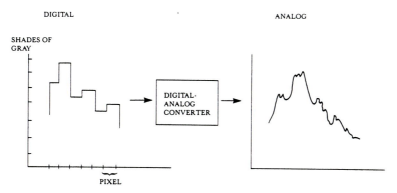

Figure 15:7. Digital-to-analog conversion. The analog signal is not reproduced faithfully as the original signal (Figure 15:6) because of a loss of detail.

ter 16). Image restoration involves algorithms to correct image noise and blurring. Image enhancement is a technique which improves the visual appearance of an image. Contrast stretching (performed on individual pixels) and weighted subtraction of image pairs are examples of image enhancement processing operations. Finally, image analysis includes those techniques which allow the operator to perform measurements (area and amplitude measurements within an image) and other quantitative analyses on the data.

It is not within the framework of this text to describe these processing operations in any great detail and therefore they will not be discussed any further.

Once processing is completed, the information can be stored onto magnetic disks or tapes or it can be displayed as a numerical printout or as an image on a television screen. In producing a television picture, it must be realized that the numerical (digital) data from the computer must be converted back to analog information.

DIGITAL-TO-ANALOG CONVERSION

The conversion of digital information to analog form is accomplished by a *digital-to-analog converter* (DAC). This conversion is illustrated in Figure 15:7. Note that the analog signal obtained is not exactly the same as the original signal (Figure 15:6). There is some loss of detail.

This analog signal goes to the television monitor (an analog device) and plays a role in generating the television picture.

CONCLUSION

In summary, digital image processing involves scanning, sampling and quantization. Essentially, scanning produces pixels or picture elements. The brightness of each pixel is measured through a process known as sampling. These brightness levels or analog signals must be converted into digital data.

This is accomplished by an apparatus known as a *quantizer* through a technique referred to as quantization, where each brightness level is assigned a numerical value. These numerical values (digital data) are then processed by the computer. Figure 15:8 shows the fundamental steps in digitizing a picture.

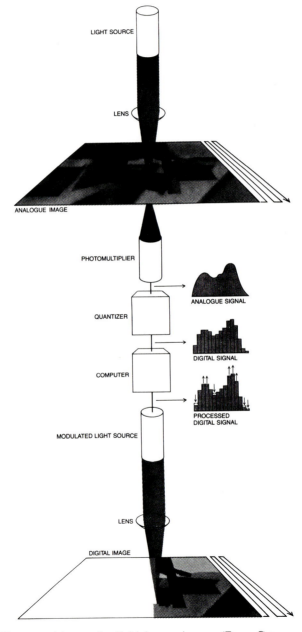

Figure 15:8. The essential steps in digitizing an image. (From Cannon, T.M. and Hunt, B.R.: Image processing by computer. *Scientific American.* October 1981.)

After computer processing, the data can either be stored in the main memory of the computer and, in this case, provide *on-line processing* as opposed to *off-line processing.* In off-line processing, data are taken from information stored on magnetic tapes and disks. On-line processing is much quicker than off-line processing.

The technology involved in digital image processing has been successful in the space program and has been extended to numerous applications which have also proven to be beneficial. Developments in computer technology have provided refinements in image processing for these applications.

Subsequent chapters will present a description of computers and focus on the imaging applications of digital image processing theory, such as in computed tomography and digital radiography.

SUMMARY

1. Digital image processing involves the use of a digital computer to process images.
2. Digital image processing was used in space studies and is still an integral part of the space program. Its success in processing images sent back from space has led to its applications in other areas such as biology and medicine.
3. Today, the technique of digital image processing has found applications in medical imaging, particularly computed tomography, ultrasound, nuclear medicine, digital radiography and magnetic resonance imaging.
4. Images can be formed by the photochemical and photoelectronic processes. Images can be represented as visible images such as a photograph or an non-visible images such as temperature and pressure. In the photoelectronic process, images can be represented as electrical signals.
5. The images formed by photochemical and photoelecronic means are analog in form, that is, they are continuous variables as opposed to discrete units such as pulses.
6. In order to process analog signals by a digital computer, they must first be converted into digital representation. This can be achieved by an analog-to-digital converter, an electronic device with complex circuitry.
7. Digital image processing is advantageous, since the computer can manipulate data to generate information that serves a more useful purpose. For imaging, the specialist can manipulate the data to give him the most beneficial results.
8. The steps in digitizing an image involve scanning, sampling and quantization.

9. In scanning, the picture is broken down into small regions called picture elements or pixels.
10. Sampling involves measuring the brightness value at each picture element location.
11. In quantization, the brightness values obtained as a result of sampling are assigned numbers. These numbers represent the gray levels which can be transformed into a gray scale bar. The final result is that the analog data are converted into digital data which are then fed into the computer for processing.
12. Image processing operations include image manipulation, restoration, enhancement and analysis.
13. After processing, the data can be stored in the computer for on-line processing which is much faster than off-line processing in which case the processed data are stored on magnetic tapes or disks.

CHAPTER 16

COMPUTER CONCEPTS — AN INTRODUCTION

COMPUTER APPLICATIONS

COMPUTERS are everywhere and their use is increasing at a rapid rate. Computers have found applications in almost every facet of human activity. They are used in business, industry, research, education, government, the

357

military, space studies, science and medicine and, finally, in the home.

More importantly and within the context of this book, computers have found increasing applications in diagnostic imaging. They are used in ultrasound and nuclear medicine, as well a in x-ray imaging such as in computed tomography and digital radiography systems. More recently, computers are used in magnetic resonance imaging techniques.

Computers have become a very significant part of our daily lives. For example, they are used in the grocery store at the checkout counter to assist in computing the cost of food as shown in Figure 16:1. Computers can process and store vast amounts of information with great speed and accuracy and, at the same time, they reduce the probability of human error. Today, computers are essential in the imaging department.

The purpose of this chapter is to introduce several concepts of computers which will enable the technologist to fully understand the role of computers in

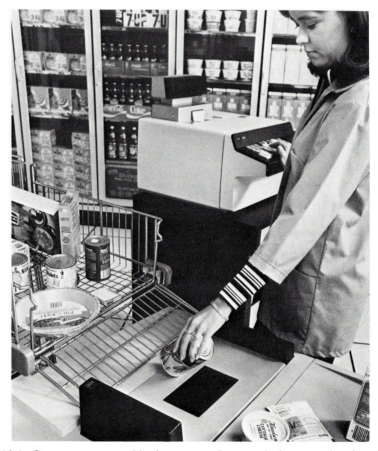

Figure 16:1. Computerss are used in the supermarket to assist in computing the cost of food and in maintaining records of inventory. (courtesy of International Business Machines Corporation.)

imaging. The chapter also introduces computer terminology to assist the reader to commence building a vocabulary necessary to understand the literature that uses the language of computer technology.

WHAT IS A COMPUTER?

A computer is a special machine for solving problems and making decisions by performing arithmetic and logical operations on data which it receives from devices that input the information to its processing unit. Once the processing is accomplished, the results can either be stored in a suitable form, in or out of the machine, or they can be displayed on output devices in a form understandable by man.

The computer can solve problems very efficiently, using a set of specific instructions (developed and outlined by man) with a great deal of speed and accuracy.

In general, a computer can be referred to as a very fast and accurate automatic computing machine.

HISTORICAL OVERVIEW

From a historical perspecitve, the computer is entering its fifth generation. The basis for this depends on definite features and components characteristic of each generation.

The first digital calculator was the *Abacus* (Figure 16:2). It operates by sliding beads on wires and found widespread use until 1642 when other computing machines such as Pascal's *arithmetic machine* and Leibnitz's (1694) calculating machine appeared. These were then followed by a host of other computers.

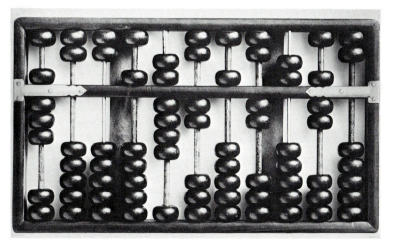

Figure 16:2. The Abacus was the first digital calculator. (courtesy of International Business Machines Corporation.)

In 1812, Charles Babbage generated the idea of an automatic computer. Babbage's machine was called a *difference engine* and was capable of automatically calculating trigonometric and logarithmic tables.

A detailed discussion of the history of computers is not practical in this text, however, the following summary is in order.

1959-1960	Second-generation computers available (solid-state devices such as transistors, smaller than first generation, less heat production and less power require-ments than first generation, reliable).
1965	Third-generation computers available (integrated circuits including magnetic cores and semiconductor, greater speed and reliability and smaller than second-generation computers).
1970	Introduction of fourth-generation, more powerful computers (advanced storage capacities [miracle chips], faster, smaller and less expensive than third-generation computers).

Today, fifth-generation computers are becoming more and more popular. These have increased storage capacities and make use of bubble memories and Josephson junctions. They can process data much faster than fourth-generation computers and miniaturization is characteristic.

TYPES OF COMPUTERS

In general, computers can be placed into two categories, namely, the analog computer and the digital computer.

An *analog computer* is one that works with data that vary continuously (for example, voltage) in time and solves problems by analogy. Physical quantities such as forces, speeds and so on can be represented in an analog computer by voltages which the computer can use to solve the problem. A good example of a simple analog computer is the *slide rule,* where length is used as the analogous quantity and distances along the rule are proportional to the logarithms of the quantities that can be represented, instead of to the quantities themselves.

A *digital computer* solves problems by counting. It operates on digital data (discrete units, such as numbers) by performing mathematical (arithmetic) and logical operations. It can perform the "four rules," namely, addition, subtraction, multiplication and division.

The remainder of this chapter will deal with the digital computer since it is commonplace in the imaging department.

DATA REPRESENTATION IN A DIGITAL COMPUTER

Since the digital computer operates on digital data, a means of representing this data appropriately is necessary. For the digital computer, the *binary number system* and other number systems are used.

The binary number system is used because most of the components in a computer (such as switches, valves, relays, transistors and semiconductors) are essentially binary, that is, they have two stable states. They can either be "on" or "off." In the binary number system there are only two ciphers (base 2), 0 and 1, as compared to the *decimal system* which has a base 10. The numbers 0 to 10 in the decimal system are represented in the binary system as follows:

Decimal	Binary
0	0
1	1
2	10
3	11
4	100
5	101
6	110
7	111
8	1000
9	1001
10	1010

These binary digits (0 and 1) are referred to as *bits* (a contraction for binary digit).

The advantage of using the binary system is that with the two-state components mentioned above, one state ("off") can be represented by a 0 and the other state ("on") can be represented as 1. Digital computers then are made up of a very large number of two-state devices which carry out operations on data by changing from one state to another in ordered groups and chains.

The binary representation of larger numbers in the decimal system can become tedious and difficult to deal with. Therefore, other number systems (hexa-decimal and octal) have been devised to represent larger binary numbers. These number systems are beyond the scope of this chapter.

THE STRUCTURE OF A COMPUTER

A computer is organized around the following essential units:

(a) Input devices
(b) A central processing unit (CPU)
(c) Storage
(d) Output devices

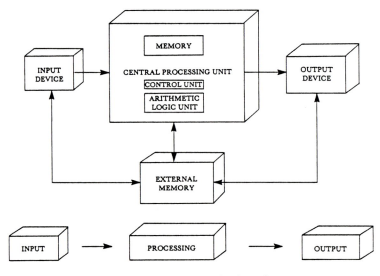

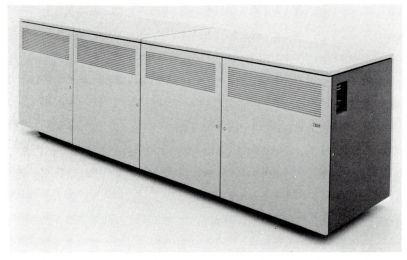

Figure 16:3. The typical organization of a computer.

Figure 16:4. The processing unit of a computer system. (courtesy of International Business Machines Corporation.)

The organization of these components is shown in Figure 16:3. The illustration also points out that computer processing involves input of information into the computer for processing followed by an output of the processed data. A processing unit is shown in Figure 16:4.

Each of the elements will now be described briefly.

Input/Output Devices

Input/output devices are often referred to as I/O devices. *Input devices* must have the capability of converting data based on the problem to be solved, into a form which is suitable for processing by the central processing unit (CPU). In a computer system, this form can be represented either as holes on cards (punched cards) and paper tape or as magnetized spots on magnetic tape and/or disks. A punched card reader is shown in Figure 16:5.

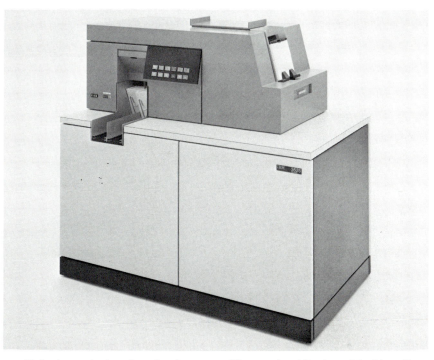

Figure 16:5. A punched card reader. (courtesy of International Business Machines Corporation.)

Input devices supply the data to the CPU for processing. Once the data are processed, the results must be displayed for interpretation by man. These results are displayed on *output devices.*

Output devices can be magnetic tape and disks, a cathode ray tube (CRT), a line printer and a plotter. If the processed information is recorded on a tape or disk, it (information) must undergo further processing before it can be displayed in visible form. Figure 16:6 shows a printer (output device), while an I/O device (CRT and keyboard) is shown in Figure 16:7.

Central Processing Unit

The CPU is the "brain" of the computer. It consists of two components: the *arithmetic/logic* unit (ALU), which performs all calculations, and the *control unit,* which coordinates the activities of the entire computer system. The CPU may also incorporate a portion of the storage or memory of the computer. The other portion of storage is usually outside the CPU.

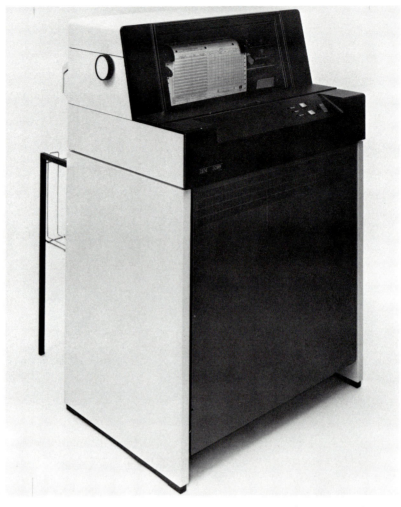

Figure 16:6. A line printer unit — an output device. (courtesy of International Business Machines Corporation.)

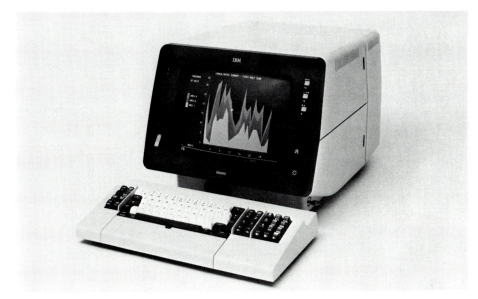

Figure 16:7. An input/output device — a CRT and associated keyboard. (courtesy of International Business Machines Corporation.)

It is clear from Figure 16:3 that there is a flow of data from I/O devices, memory or storage, to the CPU. Such flow of data is facilitated through the use of a multi-wire line called a *bus*.

Computer Storage

Storage is often referred to as the *memory* of the computer. In this chapter both terms will be used interchangeably. Computer storage are of two types: (a) main storage and (b) auxiliary storage.

In some computers the main storage is an actual part of the CPU. It is faster and more expensive than auxiliary storage. On the other hand, auxiliary storage can handle very large amounts of data compared to main storage.

Main Storage

Main storage can be of two types: magnetic core memories and semiconductor memories.

A *magnetic core memory* is made up of numerous small doughnut-shaped ferromagnetic material, where fine wires pass through each core to form a crosshatch. When a current passes through the wire, the core is magnetized, either in a clockwise direction (1) or a counterclockwise direction (0), and it is this process that results in storage.

With magnetic core memories, the information is not lost when the power supply is turned off.

Semiconductor memories are used in modern computers and they are much faster than core memories. A *semiconductor* memory is a small electronic device (transistor or diode) which functions like a switch. Again, a current flow indicates whether the switch is on (1) or off (0).

Semiconductor memories contain a vast number of tiny components arranged very neatly on a miniature chip of silicon. In this context they are referred to as *integrated circuits* (IC). A further discussion of IC technology will be given later in the chapter.

With semiconductor memories, it is necessary to have the system energized continuously in order to retain the information that they store.

More recently, other storage devices such as magnetic bubble memories have become available for use in many computers. Digital data is represented by the presence or absence of bubbles. Bubble memories ensure large storage in computers which require very little power to operate.

Auxiliary Storage

Auxiliary storage refers to storage on peripheral equipment such as magnetic drums, tapes and disks.

Magnetic disks are similar in appearance to a phonograph record, and the information is represented and stored as magnetized spots. A much smaller version of the magnetic disk is the *floppy diskette* which looks like a 45 r.p.m. phonograph record. The diskette is more suitable for use in mini and micro-computers.

The floppy diskette can also be used as an I/O device (Figure 16:8). Systems using these diskettes must incorporate a *floppy disk drive* in order to use them.

Disks can store large amounts of data which can be retrieved at a rapid rate. They are often referred to as *direct-access devices* since they permit fast access to data stored on them. Figure 16:9 shows a disk storage unit with direct-access storage unit.

A *magnetic tape* is made up of a plastic base that is coated with magnetic iron oxide. Data is put onto the tape in a similar way that music is put onto an audiotape. Magnetic tapes require a magnetic tape unit (Figure 16:10) which records the data onto the tape.

The tape unit must have a mechanism for tape movement. Such mechanism can be either a "pinch-roller" or "vacuum column." The latter is much more efficient in terms of speed and reliability.

Magnetic tapes are generally used for permanent storage and they are often referred to as *sequential-access devices* since data have to be retrieved sequentially. This is a very slow process.

Storage Capacity

The size of the memory or storage in a computer system is specified as the *storage capacity.* This is the amount of data that can be stored and is usually expressed in *bytes.* A byte (B) is a group of eight bits.

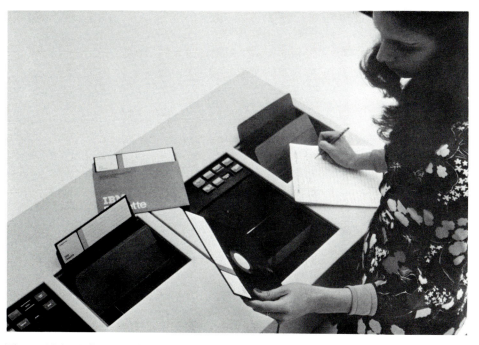

Figure 16:8. A floppy diskette unit. This is an input/output unit. (courtesy of International Business Machines Corporation.)

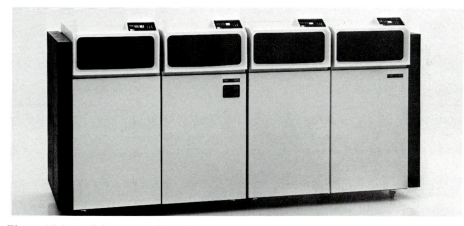

Figure 16:9. A disk storage with a direct access storage unit. (courtesy of International Business Machines Corporation.)

The size of the storage is often expressed in *K bytes,* where K represents kilo (1000). For example, computer storage can be 4K, 8K, 32K, 64K, 128K and so on. Thus a 64KB memory refers to a 6400 byte (2^{16}) memory. More recently, larger storage capacities have become available and these are expressed in mega bytes (MB), that is, 2^{20} bytes.

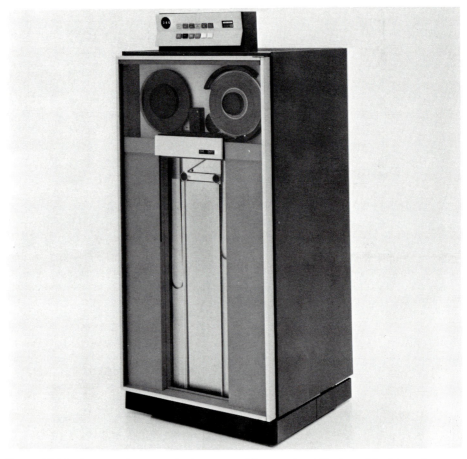

Figure 16:10. A magnetic tape unit. (courtesy of International Business Machines Corporation.)

CLASSIFICATION OF COMPUTERS

There are at least seven classes of computers. The basis for this classification depends on several parameters including cost, physical size, speed and storage capacity. Computers range from super computers, large,- medium- and small-scale computers, minicomputers to microcomputers and microprocessors. In Figure 16:11 a photograph of IBM's most powerful computer (IBM 3084) is shown.

This section will only describe the essential features of mini- and microcomputers since they are common in the radiology department.

Minicomputers

Minicomputers are inexpensive, compact and powerful computers which have become increasingly popular in government, education, business and

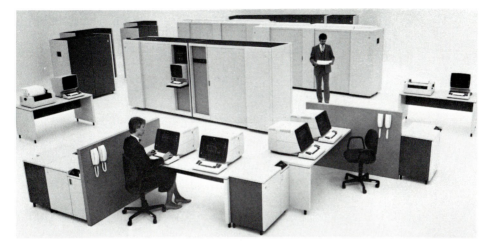

Figure 16:11. IBM's most powerful computer system. The new IBM 3084 has four central processing units and offers up to 64 million characters of main memory and 48 channels. It becomes IBM's top-of-the-line computer, with the speed and capacity to handle large data processing tasks at improved levels of price and performance. (courtesy of International Business Machines Corporation.)

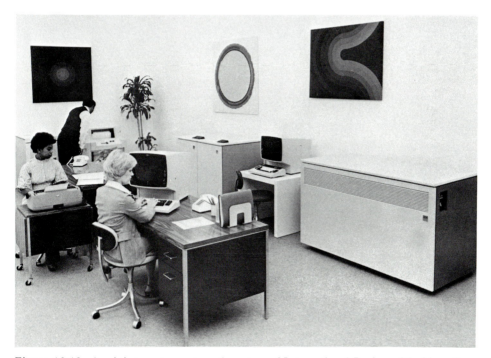

Figure 16:12. A minicomputer system. (courtesy of International Business Machines Corporation.)

health. They have also gained popularity in the radiology department and are being used in several areas including computed tomography. The operation of minicomputers is based on integrated circuit technology, and characteristic features are their circuit miniaturaization and computing power. A minicomputer system is shown in Figure 16:12.

Microcomputers and Microprocessors

Microcomputers are smaller than minicomputers and are relatively inexpensive. They have become commonplace in schools, business and even in homes (personal computers). The Apple® II and III are examples of microcomputers.

A dominant feature of microcomputers is that all functions are put onto a single chip in the form of a circuit, and, in this regard, the microcomputer chip is referred to as a *computer on a chip*. Figure 16:13 shows a thimble full of microchips.

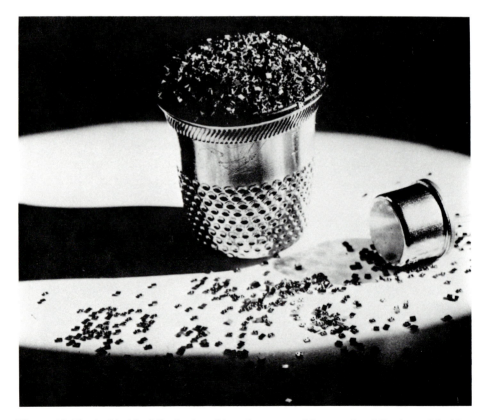

Figure 16:13. A thimble full of microchips. (courtesy of International Business Machines Corporation.)

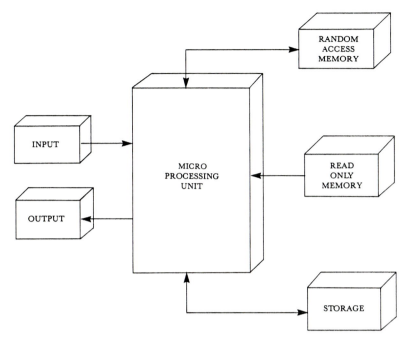

Figure 16:14. A basic organization of a microcomputer system.

The basic organization of a microcomputer is shown in Figure 16:14. The heart of the system is a *microprocessing unit* (MPU), which contains the ALU in most instances. The other two striking features are the *random-access memory* (RAM) and the *read-only memory* (ROM).

The RAM is a semiconductor memory in which programs and data are stored, that is, information can be put into or extracted out of the memory through the MPU. It should be noted that if the computer power supply is turned off, data stored in RAM will be lost.

ROM is a permanently programmed memory that cannot be erased or changed by the operator. The programs stored in ROM are referred to as *firmware*, which can be purchased from the manufacturer. For example, if one wanted to solve problems in statistics or play "Space Invaders®," then the firmware for these can be obtained at a small cost from the manufacturer.

The microprocessor can be either an 8-bit or a 16-bit system. This means that for an 8-bit microprocessor, 256 numbers (2^8) can be represented, while a 16 bit microprocessor can represent 65,536 (2^{16}) numbers. Therefore, a 16-bit microprocessor has more processing power and can perform calculations much faster than an 8-bit system.

The storage capacities for microprocessors vary from system to system. Some 8-bit microprocessors can address 64K bytes of memory, while more recent 16-bit systems can address from about 1-16 M bytes.

Microprocessors in Radiology

The use of microprocessors in the radiology department is increasing rapidly. Already they are used in the following areas:

(a) Automatic collimators. Microprocessors adjust the beam size to the film size.

(b) Selection of exposure factors (kVp, mA and time).

(c) Multi-format cameras. Microprocessors are used to position the cassette and control the exposure.

(d) Spotfilm devices. In these devices they are used to position cassettes.

(e) X-ray generators. Microprocessors control generator mA, kVp and time and also the phototimer. They are also used here to display lights on the panel and so on.

(f) Film processors. Microprocessors control the replenishing rate, development and drying temperatures, etc.

(g) Word and data processing.

(h) Image processing in CT and digital radiography.

HARDWARE, SOFTWARE AND FIRMWARE

The *hardware* in a computer system refers to the physical components that make up the computer, These include all electronic and mechanical (gears) and magnetic components. In other words, hardware forms the "nuts" and "bolts" of the computer.

In order for the computer to solve a problem, it must follow a set of precisely defined instructions. These specific instructions are called *computer programs*. The computer programs, on the other hand, are a part of the computer *software*. The term software also refers to rules, procedures (manuals) and flowcharts.

Firmware was defined preciously. In review, it refers to a programmed ROM which is fixed by the manufacturer. It is a permanent software which allows the user to communicate with the computer through the keyboard and other equipment.

PROGRAMMING AND PROGRAMMING LANGUAGES

Programming is a term which is used to indicate that the problem to be solved by the computer must be translated into a form that the computer can interpret and use. A program is usually prepared by a person who is a *programmer.*

The programmer uses a *flowchart* which consists of a set of symbols (Figure 16:15) to show how the problem will be solved. It identifies a step-by-step, detailed, logical account of the solution to the problem as shown in Figure 16:16.

SYMBOL	MEANING

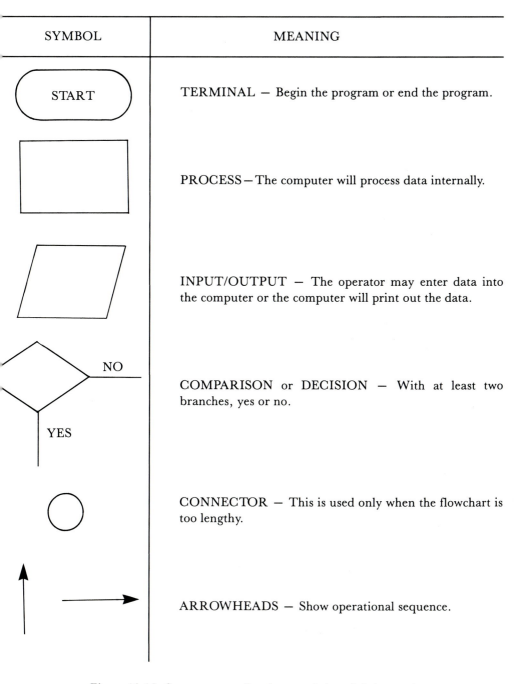

TERMINAL — Begin the program or end the program.

PROCESS — The computer will process data internally.

INPUT/OUTPUT — The operator may enter data into the computer or the computer will print out the data.

COMPARISON or DECISION — With at least two branches, yes or no.

CONNECTOR — This is used only when the flowchart is too lengthy.

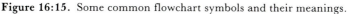

ARROWHEADS — Show operational sequence.

Figure 16:15. Some common flowchart symbols and their meanings.

FLOWCHART   PROGRAM

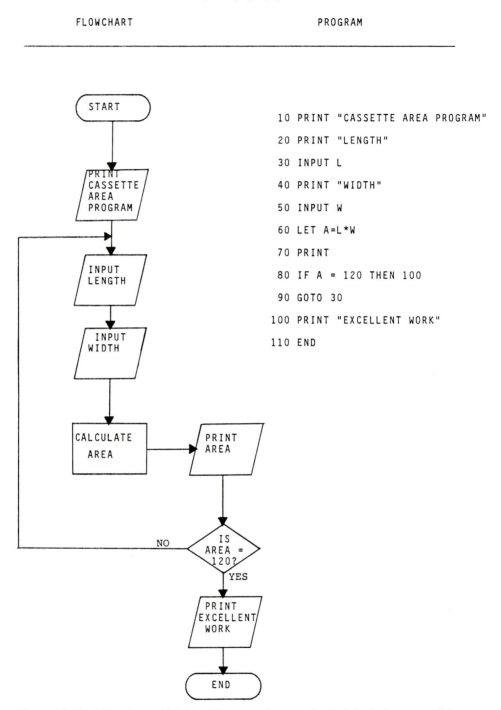

```
10  PRINT "CASSETTE AREA PROGRAM"
20  PRINT "LENGTH"
30  INPUT L
40  PRINT "WIDTH"
50  INPUT W
60  LET A=L*W
70  PRINT
80  IF A = 120 THEN 100
90  GOTO 30
100 PRINT "EXCELLENT WORK"
110 END
```

Figure 16:16. A flowchart which identifies a step by step, detailed, logical account of the solution to a problem. The associated program is shown on the right and is written in the BASIC language.

Once the flowchart is established, it must be put into a language so that the computer can process the information. Several computer languages exist and they have been divided into two groups: low-level and high-level languages.

A low-level language refers to a program written in *machine code*. This means that the instructions are coded as numbers (binary, etc.).

High-level languages include BASIC (beginners all-purpose symbolic instruction code) for general use as shown in Figure 16:16, COBOL (common business oriented language), for use in business applications, and FORTRAN (formula translator), for use in science and mathematics.

INTEGRATED CIRCUITS — A BRIEF OVERVIEW

The phraseology integrated circuit (IC) technology was mentioned previously in this chapter. The advances made in this technology have a significant impact on digital imaging techniques. In this context, therefore, a brief introduction to this topic is relevant and is of importance to the radiologic technologist.

An *integrated circuit* "consists of transistors, resistors and diodes etched into a semiconductor material" (Lenk, 1973). Usually, the semiconductor is a *silicon* wafer (a few mm in diameter) and the entire circuit on the silicon is called a "*chip*." The chip represents a complete circuit rather than separate, interconnecting components. Thus, if a series of transistors, etc., are arranged on a semiconductor, a *scale of integration* results.

Initially (late 1960s), the scale was referred to as *small-scale integration* (SSI), where at least 10-25 transistors were "etched into a semiconductor." Later, *medium-scale integration* (MSI) was introduced and included up to 1000 components on a single chip. This means that the functional capacity (ability to perform specific tasks) of the chip was increased.

In order to get a chip to perform more tasks, more components could be added onto it. This led to the development of *large-scale integration* (LSI). More recently, *very large-scale integration* (VLSI — 10,000 or more transistors on a single chip) has become available for use in modern computers and microprocessors.

For digital imaging technology, VLSI will have the following implications, as pointed out by Dr. W. R. Brody (1982) of Stanford University:

(a) VLSI circuits for storing, retrieving, displaying and transmitting images will be competitive with x-ray film, and may, when the aggregate cost of file room labor, silver storage, etc., is factored in, be considerably cheaper.

(b) VLSI circuits can be specifically fabricated for radiographic needs so that digital radiographic instruments will become competitive with conventional radiographic systems.

SPECIAL REPORT

The following special report appeared in *Radiology* in November 1982. It is reproduced here in its entirety (by the kind permission of the Radiological Society of North America and the authors) for the following reasons:

(a) To impress upon the studen the impact of computers on the practice of radiology.

(b) It presents a model of the future computerized radiology department.

The Computerized Diagnostic Radiology Department: Updated 1982. Barnhard, H. J. and Lane, G. B. Radiology, 145:551-558, November, 1982.

Abstract

"The small digital computer is becoming ever more powerful, reliable, and inexpensive. Diagnostic radiology and the computer are becoming more intertwined. During the past decade, computed tomography (CT) has achieved outstanding success. CT and other digital image systems that are capable of computer manipulation, storage, and viewing are becoming more numerous. Of increasing importance are the new and maturing reporting and operations/management systems. The many facets of newer computer and diagnostic radiology developments are discussed, and a model is presented here that integrates all applications into a single system. Many benefits in improved patient care and general operations of the department would result from its implementation. Some elements of this model exist now and can be installed with relatively little effort. Development of the entire model is within the state of current technology. A number of trends suggest that diagnostic radiology is becoming more ready to use such a model.

"If diagnostic radiology is to solve the problems of the present and meet the challenges of the future, it appears likely that we must make effective use of the computer and its allied information systems" (1). Thus began our paper a decade ago. The message appears even more valid today and the goals more easily are becomig attained. In this paper we will present a view of the future based on what has occurred in the intervening years. Certainly the star of the show has been computed tomography (CT), which has tended to obscure developments in other areas. These developments include other digitized images commonly used and those that are anticipated. In addition, there are many existing computerized reporting and operations systems that have been successfully implemented. Together with these developments the new microcomputer technology is a major force that should powerfully impact the future use of computers in diagnostic radiology.

"We have focused on these trends to develop a model of the future computerized radiology department. This model takes into account the exciting and beneficial advances that are taking place in both radiology and in the computer field, and it is most applicable in moderate-to-large hospital/clinic based departments. However, it will also be pertinent to smaller departments and those with less well defined affiliations.

WHAT'S NEW ABOUT SMALL COMPUTERS?

"The long-term trend for computers has been to gain more computing power and more memory for less money, in less space, and with greater reliability. During the past few years some significant changes have come about in computer technology that make it a more stable and affordable tool for the radiology department. These changes resulted from the same technology that broght us the poweful hand-held calculator. This revolution occurred with mass production of the silicon chip, which is now found in many aspects of our daily lives and which has recently been used in x-ray controls. We are often unaware of the chip's presence and simply accept the sophistication it brings to the end result.

"These technological trends have resulted in the development of the microcomputer, which is new in price, size, and potential. This small computer is substantially less costly than its larger predecessors, and microcomputers range in price from a few hundred dollars to twenty- or thirty-thousand dollars. It tends to be desk-top-size, which is miniscule compared to room-size giants of twenty years ago that often have no more power. The price and size point to a potential for availability in many areas of our lives, from our homes to our departments. These factors could provide a powerful stimulus for adapting the computer to uses that were out of reach earlier, and they could bring new application to the fore. Concurrent with development of the microcomputer has been the continuing decrease in costs of computer memory, an important factor because diagnostic radiology applications require large information inputs.

"Where do the minicomputer and large units fit into this new picture? The minicomputer, which was the smallest unit before the microcomputer was developed, is more expensive than the micro, and in general handles more data, more quickly than the micro. As one moves up the scale, the distinction is essentially more cost for more capacity. There is no point in paying for more capacity than is needed in the foreseeable future. Response time can be very fast on the smallest units. If a particular function, such as practice analysis, interferes with more pressing uses, it can either be done during off-hours or networked out to a larger computer. Technical differences exist between the micro- and minicomputer, but the significant differences to users are blurring as price and capacity overlap.

"Software is the term for the programs that guide and direct the computer hardware. Development of software has characteristically required much time and effort. The major limitation in the use of computers has been in obtaining software, but we are currently seeing a revolution here. Software packages increasingly are available that can be used in radiology practices with relatively minor customization. Patient billing packages, for example, have been enthusiastically prepared by a variety of entrepreneurs, from physicians to software companies. These packages are available at a fraction of the cost of custom software because development costs are shared among multiple users.

"One further step is the marketing of the so-called turnkey system that is designed to operate from day one simply by turning a key. Here, the hardware and software are so smoothly combined that their technical functioning is almost invisible to the user. These are generally stand-alone, single computers that are aimed toward specific applications. The profusion of available word processors is an excellent example of this.

"A look at the diagnostic radiology department shows that it could use a computer system that requires a number of terminals, serves several functions, and interrelates areas of application where all functions have ready access to the same information base. This can be done in several ways. The traditional approach is to select a single, general-purpose computer that is capable of meeting all anticipated needs of the department and possibly the entire hospital/clinic. But the trend now is to have a smaller dedicated radiology system with a number of links to the larger system depending upon the functions to be served. The system may use dumb terminals, which are capable only of receiving and conveying information from the central computer, or intelligent terminals, which are additionally capable of manipulating data. The latter are really microcomputers that are serving as terminals and that can have their own memory banks and software programs that rely little on the central computer. Word-processing stations linked to a central computer are in this category.

"Another approach available since the advent of the smaller computers is to link several microcomputers together using another microcomputer. At least two such networking systems are commercially available that can link up to 64 microcomputers.[2] to our knowledge this has not been tried in a radiology department, but it may have cost advantages. Another potential advantage of considerable merit is that each computer is a more or less complete unit. Therefore, each unit can function on its own even if another unit breaks down, and those that serve less critical needs can substitute for others that have broken down, or relatively inexpensive spares may be kept on hand. Thus, dependency on the ups and downs of a single, larger computer is eliminated. It must be recognized, however, that because of their recent origin, microcomputers have more limited software, particularly for

---

[2]Corvus Systems, San Jose, CA, Nestar Systems, Palo Alto, Ca.

linkage between computers. As these shortcomings are remedied during the next few years, the microcomputer network may become a very viable alternative for radiology departments.

SIGNIFICANT COMPUTER APPLICATIONS

"Several significant recent applications of computers in diagnostic radiology stand out. CT is its own success story, and it has emerged as a whole new imaging technology of revolutionary scope. In early slow tomographic equipment, CT was restricted to the head, but even then it was in demand by radiology departments. The potential for improved patient care clearly transcended all barriers, including the considerable cost of obtaining, installing, and operating the unit.

"Two new developments are digital radiography and nuclear magnetic resonance, which are showing increasing promise as ways of producing images of diagnostic quality, and are already available commercially. In nuclear medicine, the production of sophisticated images is increasingly dependent upon the computer. Since all of these images are in digital form, the potential therefore exists for viewing all of them at a common terminal.

"The glamour of these new imaging areas should not obscure the fact that other important areas of application exist. Billing and accounts-receivable packages are probably the most commonly used programs in diagnostic radiology. With the importance placed on separate billing, such computer use was a natural. Radiologists first turned to local vendors for assistance, and some have been quite successful. Others had much difficulty in many instances due to a lack of full appreciation of the differing needs of radiologists (and pathologists) from most other types of physicians. The high turnover practices of radiologists, with many open accounts, places a particular set of requirements of the system. It is not surprising then that a number of canned systems have been developed to meet these special needs. Varying degrees of overseeing are available from these commercial sources.

"Many imaginative systems have evolved in the more traditional areas of film reporting and departmental operations, with some overlap between the two. Table 16:1 reports on these systems.

"Radiographic reporting systems have developed along unstructured and structured lines. The unstructured systems do not change the way a radiologist reports; a typist inserts into the computer the free text that the radiologist speaks. The reporting function may be separate (2-5) or part of a department's computerized operating system (6-8). In this latter instance, the availability of radiology reports on terminals and prompt distribution are important functions. Information regarding the patient's passage throught the department is included in many operating systems, and if not it can be added when the diagnostic report is typed. A significant feature of these unstructured

Table 16-1

COMPUTERIZED REPORTING AND DEPARTMENTAL OPERATIONS

Reporting Method	Department Operations Computerized (number of computerized departments)	
	No	Yes
Conventional dictation without computer	(Most departments)	Cuyahoga County Hospital/Case Western Reserve University (22) Mason Clinic, Seattle (23)
Conventional dictation with input to computer	DRIS (Diagnostic Radiology Information System) (2) University of Nebraska (4-5)	Loma Linda University (6) Miami Heart Institute, FL (7) Washington University, St. Louis (8)
Structured report using computer	CLIP (Coded Language Information Processing) (11) Johns Hopkins University (12) RAPORT (20)	ARMOR (Associated Radiologists Management of Operations and Resources) (13) MARS (Missouri Automated Radiology System) (14) Massachusetts General Hospital (15-17) MAXIFILE (*) RIMS (Radiology Information Management System) (19) University of Pennsylvania (18)

*Available with RAPORT from National Computer Systems, Edina, Minnesota.

operating systems is their ability to extract and manipulate informa-tion within the diagnostic report, as well as the other information avail-able regarding the patient and departmental activities. Their outputs might include automatic diagnostic coding (9), billing, patient waiting time, diagnostic room use, and many other areas of department management. When the data to be manipulated are extensive, these reporting systems require that moderately large computers be avail-able, usually off-line at remote sites. These systems clearly have many benefits to offer, yet their potential for savings is difficult to quantify because typist time is only saved to the extent that word processing is used, and saving in other personnel time is fragmented. Other clear benefits from the improved information-capture, which results in bet-ter management, are even more difficult to quantify.

"With the structured reporting systems, the report is directly pro-duced by the radiologist without the use of a typist. The systems may use keyed input (10-14), cathode-ray tube (CRT), screen touching (16-18), bar code (18), or a penciled form (mark sense) (19,20). Usually free text may be added as the radiologist feels is necessary to ade-quately express himself. The frequency of the need for free text inser-tion varies considerably among the various systems and the radiologist who use them. Free text may be inserted by the radiologist or a typist. These systems produce an immediate report, sometimes disseminated on printers throughout the hospital. Like the autocoded unstructured reporting systems, they allow retrieval of cases based on coded infor-mation within the report, except for the uncoded free text. Despite the ingenuity and power of these systems, they have had limited acceptance even when commercially available. Cost benefits are easier to arrive at than with the unstructured systems, since typist time is clearly saved. But it is not as simple to quantify the value of a more rapidly available report and other virtues of structured systems. In addition, radiologists are reluctant to give up their traditional method of dictation. There are also some objections to repetitive reports (21) by radiologists and referring physicians.

"Departmental operation, especially with diagnostic radiology's high volume, is a natural area for computer management. As shown in Table 16:1 departmental operations may either be completely separate from a conventional unstructured dictation approach (18, 19) or be integrated with a structured or unstructured system. Departmental operation systems may include such functions as patient scheduling, file-room checkout, and practice-mangagement reports. The various systems shown in Table 16:1 have awide variety of functions that are available, and even when systems have the same functions their features may differ. Be aware that ease of transfer from one department to another varies even if the same computer is used, because of differences between departments. A simple difference might be the length of a patient's identifying code. A more complex variation would be between a completely unified department and one in which several sections operated somewhat autonomously. These differences might require some, perhaps extensive, reprogramming. Despite the need for careful analysis thcsc dcpartmcntal operating systems are often very imaginative and are well worth considering.

"Evaluation of cost effectiveness is difficult for departmental operation systems, and it usually focuses on meticulous examination of staffing requirements, as was the case in the methodology developed for evaluation of a hospital-wide information system (24). It has subsequently been shown (personal communication) that the portion of the system chargeable to diagnostic radiology will more than pay for itself in staffing needs over the life of the system. And these savings do not even attempt to include less clearly defined values such as improved patient care. Another author (25) says of a hospital-wide information system that the "primary justification for this system lies in improving quality and service levels." Regarding reduced labor costs, they would "view these cost savings as a welcome bonus" but would proceed with the system" even if none of these benefits were realized." Grann (26) has urged that "It would frequently be more advantageous to study non-dollar impacts with greater care and rigor."

"Significant advances have been made in word processing in the past few years. While not specific to radiology, word processing is a powerful aid to all typing processes. It permits easy correction of errors, insertion of new material, use of canned reports with individualization, and many other time-saving features. The output may also be saved in computer memory. Although less glamorous than other radiology appliances, it is surely one of the most dependable, is easily installed, and can provide realimprovements.

A DIAGNOSTIC RADIOLOGY COMPUTER MODEL

"The model presented here (Figure 16:17) is a blueprint for a computerized diagnostic radiology department. This model does not reflect any giant leap of the imagination. It is based on trends that are already apparent. These trends are teh increasing use of computers for information storage and transfer in the hospital/clinic setting, the presence of digital recordings already in place (CT and others), and the emerging era of additional digital images (digital radiography and nuclear magnetic resonance). Also to be recognized is the increasing sophistication and acceptance of computers by the general public as people become acquainted with computers in school, at their 24-hour banking terminal, or at home.

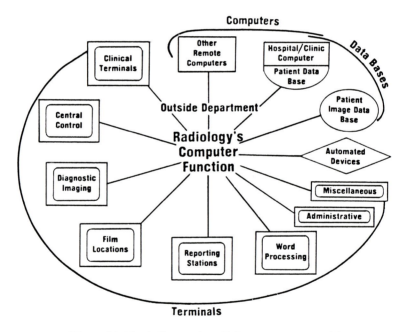

Figure 16:17. A diagnostic radiology computer model.

"The basic technology for this model does not include the important but not yet well-developed system of voice recognition by computer. Once that approach is perfected, however, its function can be integrated into a model. Clearly, turn-key systems are not available to implement the entire model at this time. Several years of additional effort will be required to accomplish the model.

"As shown in Figure 16:17, the model is grouped into categories of computers, data bases, terminals, and automated devices.

Computers

"Radiology's Computer Function refers to those computer functions that serve a radiology department's needs. The actual configuration is invisible to the user. This means that it does not matter whether the computer is in the department or serves many users throughout the hospital/clinic as long as it responds promptly and has minimum down time. The hospital/clinic computer shares information with radiology for many purposes including the main patient-data base, even if it is not the one used directly by radiology. Other remote computers might include distant computers for literature search, other hospital/clinic computers for transfer of patient inforamtion, etc.

Automated Devices

"A number of automated devices for managing film location, identification, and handling were explored in our earlier paper (1) and will not be repeated here. Included in the category of automated devices was the automatic recording of patient information from x-ray machine settings. It is noteworthy that one currently available machine [1] includes a microprocessor and is adverised as "allowing software programs to record such data as patient dosage, dosage history, department usage rate, and activity level by operator.""

Patient Image-Data Base

"The availability of various patient images on multiple terminals will be a major step forward. As noted earlier, much visual output is now computer processed. This digitized information includes CT and, increasingly, ultrasound and nuclear medicine imaging. Already available in early commercial units are the images from digital radiography and nuclear magnetic resonance. All such digitized data are readily converted to analog form for display on a CRT. Unfortunately, this viewing is now largely limited to the originating machine or its slave monitors because of variations in hardware and software design. What is urgently needed is industry agreement on a standard output. Once such a standard exists, current image-producing equipment can be fitted with "black box" adaptors and future units can adhere to that standard. Viewing terminals can be standardized and images could be made readily accessible within the radiology department and, if desired, at remote clinical terminals as well. There is a cost factor to be considered with regard to remote terminals.

"High-resolution images contain much data and therefore require expensive distribution lines and possibly special software if rapid access is to be achieved. While the cost of the lines might be acceptable

---

[1]Fischer X-ray Company, Franklin Park, Illinois.

for relatively short distances and frequent use within the radiology department, it may be viewed as excessive for long runs to infrequently used terminals. One less expensive solution would be the use of a storage tube CRT that quickly builds up and retains an image but does not require the conventional 30 frame (60 interface) changes per second to produce flicker-free images. This approach should prove quite adequate for routine viewing, and the cable could be the conventional type. It should be feasible to mix the less expensive, low-resolution units where only alphanumeric (AN) information is needed with this more costly high-resolution unit. Both alphanumerics and images will probably be transferred as a full screen image, and it would only require a software modification to send the appropriate signal to each type of terminal. Complete images could be stored at each location where they are produced, but selected images would be centrally stored in digital forms for general viewing, just as appropriate imges are photographed now. Until on-line storage media become even less expensive, long-term image storage could be on magnetic tape, including videotape. A comig option is the digital optical recorder that uses a laser beam and plastic disc.

Patient-Data Base

"This will include both diagnostic radiology reports and other information maintained within the hospital/clinic computer data bank. The physical location of the memory banks will depend upon the configuration chosen and the relative ease of access.

Terminals

"Because of the diverse yet overlapping functions of the various terminals, Table 16:2 has been provided. Each of the various terminal locations is shown with information regarding characteristics, functions, and information available to that location to meet its functios. The characteristics deserve particular mention. Almost all of the terminals display AN data. These require only low-resolution characteristics. Where images are also to be viewed, AN data may be viewed on the same screen even though that terminal is capable of the high resolution desirable for digital images (see earlier section). Machine readable (MR) methods allow easy entry, usually of patinet identification numbers, but they may be also used to identify clinicians who check out film jackets and other similar functions. The bar-code method is currently most used. Magnetic strips are an option. MR units may be stand-alone or coupled with a keyboared that allows hand entry as well.

"Each of the terminal locations will now be discussed in conjunction with Figure 16:16 and Table 16:2.

Table 16-2

TERMINALS IN DIAGNOSTIC RADIOLOGY COMPUTER FUNCTION

Locations	Characteristics AN	IM	MR	Function	Information Available
Clinical					
Nursing stations	X		X	Patient scheduling	a, c
Physicians offices	X	X	X	Report/image review, Patient scheduling	a, b, c
Central Control	X		X	Room assignment, Patient scheduling/Registration, Patient location	c, d, e
Diagnostic Imaging Rooms	X	X	X	Patient examination, Patient location	a, b, d, e, f, g, h
Film Stations				Film location	
Processing room and film jacket assembly			X	Film location, Film checkout	a, e
Film storage	X		X	Diagnostic reporting,	a, b, c, d, e, h, i, j
Reporting Stations	X	X	X	(Conventional or structured)	
Word Processing					
Patient reports	X		X	Report preparation	a, c, d
Secretarial	X			Letter-document preparation	d, e
Administrative	X		X	Billing process, Management and fiscal functions	a, c, k, p
Miscellaneous					
Radiologists office	X	X		Professional and personnel files, CME, Report/image review	a, b, j, k, e, m, p
Research area	X			Data recording and analysis	i, n, q
Library	X	X		Book/journal inventory and checkout, Continuing education	j, o
File museum	X	X	X	Image inventory/review/checkout	c, o

KEY

Characteristics

AN — Alpha numeric display
IM — Images — high resolution
MR — Machine readable input

Information Available

a — Diagnostic reports	j — Literature abstracts
b — Patient images	k — Tickler file
c — Patient data base	l — Meeting attendance
d — Staff schedule/availability	m — Interesting case file
e — Telephone/paging numbers	n — Research material file
f — Exposure factors	o — Inventory of materials
g — CPR information	p — Special files
h — Drug information	q — Statistical program
i — Reporting aids	

Clinical Terminals

"These include hospital patient areas, emergency and ambulatory clinics, and referring physician's offices whether in the hospital/clinic or more remote. Two-way communication with the radiology department allows for examination requests to be received and reports to be sent. A printer may be used at any of these external sites to permit a permanent record to be available promptly.

Central-Control Terminals

"Here the entry into and passage of the patient within the department is monitored and supervised. The reception desk schedules the appointment in the computer. Once the patient arrives, assignment to an examining room may be accomplished either at the reception desk or closer to the diagnostic rooms. Proximity of the person controlling patient flow to the diagnostic rooms becomes less important when accurate, timely information is available.

Diagnostic Imaging-Room Terminals

"A wide variety of information becomes available to both technologists and physicians. The standard display on the terminal may consist of the updated patient schedule for that particular room. Response through the terminal would indicate when a patient enters or has completed the procedure. Other information available on the terminal might include examination-exposure factors, recent patient reports and images, staff schedule and availabiltiy, telephone/paging nubmers, drug interaction, and cardiopulmonary resuscitation information. And, of course, when the image that is created in a particular diagnostic room is in digital form, the terminals will display these images.

Film-Location Terminals

"This remains an important function to the extent to which we continue to store images on x-ray film. Darkroom, film/jacket assembly, and film storage all become part of the information system to improve locatability of films. An expedited check-out and return process also improves file control.

Reporting-Station Terminals

"Whether the radiologist continues to dictate reports or uses a structured computerized method, the terminal becomes a major information source. Recent diagnostic reports that have been printed-out but have not yet been manually filed (if that method persists) become available on the CRT for review. Usage may determine that serveral viewing terminals are required at each reporting station. Diagnostic images from other areas such as CT and nuclear medicine may also be viewed. Diagnostic aids might include normal values, differential-diagnosis lists, an abbreviations list to aid in deciphering request forms, programs that establish diagnostic probability estimates, and calculation aids such as for film/distance distortion.

Word-Processing Terminals

"These will be available wherever typing is done. Personnel who type diagnostic reports will enter the patient's name or identification number. Additional information such as age, race, gender, patient location, and referring physician will be added automatically from computer memory. When corrections or additions are required, only those changes need by made and the report, letter, or manuscript is ready to be printed, eliminating the need to retype and proofread the entire document.

Administrative Terminals

"A variety of functions fall into this category, including billing and accounts receivable, which are often done from a remote office where needed information is just accessible from the computer as if it were done on the premises. Gaining access to management information is another area of considerable value to the department and may by itself warrant a terminal in the office of the radiologist-in-charge or the administrative assistant. Other administrative functions are likely to be done by the hospital/clinic when the department is closely affiliated. These include accounts payable, payroll, and inventory.

Miscellaneous Terminals

"Not otherwise addressed here are a variety of other uses including the department library's list of books and periodicals and perhaps a checkout system, and teaching film listings and lierature reference listings, which may be added to be radiologists and technologists to form private files. It is not necessary to have a separate terminal to perform each function, yet our experience is that terminals proliferate like telephones. At first they are put in relatively few places. Later the time lost in going to too few locations is recognized and more terminals are added. Once sufficient terminals are in use, electronic mail for messages and announcements may be used throughout the department and institution reducing much paperwork. Personal tickler files may be available. When a daily personnel schedule is available, it becomes simpler to schedule meetings by computer.

DISCUSSION

"The model presented here represents a powerful future tool for improving the function of diagnostic radiology departments. There are various ways the model may be applied and different results would be obtained. We are only beginning to discover the potential benefits because ever more imaginative uses evolve once such systems become widely installed. It seems reasonable to forecast that much personnel time, including that of radiologists, will be saved. More efficient operation and information transfer will benefit the patient in innumerable ways including faster passage through the department, better tools for diagnosis that will be available to the radiologists, and more accessible reports and images for the referring physician. Management tools such as trend forcasting will result in better operational decision making. Much of the drudgery and frustration of handling increasing patient loads will be relieved, making the diagnostic department a more pleasant and productive workplace for those within it and those who relate with it.

"The basic technology is here and the benefits are great, yet these systems aren't in radiology departments all over the country for a number of reasons. First, this model is more advanced than any that previously has been conceptualized, and time will be required for its development. Second, there is not universal agreement about the various components (e.g., structured reporting versus dictation), and so there will never be a single ideal system reflecting the model. Third, and critical from the cost standpoint, the new wave of microcomputer technology has not had enough time to make a major impact. Fourth, while radiologists are curious about computer developments, they have not in significant numbers seen many of the applications as worth the money and effort required. And last, external pressures for more efficient operations (translation: cost containment) have thus far only had a significant impact on the addition or replacement of major equipment, not on general operations.

"Where does that leave the department that wants to do something now? Clearly the model presented here will be available for several years. Certainly there are portions of the model available. However, these portions do not integrate readily with each other and so one is left with a much less powerful overall system. Nonetheless, let us examine these options: The most clearly definable application on the commercial market is that of word processing. This useful approach has taken root in the secretarial office as CT has in diagnostic radiology. Stand-alone word processors are readily available and are generally very easy to use because keys on the keyboard can be dedicated to specific uses. An alternative approach, and more useful learning experience, would be to purchase a small, general-purpose microcomputer and word-processing software. This minimal expenditure would also allow other programs to be run that are not essential to daily operations. For example, a general file program can be used to handle literature references or the teaching film museum. The pleasures and problems of the computer can thus be gradually introduced into the department. Later, larger scale operations will hold fewer terrors. An alternative intermediate between a stand-alone word procesor would be a word processor with capability of having other functions added.

"Billing and accounts receivable is the next area worthy of consideration. It is appealing because cost-benefit analysis is easy to make and our volume of cases often requires computer assistance. A number of software companies cater to radiologists and frequently also to patholo-

gists since we share common problems of high volume with high patient turnover. Approach with caution the company that doesn't appreciate the particuar requirements that radiologists have as contrasted
with requirements of other physicians.

"Next in availability are the structured reporting systems, which are
available both commercially and from departments whose developers
are eager to lend assistance. A visit to a using department will give one
a quick overview of the manner in which the systems work. It takes
time to become comfortable with structured reporting and this serves
as an impediment to its acceptance. This is unfortunate since these systems provide the quickest method of setting a diagnostic report to the
referring physician, thus having meaningful effect upon prompt, efficient patient care.

"Department operating systems are less evident, yet they have the
potential to work wonders in a department. Can you imagine today's
airline reservation systems functioning without computers? Certainly
the magnitude of their problem is different, but the principle is the
same. Department operating systems are more difficult to evaluate
then structured reporting systems, particularly with regard to how
much software modification will be required for the system to function
in another setting.

"It is likely then that with sufficient will, there are ways to set various parts of the model presented here going by selecting the most appropriate system available for your setting and your needs. Recognize
that some modification will be required to meet your specific requirements, and considerable software change will be needed if you do not
use the same computer.

"What is not concurrently available is any easy way to integrate the
various systems, because of various design differences including the
language used for programming, the computer(s) on which it is programmed, and different features. Each functional unit would stand
alone, quite powerful in itself, yet relative weak compared with what
might be. To use the airline reservation analogy again, it is like the earlier days when most airlines had their computer system, but to find out
about available seats on other airline, the agent had to telephone. Now
they can access each other's information and reserve seats from any airline reservation terminal. Travel agents can do the same thing from
their office terminals.

"Do you want to go the route of separate stand-alone units? If your
needs are great enough in certain areas, then each need may be met by
your choice of a separate computer system. It may be possible to plan a
sequence of system acquisitions that would integrate with each other,
but this is unlikely. It would seem prudent to meet each need now with
the least expenditure possible and relatively little expansion capability.
Such a course would be with the expectation that by the middle to late
1980s, integrated systems will be available and your earlier investment
will have paid for itself and outlived its usefulness.

"So what will take us from our present state to readily available turn-key integrated systems? The main impetus will come when there is sufficient interest within the radiologic community to stimulate commercial production. That is likely to be based on imaginative systems that will be developed by forward-looking departments. It is very important that there be standardization of interfaces so that different pieces of the model (software and hardware) can work with each other even though from different manufacturers. Then the burden of producing an entire system will not fall on any one company. There will also be more options from which to choose, so that less modification will be necessary in each department.

"It is difficult to predict what will bring about the turning point in radiologic interest. We believe business to be highly computerized, yet a recent survey of businesses with less than 500 employees revealed that only 25% had inhouse computers (27), so radiology may not be very laggard. There is nothing revolutionary about the features in the model presented here. It would create a wonderous department that many would want to emulate. Yet the thrust would not be the same as with a CT unit that might cost considerably more. Certainly CT has more dramatic medical impact, even though the day-to-day effect of a computerized department would likely be greater in terms of its influence on overall patient care and costs. The final shove may be an external one, when the pressures of cost containment and record keeping become such that no other answer suffices. We hope that we can more gracefully cloak ourselves in the benefits that the computer has to offer without such outside pressures.

REFERENCES

1. Barnhard, H.J., Dockray, K.T. Computerized operation in the diagnostic radiology department. AJR 1970; 109:-628-635.
2. Barnhard, H.J., Jacobson, H.G., Nance, J.W. Diagnostic radiology information system (DRIS). Radiology 1974; 14:314-319.
3. Gell, G., Oser, W., Schwarz, G. Experience with the AURA free-text documentation system. Radiology 1976; 119:105-109.
4. Wilson, W.J. An automated system for coding radiology reports. In: Computer applications in radiology: Proceedings of a conference held at the University of Missouri, Columbia, Sept 23-26, 1970. Columbia:University of Missouri, c1972, pp. 319-328, DHEW Publications no. (FDA) 73-8081.

Acknowledges: We wish to thank James R. McConnel, Research Associate, University of Arkansas Graduate Institute of Technology, and Mike Oglesby, Systems Analyst, Department of Behavioral Sciences University of Arkansas for Medical Sciences, for their technical assistance in the preparation of this manuscript.

5. Jahn, E., Howard, B.Y. Computers serve radiology at the University of Virginia Medical Center. J Appl Radiol, 1978; 7:46-48.

6. Stone, D.A. Loma Linda University's computerized radiology information system. J Appl Radiol 1978; 7:49-53.

7. Katz, A., Budkin, A., Shupler, R. An automated radiology information system. Radiology 1977; 124:699-704.

8. Jost, R.G., Trachtman, J., Hill, R.L., Smith, B.A., Evens, R.G. A computer system for transcribing radiology reports. Radiology 1980; 136: 63-66.

9. Barnhard, H.J., Long, J.M. Computer auto-coding selecting and correlating of radiologic diagnostic cases. A preliminary report. AJR 1966; 96:854-863.

10. Brolin, I. MEDELA: an electronic data-processing system for radiological reporting. Radiology 1972; 103:249-255.

11. Leeming, B.W., Simon, M., Jackson, J.D., Horowitz, G.L., Bleich, H.L. Advances in radiologic reporting with computerized language information processing (CLIP). Radiology 1974; 133:349-353.

12. Wheeler, P.S., Simborg, D.W., Gitlin, J.N. The Johns Hopkins radiology reporting system. Radiology 1976; 119:315-319.

13. Bauman, R.A. Computer information systems for radiology. In: Sixth conference on computer applications in radiology and computer/aided analysis of radiological images held at Newport Beach CA, June 18-21, 1979. IEEE Catalog No. 79CH 1404-3c; 181-187 (available from IEEE Service Center, 445 Hoes Lane, Piscataway NJ 08854).

14. Lodwick, G.S., Wickizer, C.R., Dikhaus, E. MARS — its tenth anniversary of operation and its future. Methods Inf Med 1980; 19:125-132.

15. Bauman, R.A. Computer information systems for radiology. In: Sixth conference on computer application in radiology and computer/aided analysis of radiological images held at Newport Beach CA, June 18-21, 1972. 181-187 IEEE Catalog No. 79CH 1404-3C (available from IEEE Service Center, 445 Hoes Lane, Piscataway, NJ 08854).

16. Pendergrass, H.P., Greenes, R.A., Barnett, G.O., Poitras, J.W., Pappalardo, A.N., Marble, C.W. An on-line computer facility for systematized input of radiology reports. Radiology 1969; 92:709-713.

17. Lazarus, C.B., Poitras, J.W., Mitchell, W.P., et al. Automation of scheduling and file room functions of a diagnostic radiology department. VOl I and II. DHEW Publication #(DA)75-8020, 1975.

18. Arenson, R.L., London, J.W. Comprehensive analysis of a radiology operations management comptuer system. Radiology 1979: 133:-355-362.

19. Leslie, E.V., Mazur, J., Suess, C.A. RIMS-1979. In: Sixth conference on computer application in radiology and computer/aided analysis of radiological images held at Newport Beach CA, June 18-21, 1979. 403-413, IEEE Catalog No, 79CH 1404-3C (available from IEEE Service Center, 445 Hoes Lane, Piscataway, NJ 08854).

20. Mani, R.L. RAPORT radiology system: results of clinical trials. AJR 1976; 127-811-816.

21. Seltzer, R.A., Reimer, G.W., Cooperman, L.R., Rossiter, S.B. Computerized radiographic reporting in a community hospital: a consumer's report. AJR 1977; 128:825-829.

22. Bellon, G.M. Computerized information management: a ten-year experience in a hospital based radiology department; In: Sixth conference on computer application in radiology and computer/aided analysis of radiological images held at Newport Beach CA, June 18-21, 1979, 391-402, IEEE Catalog No. 79CH 1404-3C (available from IEEE Service Center, 445 Hoes Lane, Piscataway, NJ 08854).

23. Burnett, L.L. A clinic-hospital radiology information system. In: Sixth conference on computer applications in radiology and computer/aided analysis of radiological images held at Newport Beach, CA, June 18-21, 1979, 377-379, IEEE Catalog No. 79CH 1404-3C (available from IEEE Service Center, 445 Hoes Lane, Piscataway, NJ 08854).

24. Bunnell, P., Lemons, L.F., Shapin, P.G. AHIS cost effectiveness. In: Fourth annual symposium on computer applications in medical care held at Washington, D.C., Nov 2-5, 1980. 665-672, IEEE Catalog No. 80CH 1570-1 (available from IEEE Service Center, 445 Hoes Lane, Piscataway, NJ 08854).

25. Pfeiffenberger, R.G., Moehring, R.L. Patient care system — Good Samaritan Hospital, Cincinnatti, Ohio. In: Fourth annual symposium on computer applications in medical care held at Washington, D.C., Nov 2-5, 1980, 8-12, IEEE Catalog No. 80CH 1570-1 (available from IEEE Service Center, 445 Hoes Lane, Piscataway, NJ 08854).

26. Grann, R.F. Failure to learn from failure: evaluating computer systems in medicine. In: Fourth annual symposium on computer applications in medical care held at Washington, D.C., Nov 2-5, 1980, 480-484, IEEE Catalog No. 80CH 1570-1 (available from IEEE Service Center, 445 Hoes Lane, Piscataway, NJ 08854).

27. Rosenberg, R. Study finds vast market for small business computers. Mini-micro Systems 1980, 13:43-49.

SUMMARY

1. Computers are used in almost every facet of human activity. They can process and store vast amounts of information with great speed and accuracy and reduce the probability of human error.

2. A computer is a special machine for solving problems and making decisions by performing arithmetic and logical operations on data.

3. The history of computers is traced from the abacus to Babbage's difference engine, through second- and third-generation computers to the introduction of fourth-generation machines. The characteristic features of fifth-generation computers are mentioned briefly.

4. There are two types of computers: the analog computer and the digital computer. The analog computer solves problems by analogy and works with data that vary continuously in time, such as voltage. A digital com-

puter solves problems by counting, hence operates on, digital (numerical) data.

5. The binary number system (base 2) is used in the digital computer since electronic devices in the computer work on two states, that is, they can either be "on" or "off." Other number systems, such as the hexadecimal, have been devised to represent larger binary numbers.

6. The binary digits (0 and 1) are referred to as bits.

7. The units in a computer system are input, processing storage and output. Input devices supply data to the processing unit and the results of processing are displayed on output devices such as a television monitor or a line printer.

8. The central processing unit consists of an arithemtic/logic unit which performs calculations, and a control unit which coordinates the activities of the entire computer.

9. Storage is often referred to as memory and may be main storage or auxiliary storage. Main storage involves the use of magnetic core memories and, more recently, semiconductor memories. Auxiliary storage is accomplished on magnetic disks and tapes.

10. The storage capacity is expressed as the amount of data that can be stored. This is expressed in bytes where one byte is a group of 8 bits.

11. There are at least seven classes of computers. The basis for this classification depends on cost, physical size, speed and storage capacity.

12. The minicomputer and microcomputer are described since they are commonly used in x-ray imaging. The microcomputer is referred to as a "computer on a chip."

13. The areas in which microprocessors are used in radiology are listed.

14. The terms hardware, software and firmware are described. Software refers to the programs that direct the operation of the computer, while hardware refers the physical components (such as electronic and mechanical devices). Firmware is a programmed read-only memory fixed by the manufacturer. It is permanent software.

15. Programs are a specific set of instructions which the computer must follow in order to solve a problem. Programs are written in several languages (such as BASIC) so that the computer understands the problem to be solved.

16. Integrated circuit technology is important to the technologist. This circuit consists of "transistors, resistors and diodes etched into a semiconductor material." The arrangement of these transistors, etc., on a semiconductor results in a scale of integration. Small-, medium- and large-scale integration are highlighted.

17. The use of very large-scale integration has implications for x-ray imaging with particular applications in storage, retrieval, display and transmission of images.

Section D

DIGITAL IMAGING APPLICATIONS

CHAPTER 17

COMPUTED TOMOGRAPHY

THE introduction of computed tomography (CT) marks the beginning of a new activity for the radiologic community. So remarkable is CT that it has been hailed as a revolutionary breakthrough in the history of medicine, as was the discovery of x-rays in 1895.

The basic concepts of CT have been extended to generate other imaging methods such as digital radiography and magnetic resonance imaging.

This chapter will introduce the relevant concepts of CT and will indicate how the fundamental principles of digital image processing have been incorporated into the acquisition of the CT image.

CT — A DEFINITION

The term computed tomography (CT) implies that a computer (hence the term computed) is used in the acquisition of the image. It also means that some basic theory of tomography is used to produce the image. In essence, this theory involves the production of an image of specific layer of the body. For CT, the layer of interest is a *cross-sectional* layer that is totally free of superimposition of structures above and below the desired cross section. Such superimposition is one of the primary shortcomings of radiography.

Conventional tomography (*geometric tomography*) can be used to eliminate the problem of superimposition of structures. However, there are other limitations imposed by conventional tomographic methods, such as image blurring which still persists and poor contrast resolution caused by the presence of scattered radiation due to the *open beam geometry* of the system.

In CT, these shortcomings are completely removed through the use of the following:

(a) Special detectors.
(b) Highly collimated x-ray beams.
(c) Multiple x-ray transmission readings obtained through specific scanning (x-ray tube and detector motion) sequences.
(d) Complex mathematical techniques for reconstructing a cross-sectional image through the use of a computer.

In general, CT is a *digital imaging technique* based on similar steps involved in digital image processing theory. These steps involved:

(a) Scanning the patient, through special motions of the x-ray tube and detectors.
(b) Sampling each portion of the anatomy scanned by using special detectors to measure transmitted x-rays and converting them into electrical signals (analog data).
(c) Quantization, where each measurement in (b) above is assigned a numerical value (digital data).
(d) Processing the digital data with a digital computer.
(e) Display and storage of the computer-processed image.

HISTORICAL BACKGROUND

Various aspects of the CT technique go back as far as 1917, when Radon introduced the idea of using mathematics based on projection data to solve problems relating to the theory of gravity. Other workers then focussed their efforts on a basic theorem which dealt with reconstruction of an object by means of multiple projections of the object (*image reconstruction from projections*). This work led to the development of techniques which proved successful in astronomy, electron microscopy, optics and medicine (isotope and diagnostic radiology).

In 1961, Oldendorf, Kuhl, Edwards and Cormack applied reconstruction techniques to solve medical problems. From 1967 to 1972, Hounsfield, working in England, developed and introduced the first clinically useful CT scanner.

Hounsfield and Cormack — A Short Biography

In 1972, Godfrey Newbold Hounsfield receive the equivalent of the Nobel Prize in Engineering for his work on CT. Hounsfield was born in England in 1919. He studied electronics at the Royal Air Force in Cranwell. Later, he attended Faraday House where he graduated in electrical and mechanical engineering.

In 1951, he joined the staff at EMI (Electric and Musical Industries) and in 1967 he began working on pattern-recognition techniques which later gave birth to CT scanning.

In 1979, Hounsfield shared the Nobel Prize in Medicine and Physiology with Allan MacLeod Cormack, a physics professor at Tufts University in Medford, Massachusetts. Cormack was born in South Africa in 1924 and studied nuclear physics at Cambridge University. He is recognized for his contribution to CT, since he developed solutions to some of the mathematical problems involved in CT.

Today, the clinical usefulness of CT is well established for the central nervous system and other parts of the body. Hounsfield should therefore be recognized as the man who opened up a whole new area of interest for technologists, radiologists, medical physicists and other related health professionals.

THE PROBLEM IN CT

The fundamental problem in CT is to calculate all absorption coefficients (μ's) for the anatomy of interest knowing a large set of x-ray transmission measurements. This problem is essentially reduced to solving a large number of simultaneous equations. To do this requires mathematical solutions and a computer for quick calculations. The solutions have been referred to as *reconstruction algorithms*. These algorithms have been classified into three groups with each group having specific advantages and disadvantages. A discussion of these algorithms is beyond the scope of this chapter. Readers interested in a fundamental discussion of these methods may refer to the text by Seeram (1982).

DATA ACQUISITION

The term *data acquisition* is one that has found common usage in present-day imaging trends. The term relates to the method by which information (usually analog, in this context) is collected from the patient and transformed into digital information before it is sent to a comptuer for processing.

For CT, a typical data acquisition scheme is shown in Figure 17:1. It consists of the x-ray tube and collimation, imaging object (patient), detectors and the detector electronics. The unit which houses the tube and detectors and associated electronics is called the *gantry*. The gantry and patient couch are shown in Figure 17:2. The opening in the gantry is referred to as the *gantry aperture*.

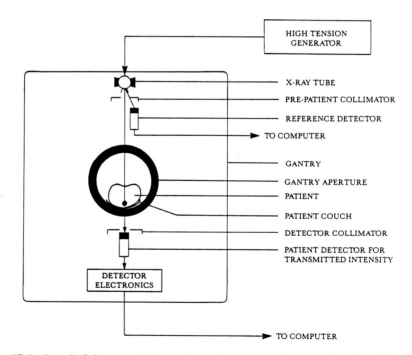

Figure 17:1. A typical data acquisition scheme for computed tomography. The information collected from the patient (analog data) is converted to digital data through the detector electronics before it is sent to a digital computer for processing.

X-ray Tubes

X-ray tubes for CT are essentially similar to those described in Chapter 5, however, certain modifications are necessary for CT operation. X-ray tubes for CT are of two types: the stationary anode and the rotating anode.

Stationary-anode Tubes

Earlier CT scanners (first and second generation) used stationary-anode x-ray tubes because of their typical long scan times. These tubes have the capability of higher power output and higher x-ray intensity for long exposure times, compared to rotating-anode tubes. These tubes are, therefore, used in CT scanners with scan times ranging from about 10 seconds to several minutes.

The target is made of tungsten and they have a 20° angle of bevel with focal spot sizes ranging from 1 to 4 mm × 10 to 20 mm. They are rated at 120-150 kVp maximum and operate typically at 80-140 kVp at 20-35 mA.

Rotating-anode Tubes

For CT machines with faster scan times (below 10 sec), the rotating-anode x-ray tube is used since it provides a higher intensity and higher power output for short exposure times than stationary-anode tubes.

These tubes are air cooled and are pulsed in operation or they can be energized continuously for short exposure times. High heat-storage capacities (anode and housing) as well as small focal spots (about 0.6 mm) are also characteristic features of rotating-anode tubes for CT.

One of the problems with operating x-ray tubes for CT is that of stabilization of the kVp because of the high voltages used. This is of vital importance, since voltage fluctuations may result in poor image quality. Stabilization is accomplished by making a larger insert envelope to increase the distance between the anode and cathode and also the distance between these electrodes and the glass envelope.

X-ray tubes get very hot during their operation for CT work; therefore, ample time should be allowed between exposures for sufficient cooling. In this regard, the computer informs the operator to wait for such cooling to occur.

Collimation

The influence of collimation on image quality and radiation dose is well known for conventional imaging. In CT, collimation also has an effect on image quality and dose.

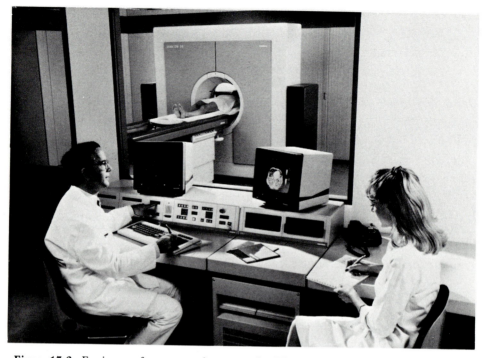

Figure 17:2. Equipment for computed tomography. The patient couch and gantry are shown in the background while the operating console is shown in the foreground. The opening in the gantry for the patient is referred to as the gantry aperture. (courtesy of the Siemens Corporation.)

In Figure 17:1, two collimation schemes are apparent. They are (a) pre-patient collimation and (b) post-patient collimation or predetector collimation.

Pre-patient collimation implies that the radiation beam is collimated at the x-ray tube. This is sometimes referred to as *source collimation.* The *thickness of the slice* (sensitivity profile) to be imaged depends on the collimator at the x-ray tube. Therefore, for different slice thicknesses, different collimators must be used. In general, thicknesses between 10 mm and 15 mm are not uncommon. In some cases, thinner slices may be obtained through the use of auxiliary collimators. It should be realized that as the slice thickness decreases, radiation dose must be increased to reduce noise and to maintain image quality.

The choice of slice thickness is usually dependent on the patient's clinical data and the structure of interest to the radiologist.

Post-patient collimation, on the other hand, refers to the collimation at the detectors. These collimators reduce scatter much the same as a grid in conventional imaging. The opening of the detector collimator is called the *detector aperture width or size.* Such size influences the inherent spatial resolution of the machine such that the smaller the aperture width (size), the greater the spatial resolution.

In order that radiation is not wasted and dose to the patient is not increased, the detector aperture width is somewhat larger than the pre-patient collimator width.

Alignment of pre- and post-patient collimators is of vital importance, since misalignment will produce streak artifacts on the image.

Detectors

The purpose of the detectors in CT is to detect and measure transmitted x-rays and convert them into electrical signals. The detectors are coupled to a special electronic box referred to as the *detector electronics* or the *data acquisition system* (DAS) (Figure 17:1), which convert electrical signals to digital data.

Presently, CT detectors fall into two categories: scintillation detectors and gas-ionization detectors.

The *scintillation* detector was first used by Hounsfield in his original experiments. A scintillation detector consists of a scintillation crystal coupled to a photomultiplier (PM) tube. The crystal most commonly used is *sodium iodide* (NaI), although other crystals such as *calcium floride* (CaF_2), *bismuth germanate* (BGO), *cesium iodide* (CsI) and cadmium tungstate ($CdWO_4$) have been used.

The crystal has the property of converting the radiation into light photons in proportion to the energy of the x-rays it absorbs. The light photons are in turn converted into electrical signals by the PM tube. These signals then go to the DAS for conversion into digital form.

In the *gas-ionization* detector, a volume of gas is ionized by the radiation beam falling on the detector, to produce an electrical signal. The gas which has found widespread use is *xenon* which is pressurized to about 20 atmospheres. Different CT systems use different detectors of either category. In the future, *solid-state detectors* (semiconductors) may become availabe for use in CT.

One of the advantage of NaI detectors is that they have a higher detector efficiency than CaF_2, but NaI suffers from the problem of afterglow (emits light for several seconds after the exposure) which can destroy the detector signal. This afterglow problem is removed by BGO, however, BGO has a lower light output than NaI.

Xenon gas detectors experience no afterglow problems. They are simple and compact compared to NaI, however, xenon has a low absorption efficiency and exhibit other problems.

There are several properties of detectors which are important to CT scanning. It is not within the scope of this chapter to discuss them all, however, the few which deserve mention here are efficiency, stability, and dynamic range.

Detector *efficiency* refers to *photon capture ratio* (how many photons are detected) and *photon conversion efficiency* (how many photons are converted into electrons). For scintillation detectors, the conversion ratio is higher than for xenon detectors, but xenon detectors have a higher capture ratio than scintillation detectors. Therefore, the total efficiency for both detector types is about the same.

If a detector response is not steady, the detector is said to exhibit poor *stability* which ultimately degrades image quality. Hence, frequent calibrations may be necessary to correct the instability.

The *dynamic range* of a CT detector is expressed as a ratio of the largest signal to the smallest signal to be measured to a certain precision (say 0.1%). NaI detectors have a limited dynamic range.

Measurement of Radiation

From Figure 17:1, it is apparent that two sets of x-ray measurements are taken. The first one is taken by the *reference detector* which measures the intensity of the beam leaving the x-ray tube. The second measurement is recorded by the detector below the patient, which detects the intensity of the transmitted photons.

These two measurements are used to calculate *relative transmission values* (RTV) such that:

$$RTV = \log \frac{\text{Intensity of x-rays at source}}{\text{Intensity of x-rays at detector}}$$

These values are used to calculate *CT numbers*. CT numbers are in turn related to the linear attenuation coefficients (μ's) of the anatomy to be imaged by the following relationship:

$$\text{CT number} = \frac{\mu_{\text{tissue}} - \mu_{\text{water}}}{\mu_{\text{water}}} \times C$$

where C is a manufacturer's *scaling factor* or *contrast factor* and is usually assigned the value of 500 or 1000.

In the original EMI scanner, a value of 500 was used and resulted in a scale of values varying from +500 for bone and -500 for air, with water being zero. (These values are assigned arbitrarily for convenience.) Such a scale is referred to as the *EMI scale* and the CT numbers are referred to as EMI units (EMU). Recently, most manufacturers have set the value of C to be 1000, in which case the scale now extends from +1000 for bone to -1000 for air, with water still at zero. This scale is referred to as the *Hounsfield scale* and the CT numbers are called Hounsfield units (Hn units), in honor of the inventor. The advantage of the Hounsfield scale is that it expresses μ more accurately than the other scale. Figure 17:3 shows the two scales with tissue values of clinical significance.

Once CT numbers are obtained, they are fed to the computer for processing to reconstruct the image. When reconstruction is completed, the *reconstructed image*, as it is now called, can be displayed as a numerical printout as shown in Figure 17:4. Since this number printout is difficult to interpret, another means

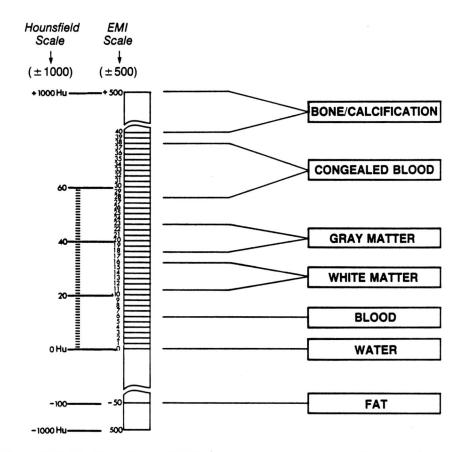

Figure 17:3. The Hounsfield and EMI scales, showing tissue values of clinical significance in CT scanning. (From Seeram, E.: Computed Tomography Technology. W.B. Saunders Co., Philadelphia. 1982.)

of image display is necessary. The CT numbers must now be converted to shades of gray. Such conversion of digital data is accomplished by a *digital-to-analog* (DAC) converter, and the analog signal can now be displayed as shades of gray (or color) on a TV monitor (Figure 17:5).

The CT number display is a display of the cross section of interest. The number display is usually arranged in rows and columns. Such arrangement is called a *matrix* (matrix sizes of 160 × 160, 256 × 256, and 512 × 512 are common to CT machines.)

The matrix consists of a set of small regions (squares) called picture elements or *pixels* (Chapter 15). Each pixel is a representation of the CT number computed for a specific volume of tissue (such as 1.5 mm × 1.5 mm × 13 mm) referred to as a *voxel*. In general, the CT number is proportional to the average attenuation of all structures contained in the voxel, and this is called *partial volume averaging*. Figure 17:6 shows the relationship between matrix, pixel and voxel.

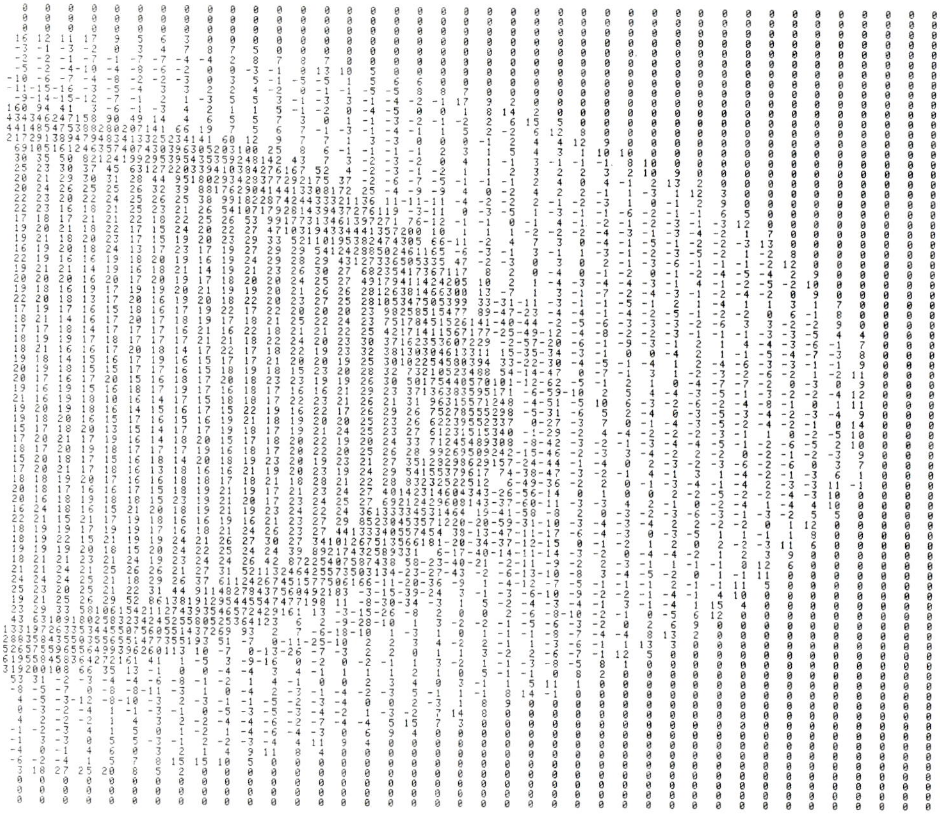

Figure 17:4. A portion of a reconstructed image, displayed as a numerical printout.

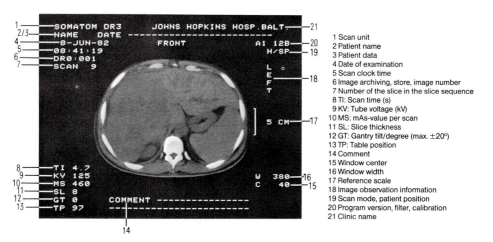

1 Scan unit
2 Patient name
3 Patient data
4 Date of examination
5 Scan clock time
6 Image archiving, store, image number
7 Number of the slice in the slice sequence
8 TI: Scan time (s)
9 KV: Tube voltage (kV)
10 MS: mAs-value per scan
11 SL: Slice thickness
12 GT: Gantry tilt/degree (max. ±20°)
13 TP: Table position
14 Comment
15 Window center
16 Window width
17 Reference scale
18 Image observation information
19 Scan mode, patient position
20 Program version, filter, calibration
21 Clinic name

Figure 17:5. A CT image displayed on a television monitor as shades of gray. Image identification is also given. (courtesy of the Siemens Corporation.)

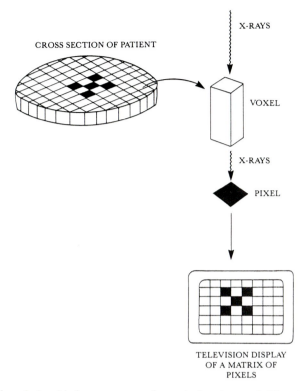

Figure 17:6. The relationship between a matrix, a pixel and a voxel. The pixel is a representation of a voxel which is displayed on a two-dimensional television screen.

COMPUTER PROCESSING AND STORAGE

The computer in CT is a digital computer, that is, it operates on digital data which it receives from an analog-to-digital converter. More specifically, the computer is a minicomputer system which is capable of several functions, the most important being that of image reconstruction.

Image reconstruction involves the use of specific computational methods to solve the problem in CT. These methods are referred to as *reconstruction algorithms*. An *algorithm* is a specific set of rules to solve a problem using a finite number of steps. Reconstruction algorithms form part of the software of the CT system. Such software is usually protected by manufacturers through the use of license agreements. Image reconstruction may be done either by *array processors* (electronic circuitry for doing calculations on digital data) or by *hard-wired electronics* or sometimes by a combination of both.

Some CT scanners have microprocessors and/or hard-wired electronics for handling other specific functions. A system which uses microprocessors is much more flexible than a hard-wired system, in that updated equipment can easily be added to a microprocessor system. On the other hand, the hard-wired system does not allow for the addition of update parameters, but it is much faster than the microprocessor approach.

Two other computer functions which deserve mention are *machine control functions* and *display functions*.

Machine control functions refer to control and operation of the gantry and patient couch, selection and accurate positioning of slices, monitoring exposure factors (kVp and mA) and the heat load capacity of the x-ray tube.

Display functions, on the other hand, refer to image magnification and measurements (distances, angles, mean, standard deviation), labelling with letters and/or numbers, *reformatted images* (sagittal and coronal images) which are generated by the computer using the data obtained from the axial scan and computer graphics. Some of these display functions are done by microprocessors.

Computer storage in CT consists of two types: primary and secondary. In primary storage, data (CT numbers) are stored in the central processing unit mainframe memory. Secondary storage refers to storage of data on magnetic tapes, disks and floppy diskettes.

DATA COLLECTION SCHEMES

A *data collection scheme* refers to the type of beam geometry, scanning mode and the number of detectors used to acquire transmission readings. Presently, several schemes are available for clinical use, resulting in five categories of CT scanners.

First-generation Scanners

These are scanners which use a *single pencil beam* with one or two detectors and a scanning mode based on the *translate-rotate* principle. The x-ray beam is highly collimated. The x-ray tube and detector move across the patient (translate) to collect a set of transmission readings. After one translation, the tube and detector rotate 1° and translate across the patient to collect another set of transmission readings (Figure 17:7). This sequence of events is repeated so that the gantry rotates through 180°. This is necessary in order to collect an adequate number of readings to perform the reconstruction.

The total scan time for this type of scanner ranges from 4-5 minutes. The *scan time* is defined as the time needed to collect an adequate number of x-ray transmission readings in order to perform the reconstruction. An insufficient number of transmission readings will result in poor reconstruction and loss of information in the image, leading to image artifacts. The scan time is inversely proportional to the number of detectors. Therefore, an increase in the number of detectors decreases the scan time.

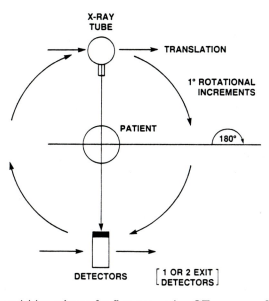

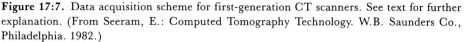

Figure 17:7. Data acquisition scheme for first-generation CT scanners. See text for further explanation. (From Seeram, E.: Computed Tomography Technology. W.B. Saunders Co., Philadelphia. 1982.)

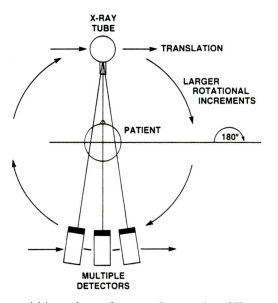

Figure 17:8. Data acquisition scheme for second-generation CT scanners. See text for further explanation. (From Seeram. E.: Computed Tomography Technology. W.B. Saunders Co., Philadelphia. 1982.)

First-generation scanners used about two scintillation (NaI) detectors and stationary-anode x-ray tubes. The first EMI brain scanner (Mark I CT 1000) also employed a *water bath* around the patient's head to ensure more accurate readings and to provide water as a reference for transmission readings.

Second-generation Scanners

These scanners feature *multiple pencil beams* with multiple detectors (3 to 60) of the scintillation type. Different scanners use different detectors such as NaI, CaF_2, and BGO.

The scanning mode is still based on the rotate/translate principle with larger rotational increments ranging from 3°-30° (fan) for 180° (Figure 17:8). The advantage of multiple pencil beams and detectors is that more transmission readings can be collected for each translation. The scan time for these scanners range from about 20 seconds to 3-5 minutes.

Third-generation Scanners

Third-generation scanners have a beam geometry that describes a fan (fan beam geometry) and consist of a multiple detector array. The scanning mode is purely rotational (Figure 17:9). The x-ray tube and detector array are coupled so that they both rotate around the patient to collect transmission readings.

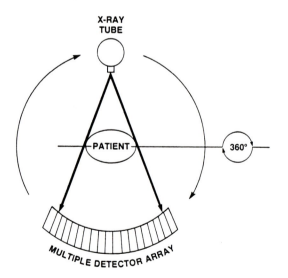

Figure 17:9. The method of data collection for third-generation CT scanners. See text for further explanation. (From Seeram, E.: Computed Tomography Technology. W.B. Saunders Co., Philadelphia. 1982.)

These scanners are much faster than first- and second-generation scanners with a scan time of 5-10 seconds. Such fast scan time is advantageous from the standpoint of reducing artifacts due to patient motion.

The radiation beam is a pulsed fan beam with a detector array ranging from 128 (Atronix 1110) to 600 (American Science and Engineering). Most of these scanners use xenon gas detectors.

Fourth-generation Scanners

The principle of data collection for fourth-generation scanners is somewhat different than first-, second- and third-generation scanners, in that the beam geometry is now a *wide fan beam.*

The detectors form a *stationary ring* around the patient so that the scanning mode is now *purely rotational* with a continuous fan beam of radiation as opposed to a pulsed fan beam.

The detectors in the circular array can range from 600 to 2000, which make the scan times for these scanners vary from 2-10 seconds. In most cases xenon is used.

There are several limitations imposed by this arrangement of tube and detectors (Figure 17:10). For example, the tube-to-object distance is less than the object-detector distance and this may increase patient dose.

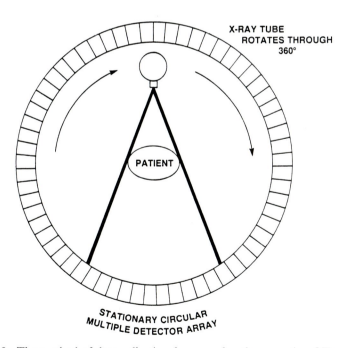

Figure 17:10. The method of data collection for some fourth-generation CT scanners. See text for further explanation. (From Seeram. E.: Computed Tomography Technology. W.B. Saunders C., Philadelphia. 1982)

Another type of fourth-generation scanner which has become commercially available is one that utilizes a *nutating sensor geometry*. This means that the ring of detectors is arranged in such a way that the detectors closest to the x-ray tube will move out of the path of the x-ray beam so that the beam may fall on the "far away" detectors.

The advantage of this data collection scheme is that it reduces the limitations imposed by the stationary detector ring with rotating tube design.

IMAGE DISPLAY AND DOCUMENTATION

Once the reconstruction process is complete, the image can be stored for use at a later time or it must be displayed in a suitable form for viewing and interpretation by the radiologist.

Historically, the CT image was first displayed as a numerical printout where the numbers represent CT numbers. Since this image was not suitable to the radiologist, it was converted to a gray scale image for display on a television monitor and for recording by photographic means.

CT manufacturers have provided display/viewing/recording facilities in the form of attractive consoles. These consoles are of two types, namely, the *operator console* and the *physician console*. Essentially, both have similar features.

In Figure 17:11, a typical control console for CT is shown. The common elements include a television monitor for image display, photographic recoding equipment, window width and window level controls, kVp, mA and other technical factors, an alpha numeric keyboard and floppy disk drives.

The television monitor has controls for adjusting the brightness and contrast of the image. On one side of the picture tube is displayed a *gray scale bar* which shows about 8 to 16 shades of gray. This bar has no direct relationship to the CT image itself but rather assists the viewer to familiarize himself with the range of the gray scale. It also indicates that the television monitor has been appropriately set to include the entire range of the gray scale to be shown.

Photographic recording may take two approaches. First, the image can be recorded by instant photography, in which case an instant camera (e.g., Polaroid®) is coupled to another monitor on which the CT image is displayed. The shades of gray that can be displayed on instant photographic film is somewhat limited and may range from 10-16 shades.

In the second approach, the CT system may include a *multi-image multi-format camera* which records CT images onto x-ray film. Image formats will differ for different film sizes, for example, 4 images on an 8 × 10 is not uncommon. With x-ray film, the number of shades of gray displayed is greater than in instant photography.

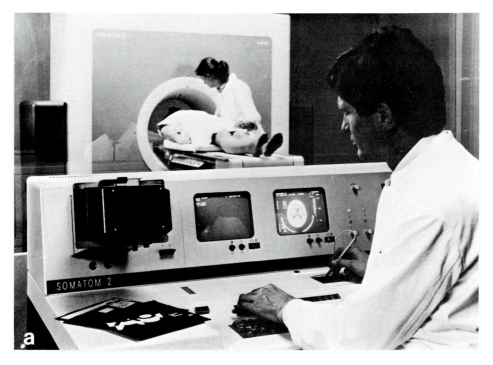

Figure 17:11. A control console of a CT unit. In (a) the alphanumeric keyboard, photographic recording equipment, television monitors and other controls are shown. In (b) the operator is loading the floppy disk drive with a floppy disk. (courtesy of the Siemens Corporation.)

An *alpha numeric keyboard* is provided on the console to allow the operator to communicate with the computer. The keyboard consists of letters and numbers (numeric) and is similar in appearance to a typewriter keyboard. Various codes are established by manufacturers to allow for this communication.

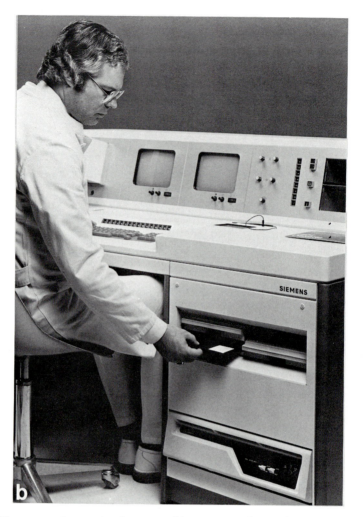

All CT systems have another set of keys apart from the ones on the alpha numeric keyboard. These keys are referred to as *interactive function keys*. They allow the operator to perform other tasks such as highlighting certain structures, obtaining certain statistical data (mean, standard deviation), magnification, labelling, and so on.

Storage of data was discussed previously and included the use of magnetic tapes, drums, and floppy diskettes. Disk drives are therefore provided on consoles, and disks are simply inserted into the drive for recording images. The image on the disk can be erased so that the disk may be used again or it can form a part of the patient's record.

Two other controls that deserve special mention are the window width (WW) and window level (WL) controls. These are found on the consoles and operate in a similar fashion as television brightness control knobs.

Recall the acquisition of the CT numbers. When reconstructing an image of a slice, a range of CT numbers are contained to represent various tissues. This range of CT numbers is defined as the *window width*, while the center of the range is called the *window level*. A CT unit using the 1000 Hn scale has a range of CT numbers equal to 2000 with the center of range being 0. The WW and WL controls thus allow the radiologist to examine specific tissues that are of interest to him. They also vary the "contrast" of the image.

BASIC CONFIGURATION OF A CT SCANNER

The elements of CT have been discussed in terms of data acquisition, collection, processing, viewing and display. The components of the CT system have been described and range from the x-ray tube and generator, collimation, detectors, detector electronics, computer processing and storage to the consoles for display, viewing and recording of images.

The functional relationship of these components is shown in Figure 17:12.

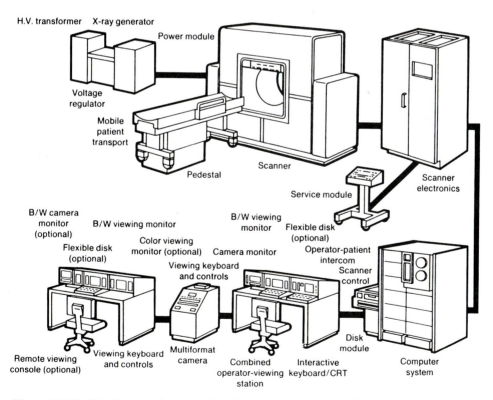

Figure 17:12. The functional relationship of the components of a CT scanner. (courtesy of Picker International.)

RADIATION DOSE

The radiation dose for CT studies depends on several factors and in general ranges from 2 to 10 rads.

In order to fully appreciate dose in CT, one must first refer to doses for conventional imaging procedures. For example, the surface radiation doses for a skull series (4 films), abdomen (1 film), angiogram (11 films/biplane) and pneumoencephalography (18 films) are 0.5 rads, 0.2 rads, 10 rads and 30 rads, respectively.

In CT, the factors which affect dose relate to the design of the scanner as well as the operating technique. In terms of scanner design, the scanner geometry (generation), rotation angle, x-ray tube focus, collimation and filtration, and detectors are important. For example, the radiation dose distribution from a 180° translate/rotate scanner is generally asymmetric, that is, the dose is greater on one side of the patient compared to a 360° rotate scanner, where the dose is more evenly distributed over the patient.

The x-ray tube focal spot size influences the dose, in that larger focal spots produce larger penumbra and hence higher doses will be delivered to the patient for multiple scans. Higher filtration will lower the patient dose.

The operating parameters, on the other hand, are several and vary from scanner to scanner. Such parameters include kVp, mA, scan time, patient orientation (supine or prone), slice thickness (decreasing slice thickness increases the dose for the same image quality), spacing of the slice (dose increases if profiles overlap) and the number of adjacent slices. Others include repeat scans, dynamic scanning, the size of the pixel and the reconstruction algorithm. The latter two affect dose in an indirect manner (that is, when mA-secs must be increased to give some specified image quality).

In order to reduce dose in CT, attention must be focussed on the design and operating parameters. For example, optimizing x-ray tube collimation, detector efficiency and filtration can result in decreased doses. With regards to the operating parameters, dose can be reduced by performing fewer scans, increasing the separation of slices, decreasing the mA-secs or scan times, and increasing the pixel size.

ARTIFACTS

Artifacts in CT are numerous and can arise from several factors such as the patient, metal objects and the CT scanner itself. Artifacts which may appear on a CT image can range from *streaks, rings, increased noise* to *shading, cupping* and *capping*. A discussion of all artifacts is beyond the scope of this chapter, however, only the more common ones will be described.

Rings appear as concentric circles on the image. The cause for such rings may be related to several factors such as a "dead" detector cell, loss of pressure

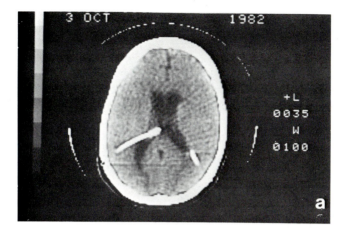

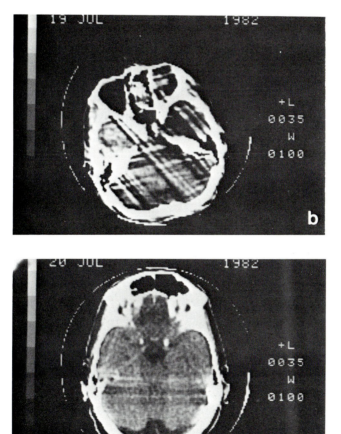

Figure 17:13. Streak artifacts produced by (a) metal, (b) motion of patient and (c) sharp interfaces such as the petrous bones.

in gas-ionization detectors, and unbalanced detectors. Ring artifacts tend to occur on third- and fourth-generation scanners, since their data acquisition schemes involve a circular motion of x-ray tube and detectors.

Streaks on CT images may appear as a star (starlike) array or as lighting bolts. They are caused by metal structures (such as needles, shunts, zipper, buttons), dense bone (petrous) and sharp interfaces (such as contrast media/air). Motion of the patient also produces streak artifacts. Figure 17:13 shows streak artifacts from metal, patient motion and sharp interfaces.

Shading, cupping and capping are terms used to refer to artifacts arising from a general variation of CT numbers in the image.

In a shading artifact, CT numbers are higher on one side of the image compared to the opposite side. In cupping and capping, CT numbers around the outer edges of the image are higher (increased density) and lower, respectively, than those numbers in the center of the image.

The causes for such variations are several and include poor patient centering in the gantry aperture, beam hardening, detector problems, generator calibration problems, and so on.

Noisy images, on the other hand, can be due to insufficient photons at the detector, reduced pressure in gas-ionization detectors, too low an mA setting or a decrease in x-ray tube output.

Motion artifacts can be reduced by immobilization and sedation fo the patient, as well as by decreasing the scan time. Other artifacts (equipment-related) are usually eliminated by computer algorithms and, in some cases (ring artifacts), by stabilizing circuitry and calibration protocols.

IMAGE QUALITY

The quality of the image in CT can be described in terms of spatial resolution and contrast resolution.

Since image quality is a broad topic, only relevant details will be mentioned here.

Contrast resolution is defined as the ability of the scanner to discriminate tissues which differ only slightly in density. The factors which influence contrast resolution are listed and explained in Table 17:1.

Spatial resolution is defined as the ability of the scanner to discriminate very small objects and there are a number of factors which affect such resolution. These factors are listed and explained in Table 17:2.

FUTURE TRENDS

The development of more efficient CT scanners has progressed at a rapid rate since the introduction of the first EMI brain scanner. These changes have been described and a number of features have been highlighted.

Table 17-1

FACTORS INFLUENCING CONTRAST RESOLUTION IN CT

FACTOR	EXPLANATION	GENERAL RELATIONSHIP
Photon Flux	This is the amount of transmitted photons through the patient. This is determined by the exposure factors (kVp, mA and time) and by the thickness of the slice.	The higher the exposure factors, the greater the x-ray quanta. Higher kVp (120-140) produces good contrast resolution. Higher mA increases the number of photons. Increased time increases the amount of transmitted photons.
Slice Thickness		Increased slice thickness results in increased number of photons detected.
Detector Efficiency	In general, this refers to the *capture efficiency* (ratio of the number of photons incident on detectors to the number of photons captured) and the separation between detectors.	Gas-ionization detectors have lower capture efficiency than solid state detectors.
Reconstruction Filter	This can be used to improve contrast resolution by reducing noise through a process known as *smoothing* (elimination of high spatial frequencies).	

Table 17-2

FACTORS INFLUENCING SPATIAL RESOLUTION IN CT

FACTOR	EXPLANATION	GENERAL RELATIONSHIP
Width of the beam	The width at the center of the beam is of importance in this regard. This width depends on the focal spot size, detector aperture size and the source-to-object distance in relationship to the source-to-detector distance (magnification factor).	Larger detector aperture produces blurring. If the object is scanned in a wider beam, it will be more blurred than if object is scanned in a less wide beam. Smaller focal spot sizes gives better definition.
Slice thickness	This is related to the longitudinal size of the focal spot and the prepatient collimation.	Wider slices produces poor axial resolution.
Reconstruction algorithm filter	This filter is a mathematical formula which is used to eliminate the blurring characteristic of the simple back projection algorithm through a process called *spatial filtration.*	Filtered back projection (convolution technique) produces sharper images than iterative techniques and the simple back projection.
Image matrix	Two such matrices are important. The *reconstruction matrix* (computer) and the *display matrix* (CRT screen).	Smaller pixels in the matrix tends to produce a sharper-looking image. A 512 x 512 matrix will produce a picture that appears sharper than say a 256 x 256 matrix.

In the future, the following may appear:

A. (1) More work on *dynamic scanning* (method used to obtain multiple images at a rapid rate) in CT.
   (2) Improved collimation schemes.
   (3) Improved image quality.
   (4) Development of quality assurance protocols for CT.
   (5) New x-ray sources and detector arrays.
   (6) Computer software for additional functions such as *multiple imaging* (display of four to six images at one time) and *high-resolution technology* (display of raw data on smaller pixels).
B. (1) Three-dimensional CT scanning.
   (2) Quantitative CT.
   (3) Fast CT scanning.

In *three-dimensional CT*, volume scanning is characteristic and computer software allows for viewing the image in three dimensions.

Quantitative CT involves the "study of accuracy, precision and consistency of CT value measurements" (Parker and Stanley, 1981). It includes methods used to study area, volume, linear measurements of the anatomy of interest and densitometry. In densitometry (measuring the distribution of densities), mineral content of bone and blood flow measurements can be determined.

Fast CT scanning refers to those scanners which have the potential for imaging, at high speeds, structures such as the heart, with three-dimensional display. An example of one such scanner is the *dynamic spatial reconstructor* (DSR) unit, which is under study at the Mayo Clinic. The DSR consists of multiple x-ray tubes coupled to multiple image intensifiers (28) to generate a 10 msec scan speed.

CINE COMPUTED TOMOGRAPHY

Recently, a high-speed CT scanner has become commercially available after years of intensive research at the University of California, San Francisco. The scanner has been referred to as a *cine computed tomography* machine (C-100) capable of multiple slices at scan speeds more than 30 times faster than conventional CT scanners.

The following account which includes a background and technical descirption of the Cine CT Scanner is taken from information provided by *Imatron Inc.* in San Francisco.

Clinical Significance of Cine CT

Background

"During the ten years since the clinical introduction of computed tomography, scan times have been reduced by two orders of magnitude

— from 4½ minutes to a few seconds. This improvement, combined with that in spatial resolution, has enabled increased applications in the imaging of body organs and some simple methods for examining flow of injected contrast media. Although x-ray tube technology and the mechanical scanning systems have been pushed to their limits, many practical problems remain which require patient sedation, glucagon and breath-holding in order to minimize motion artifacts, especially those from high-contrast objects.

The Advantages of Cine-CT

"The advent of cine computed tomography, with scan times a further two orders of magnitude shorter, now permits not only the elimination of artifacts but also the opportunity to image motion and obtain additional data concerning function and flow. The use of non-mechanical, electron beam scanning gives flow studies and repeatable volume examinations in a fraction of a second. For the first time, successive images in a movie display enable true visualization of motion. In contrast, gated scans, which are made up of many incomplete projections acquired over several seconds, are reconstructed to provide a set of composite images.

Performance Characteristics

"The C-100 system provides scan rates up to 24 per second, scan times between 33 ms and 100 ms, interscan delays as short as 8 ms and repeatable multi-slice volumes without moving the patient. Thus, high patient throughput is achieved with competitive spatial and contrast performance and the added capability of trading off contrast resolution for temporal resolution.

Clinical Modes of Operation

"The three prime modes of operation — continuous, triggered and volume — can be applied singly or together to provide a comprehensive examination of any part of the anatomy.

The continuous mode is used for imaging moving organs or contrast media with optimum temporal resolution. In the triggered mode a lower repetition rate is used, but the fast (typically 50 ms) scan times provide a full, multi-slice examination of flow in only a few seconds. Volumes can be imaged rapidly either by using the multiple target rings (8 cm in 225 ms) or by incrementing the couch continuously while scanning, up to 17 cm per second. Thus, much of the time and patient discomfort from lengthy conventional procedures can be eliminated. In contrast studies a single injection can usually be used for the total study and dynamic charactgeristics can be evaluated using a bolus rather than a drip infusion. There are no artifact problems even without sedation, in trauma cases, pediatric cases, or while the patient is breathing normally.

C-100 Benefits in Conventional Applications

"Full lung studies may be completed in a few minutes. Lesions adjacent to the heart wall will not be obscured by motion. Anatomy within the lungs is not degraded by cardiac motion nor by breathing.

"Abdominal studies, even those involving 20 or more slice levels, can be rapidly performed. Additionally, the superior temporal resolution permits liver and renal flow studies to be performed using bolus injections.

"Trauma cases, requiring a fast evaluation of a frequently uncooperative patient, should be straightforward.

"Pediatrics can typically be scanned without sedation and these patients will not be alarmed by any mechanical vibration or noise.

"Volume studies, using continuous incrementation of the couch, can be run with minimum patient discomfort and no requirement to maintain one position for more than a few seconds. Any subsequent multiplanar reconstructions will not be distorted by misregistration.

New Applications Enabled by Cine CT Technology

"The C-100 was developed with the prime requirement of providing optimum imaging of the heart. The unique multiple ring target, short scan time and minimum interscan delay now allow repeatable, triggered volume studies from a single contrast injection. From these triggered studies quantitative data is simply extracted using flow curves of CT number versus time. This perfusion data, combined with the dynamic imaging of cardiac motion, makes cine CT the preferred investigative technique for screening or follow up of a broad range of clinical conditions.

"Motion studies in orthopedic applications have also shown early promise. Continuous scan sequencing while flexing a joint (knee, shoulder, elbow, temporo-mandibular, for instance) shows in exceptional detail the relationship of bone, cartilage and tissue — either in a single plane or in 3 dimensions using the volume mode.

"Flow studies outside the heart are enabled by the rapid sequence capability. Areas of clinical interest are the liver, renals, carotid arteries and, ultimately, the brain.

Cardiac Applications on Cine CT

"The low radiation dose and small amounts of intravenous contrast required will make it economically feasible to screen adult and pediatric patients with acquired congenital heart disease prior to angiography. Normal flow measurements by cine CT would preclude the necessity for a more invasive and expensive examination.

"Follow-up scans to monitor drug therapy and to evaluate patients after open-heart surgery will also be applicable to a broad range of clinical conditions.

"Measurements of myocardial perfusion, now being corroborated in animal and other studies under clinical research programs, promise to revolutionize the early diagnosis of cardiac disease. Correlation of the wall and valve motion revealed by the C-100 with the flow measured at corresponding slice levels should add significantly to our understanding of disease processes.

"While other studies will not necessarily be replaced by cine CT, the addition of this powerful technique to the diagnostic arsenal is likely to limit the number of procedures necessary and will frequently reduce the average cost of care per patient.

Technical Description

"The Cine-CT system (C-100) consists of an innovative scanning electron beam x-ray tube, a stationary detector array, and computer system for data acquisition, reconstuction, and display. Figure 17:14 and Figure 17:15 illustrate the design of the system schematically. An electron beam is accelerated and focussed along the axis of the x-ray tube. Coils magnetically steer the beam along a 210° curved target. Four target rings are available and are typically scanned serially to obtain a multiple slice examination. Ring collimators near the source restrict the x-ray beam to a wide fan, 2 cm thick. An approximately 30° fan-shaped sector of the x-ray beam is attenuated by the scanned object and the resulting intensity distribution is measured by a curved detector array. The digitized detector output is stored in a bulk memory and used for computerized reconstruction. Overlap of the detector and target rings assures that a complete set of data is obtained.

"Since the detector array actually consists of two contiguous rings of 216°, a single scan will produce a pair of side-by-side tomographic slices. Figure 17:16 illustrates the multiple slice configuration obtained by serial scanning of the four target rings in combination with the dual detector ring. For each traverse of the electron beam on any one of the four x-ray targets, a pair of 8-mm thick slices are imaged. The collec-

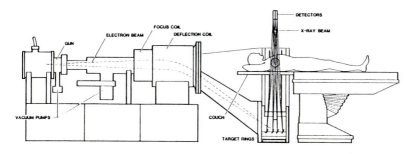

Figure 17:14. A high speed CT scanner design. Shown here is the CINE-CT system (C-100). See text for further explanation. (courtesy of Imatron Inc., San Francisco, California.)

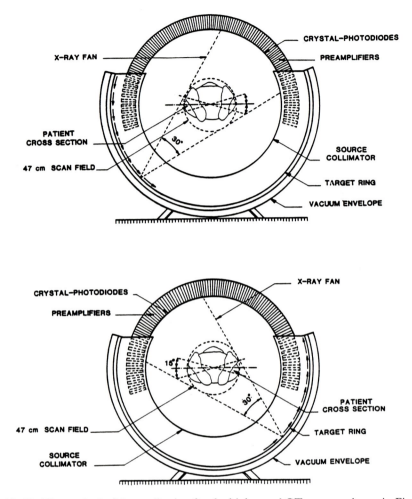

Figure 17:15. The method of data collection for the high speed CT scanner shown in Figure 17:14. See text for further explanation. (courtesy of Imatron Inc., San Francisco, California.)

tion of eight slices covers a region approximately 8 cm thick, large enough to encampass all of the left ventricle and virtually all of the heart of typical patients.

"The scanning electron beam x-ray contains an electron gun which produces a beam current of 300 to 800 mA at 130 kV. After leaving the gun, the beam expands because of the mutual repulsion of the electrons and is focussed by a magnetic lens. A bending magnet deflects the converging beam through a fixed angle as indicated in Figure 17:14. A time variation of the magnet coil currents causes the plane of bending to rotate. At the base of the conical section, the focussed beam strikes one of the four target rings.

"In all medical x-ray tubes, the dissipation of heat at the target is an important factor, because less than one percent of the incident electron

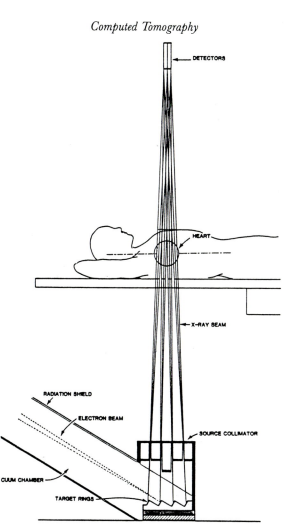

Figure 17:16. The method of obtaining multiple slices from the high speed CT scanner shown in Figure 17:14. See text for further explanation. (courtesy of Imatron Inc., San Francisco, California.)

energy is converted into energy in the form of x-rays. The remaining energy heats the target surface localized at the focus, and the heat is dissipated into the surrounding target structure. Generally, a high instantaneous x-ray output is required for short exposures, and a high average of x-ray output (a large "duty-cycle") allows many exposures to be made in a given time. Two circumstances render the scan tube ideal for achieving high instantaneous as well as high average x-ray output; the focal spot travels with a speed of typically 66 meters per second, and the heat input is "diluted" over a focal track length of 330 cm. The average x-ray output can be increased beyond the corresponding value of rotating-anode x-ray tubes because the total mass of the target structure, acting as a heat sink, is a factor of 100 higher than the largest conventional tubes.

"Each detector ring is equipped with 432 individual x-ray-sensitive elements. Each element consists of an x-ray-to-light converter crystal, a light-to-current converting silicon photodiode, and a preamplifier. All three components (crystals, photodiodes, and amplifiers) form an optimized matched system in order to achieve the stringent requirements of quantum limited detection, stability, and accuracy.

"The data acquisition system digitizes and stores the detector data. This data is stored in a random access memory system that can hold ECG triggered data for 38 consecutive heartbeats (76 slices, 2 slices per heartbeat) prior to disc transfer. For a multi-slice sequence, double-CT slices can be selected by switching between the four target rings; thus flow phenomena can be studied over 8 cm of the heart. Cine scanning sequences are performed such that up to 2 seconds of continuous scan data are collected prior to disc transfer. 50 msec scans, with an 8 msec interscan delay, proceed at 17 scans/second for a dual-slice study. In a multi-slice study, an 8 slice volume is covered by consecutive scans on each of the 4 target rings in approximately 250 msec.

"The patient table is designed to provide optimal positioning of the patient within the scan field. The patient table can move forward or backward, move up or down, angulate up to 25°, and swivel up to 25° in each direction. The large degree of freedom offered in selection of the patient position enables the scanner to image areas often considered difficult, such as the posterior and anterior walls of the heart and the heart valves. Controls on both sides of the table make contact with the patient simple for both the technician and the physician. The operator can control the table from the scanner room or from the operator's console.

"The scan control computer is programmed to provide safety interlocks, protecting the scan tube, the patient,and the staff from any unusual conditions in beam position or intensity. The beam can be shut down in less than millisecond after receiving an abort instruction from the computer.

"Cine-CT has the capability to collect many images in a short time period, so there are unique requirements on the display system. The system is equipped with conventional as well as specialized display and analysis functions. The display system consists of a CRT display screen, a trackball, window and level control knobs, an identify button, and function keys for processing of data.

"The system has features to enable tailoring of the image for optimal diagnostic value. Images can be reformatted into oblique, sagittal, and coronal views. The CT number range extends from -1000 to +1000 with a continuous viewing window range from 1 to 2000. For visualization of small structures magnification of images up to fifteen times is possible. For quantitative analysis, several regions-of-interest (ROI) shapes are available to provide versatility in types of quantitative measurements: ellipse, rectangle, and irregular. The average, standard deviation, area, and number of pixels are determined for any

ROI. Other conventional diagnostic features are available including a histogram display, multiformat display, gray scale band display, CT number display, mark display (grid and scale), measurement function, erase graphics function, annotation, zoom, pan, screen save, and blink/identify.

"Many specialized display programs are available to satisfy all the needs of the physician. For real-time visualization of the beating heart or visualization of the progression of contrast through the heart at the same point in the cardiac cycle, movie-mode displays are performed. The flow of contrast within the heart chambers and myocardium can be studied through the use of the flow study program, resulting in myocardial perfusion measurements. If additional analysis of myocardial perfusion is desirable, other programs are available. Volume study programs determine the volume of a heart chamber, a vessel, or any other region of interest. The motion of the walls of the heart, including the thickening of these walls, can be studied quantitatively to obtain a variety of measurements, including regional or total ejection fraction. The high speed of the C-100 makes all of these measurements very accurate. For studies involving parts of the body not subject to significant amounts of involuntary motion, several images obtained in a short amount of time may be averaged to improve image quality. Thus quality, motion-artifact free, body and head images can also be produced with very short examination times.

Conclusion

"Continuing clinical research is revealing ever-increasing application for this unique scanner. The competitive imaging performance of the C-100 provides high throughput, straightforward examinations. The dose flexibility and flow measurement capability are now being exploited in a broad range of cardiac and non-cardiac examinations.

"The C-100 scanner, which reveals accurate data of blood flow and cardiac function in three dimensions, provides a cost-effective, non-invasive but comprehensive examination. Extensive clinical research centered around this new technology will further underline its important place in evaluation of cardiac disease.

SUMMARY

1. Computed tomography (CT) is a technique in which a computer is used to reconstruct cross-sectional images, from transmission (x-ray) data obtained from the patient.
2. The shortcomings (such as the problem of super imposition) of radiography and tomography (conventional) are removed by CT through the use of special detectors and complex mathematics for reconstructing images.

3. The steps in digitizing an image as used in CT involve scanning, sampling and quantization.

4. Historical perspectives are discussed with special reference to Hounsfield, who developed the technique for clinical applications, and to Cormack, who provided a mathematical solution to the problem in CT.

5. The problem in CT is to calculate the linear attenuation coefficients for the anatomy under study knowing a large set of x-ray transmission measurements.

6. The data acquisition scheme in CT consists of the x-ray tube, collimatior, imaging object, detectors, and detector electronics. The unit which houses the x-ray tube and detectors is the gantry.

7. X-ray tubes in CT may be of the stationary-anode type or the rotating-anode type. Stationary anode tubes have higher power output and higher x-ray intensity for long exposure times. Rotating anode tubes, on the other hand, provide higher intensity and power for short exposure times.

8. Collimation influences the thickness of the slice.

9. The opening of the detector collimator is the detector aperture width. This width influences the inherent spatial resolution such that smaller widths provide better spatial resolution.

10. The detectors and associated electronics are referred to as the data acquisition system (DAS). The DAS convert x-rays into electrical signals which are subsequently converted into digital data.

11. Detectors may be scintillation detectors or gas-ionization detectors. The former consists of a scintillation crystal coupled to a photomultiplier tube, while the latter is a volume of gas in a chamber.

12. Detector efficiency, stability and dynamic range are defined.

13. Relative transmission measurements are used to calculate CT numbers. The old and new CT number scales are discussed.

14. A matrix is a display of CT numbers which are arranged in rows and columns. The matrix consists of a set of small regions called pixels (picture element). Each pixel is a representation of the CT number computed for a specific volume of tissue called a voxel (volume element).

15. The minicomputer system is used in CT. It is capable of several functions including image reconstruction. Image reconstruction may be done by array processors or by hard-wired electronics or sometimes by a combination of both. Some CT scanners have microprocessors for handling other specific functions.

16. Two other computer functions include machine control functions and display functions. The former refers to control and operation of the gantry, patient couch, selection and positioning of slices, monitoring exposure factors and the heat load capacity of the x-ray tube. Display functions refer to magnification, measurements, labelling and image reformation and computer graphics.

17. Computer storage in CT refers to both primary (data stored in the CPU mainframe memory) and secondary (data storage on disks and diskettes).

18. The data collection scheme in CT refers to the type of beam geometry, scanning mode and the number of detectors used. Five data collection schemes are described.

19. First-generation CT scanners are based on a single pencil beam with one or two detectors. The scanning mode describes the translate-rotate principle. After one translation, the tube and detectors rotate 1° and translate across the patient again. This is repeated until the gantry rotates 180°. The scan time is about 4-5 minutes.

20. Second-generation CT scanners are based on multiple pencil beams with multiple detectors. The rotational increments range from about 3°-30° for some scanners. The scan time ranges from 20 seconds to 3 minutes.

21. Third-generation scanners have a beam geometry that describes a fan. A multiple detector array is used and the scanning mode is purely rotational. The scan time ranges from 5-10 seconds.

22. The beam geometry for fourth-generation scanners is a wide fan. The detectors form a stationary ring around the patient and the scanning mode is purely rotational. The scan time ranges from 2-10 seconds.

23. Another type of fourth-generation scanner is one based on a nutating sensor geometry. This scheme reduces the limitations imposed by the stationary detector ring with rotating tube design.

24. Image display and documentation are discussed with respect to the operator and physician consoles. A typical console consists of a television monitor, photographic recording equipment, window width and window level controls, an alphanumeric keyboard and floppy disk drives.

25. The window width is the range of CT numbers while the window level is the center of the range.

26. Factors affecting radiation dose in CT include the scanner geometry, rotation angle, x-ray tube focus, collimation, filtration, type of detectors and so on.

27. Artifacts appearing on CT images may range from streaks, rings, increased noise to shading, cupping and capping. These are described briefly.

28. Streaks arise from metals and patient motion. Rings may be attributed to a malfunctioning detector cell in third- and fourth-generation scanners.

29. Shading, cupping and capping arise from a general variation of CT numbers in the image. Each is described.

30. Noisy images arise from insufficient photons arriving at the detector, reduced pressure in gas-ionization detectors, too low mA and a decrease in x-ray tube output.

31. Image quality is described in terms of spatial and contrast resolution. Each term is defined and the factors influencing both are given in the form of a table.

32. A discussion of future trends identifies a number of developments. These include dynamic scanning, improved collimation schemes, quality assurance protocols, new x-ray tubes and detector arrays, computer software, three-dimensional CT, quantitative CT and high-speed CT scanning. A high-speed CT scanner, the cine CT scanner, is described.

CHAPTER 18

DIGITAL RADIOGRAPHY

THE fundamental concepts of digital image processing were described in Chapter 15. The task of digitizing images requires a computer and therefore computer concepts, and the role of computers in imaging were identified and discussed in Chapter 16. One such application, CT, was later described in some detail in Chapter 17. CT is clearly an example of a digital imaging technique which is based on digital image processing theory and computer technology.

Significant developments and clinical work in CT proved its potential as an imaging tool. As a result of the success of pre-scan localization images (computed radiography) in CT, another technique was introduced and it gained popularity, particularly in intravenous angiography. This technique is referred to as *digital radiography*.

DEFINITION OF DIGITAL RADIOGRAPHY

In conventional radiography, x-rays pass through the patient and fall upon a film/screen cassette to form a latent image on the film. This image is rendered visible through chemical processing of the film, and the image is usually viewed with the aid of a viewbox or illuminator.

In digital radiography, the data collected from the patient (analog data) is converted into digital form so that it is suitable for processing, storage and retrieval by a digital computer (Brody, 1979). This concept is illustrated in Figure 18:1.

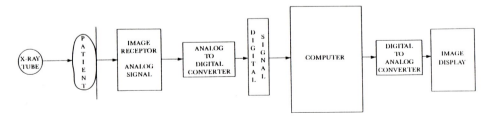

Figure 18:1. The concept of digital radiography. The data collected from the patient is converted into digital form for input into a digital computer.

Terms Synonymous with Digital Radiography

Other terms have been used to describe the technique of digital radiography. The terms are descriptive and emphasize the method of data collection characteristic of the technique together with their specific clinical application. These terms include: *digital fluoroscopy* (DF), *digital subtraction angiography* (DSA), *digital vascular imaging*, (DVI), *computerized fluorography* (CF), *digital video angiography* (DVA), *digital video subtraction angiograhy* (DVSA), *intravenous video arteriography* (IVA), and *scanned projection radiography* (SPR).

In this chapter, the term digital radiography will be used to emphasize that the technique is based on non-tomographic principles and to ditinguish it from computed tomography.

ADVANTAGES OF DIGITAL RADIOGRAPHY

Limitations of Radiography, Fluoroscopy and Computed Tomography

The primary limitations of conventional radiography and fluoroscopy are poor demonstration of low contrast structures and the problem of superimposition. The latter problem imposes a limitation on the detection of specific structures such as a lesion. In addition, radiography is limited in its ability to display, store, and retrieve and manipulate images.

Apart from its excellent frame rate (30-60 frames per second) and good temporal (0.1 to 100 m sec) and excellent spatial resolution (1.5 line pairs for television), fluoroscopy also suffers from inflexible display of its images.

CT, on the other hand, provides excellent low contrast resolution and removes the problem of superimposition by utilizing a tomographic approach (cross-sectional images) coupled to computer processing of images. The CT principle also allows the operator to "window" the image displayed on the television monitor to the desired contrast. However, CT imposes limitations as well. One such limitation is the time taken to scan the patient, particularly when a large area of the patient is to be examined, and therefore CT is not suitable for screening purposes.

CT is also limited by the *signal-to-noise ratio* (SNR), that is, the ratio of the signal strength to the fluctuations in the signal, and finally by its poor frame rate.

Advantages

The limitations imposed by radiography, fluoroscopy and computed tomography may be removed by digital radiography. Such removal is made possible by the application of computer technology and digital image processing theory to the present concepts of radiography and fluoroscopy.

One of the main advantages of digital radiography is its improved (or optimum) detectability of low contrast structures because of the high efficiency detectors used and the improved signal-to-noise ratio.

Since the digital computer is used in digital radiography, other advantages include:

(a) Quantitative analysis. Distances, areas and volume can be calculated rapidly and image features can be distinguished quite readily.

(b) Data can be stored for retrospective reanalysis of images. Storage is accomplished through the use of magnetic tape or disks.

(c) The use of window width and window level controls allows greater flexibility in image display.

(d) Image manipulation and enhancement are possible through the use of special computer programs.

(e) Image transmission. Digital images can be transferred via the telephone (or by microwaves) without the loss of image quality.

(f) Fast and accurate procesing of information collected from the patient.

HISTORICAL PERSPECTIVES

The development of digital radiography is attributed to several groups and it is particularly based on previous works on digital video image processing done in other areas such as in astronomy.

A description of video image processing is given by Dennison in a National Aeronautics and Space Administration (NASA) paper published in 1974.

A complete account of the history of digital radiography is not within the scope of this chapter and therefore only a brief identification of some of the pioneers will be given.

Within the last decade, the first applications of computer processing of x-ray television images through digital subtraction methods have been under investigation by a number of research teams. In the 1970s, Heintzen et al., Frost et al., and Hohne et al., published their initial results on digital radiography.

Later, the technique gained momentum and other studies in intravenous angiocardiography and carotid angiography were conducted to assess the potential of digital angiography. Significant work in this area was also done by the University of Wisconsin and the University of Arizona working groups. A digital video image processor was developed at the University of Wisconsin by Kruger and Mistretta et al. (1978, 1979), while digital video image programs were implemented at the University of Arizona by groups such as Ovitt et al. (1978, 1979, 1980).

Patient investigations were reported by Strother, Crummy and Sackett in 1980. Other workers such as Brody et al. (1980, 1981) also reported findings using digital scanned projection radiography.

Today, numerous x-ray equipment manufacturers are involved in developing and marketing digital radiography units. Investigators continue to report their clinical findings in imaging journals and national and international symposia.

THE CONCEPT OF DIGITAL RADIOGRAPHY

The concept of digital radiography in a broad sense is illustrated in Figure 18:1. The data collected from the patient (analog data) must first be digitized so that the information can be processed and stored by a digital computer.

Digitization is fundamental to digital radiography and is necessary, since it is more advantageous to collect, transmit and store digital data as opposed to analog data.

The concept of digital radiography is further expanded in Figure 18:2. In this case, the image produced by the television chain is digitized and processed by a digital computer. Another important point about the figure is that it illustrates a non-tomographic technique (fluoroscopy) and therefore the problem of superimposition immediately comes to mind. Recall that in CT, this problem is eliminated by the cross-sectional imaging format.

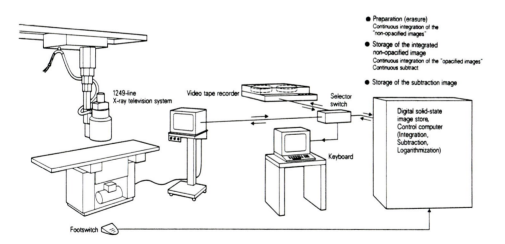

Figure 18:2. A digital fluoroscopic scheme. The information collected from the patient falls on the image intensifier. The image received by the television chain is digitized and then processed by a digital computer. (From Baert, AL et al.: Computer angiography — Intravenous arteriography. *Electromedica* 2-1981.)

In digital radiography, the problem of superimposition makes it difficult to image desired structures, such as blood vessels, for example, and therefore it must be eliminated. This is usually accomplished by some form of subtraction technique in which images are subtracted in time (temporal subtraction) and also with respect to energy (energy subtraction). The advantages of digital radiography are therefore made possible through these subtraction techniques.

METHODS OF SUBTRACTION

The methods of subtraction in digital radiography are:
  (a) Temporal subtraction
  (b) Energy subtraction
  (c) Hybrid subtraction

Temporal Subtraction

The term *temporal subtraction* describes a technique which uses the element of time in the subtraction process. Temporal subtraction (also referred to as "mask mode" subtraction) is somewhat similar to screen-film subtraction, in which a pre-contrast image is obtained and post-contrast images subtracted from it. The pre-contrast image is referred to as the *mask image.*

In comparison to screen-film subtraction, temporal subtraction in digital radiography is accomplished by the computer with greater speed and accuracy.

There are several modes of temporal subtraction and the fundamental difference among them depends on the method in which the x-ray beam is utilized in the production of images. These modes are: (a) serial mask mode, (b) continuous mode, (c) time interval difference mode, and (d) the post-processing mode.

Serial Mask Mode

The *serial mask mode* is shown in Figure 18:3. It is similar to subtraction in film radiography but differs in several ways:

  (a) The mask image is obtained and stored in digital form before the contrast is injected
  (b) The contrast is injected (either in the basilic or cephalic vein)
  (c) Other images (post-injection images) are collected from the image intensifier television chain and are subtracted at rates of about 1 to 2 per second from the mask image and are stored in digital form or they can be recorded on tape or disk.
  (d) The results of (c) above are difference images which show only the opacified vessels. The contrast in the subtracted images can be altered by changing the window width.

In the serial mask mode subtraction process, the radiation is pulsed at several hundred mA and usually the kVp setting is around 60-80 kVp, so that the

UNSUBTRACTED IMAGE   SUBTRACTED IMAGE

MASK

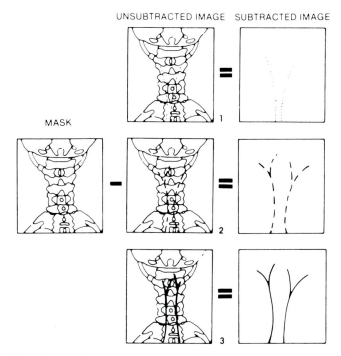

Figure 18:3. The serial mask mode of temporal subtraction in digital fluoroscopy. See text for further explanation. (courtesy of Philips Medical Systems.)

x-ray spectrum is kept close to the K-edge of iodine (33 keV).

This mode of subtraction is useful in visualization of carotid arteries, peripheral vessels (including grafts), and abdominal and renal arteries.

Continuous Mode

The fundamental approach to *continuous imaging* is illustrated in Figure 18:4. This mode is also referred to as *fluoroscopic mask mode* and it differs from serial mask imaging in that:

(a) the mask image is stored prior to the contrast injection.
(b) Real time fluoroscopic images of opacified vessels are then subtracted from the mask to eliminate common elements.
(c) The operation of the fluoroscopic unit is continuous at mA values higher than in conventional fluoroscopy (up to 15 mA).

This mode of subtraction in digital radiography is useful in evaluating heart wall motion, bypass graft patency, and pulmonary arteries.

Time Interval Difference

In *time interval difference* (TID) imaging, a mask is first obtained, then a difference image or a subtracted image is created from two images recorded while contrast is distributed in the vessels. This is done through subtraction of se-

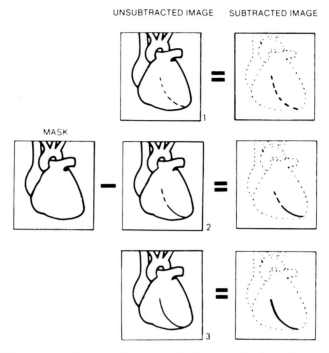

Figure 18:4. The concept of the continuous mode of temporal subtraction in digital fluoroscopy. See text for further explanation. (courtesy of Philips Medical Systems.)

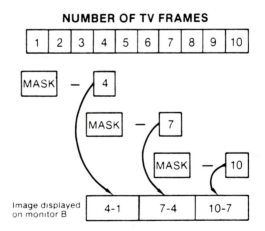

Figure 18:5. The idea of time interval difference imaging in digital fluoroscopy. See text for further explanation. (courtesy of Philips Medical Systems.)

quential images separated by selectable time intervals as shown in Figure 18:5. The subtracted image only displays short-term changes in the contrast distribution.

TID was developed to image moving structures and to deal with problems arising from respiratory motion. It is useful for application in cardiac work, particularly in assessing the cardiac chambers.

Post Processing

This mode is primarily used in off-line subtraction and enhancement of images. The technique allows the operator to recall previously stored images for retrospective reanalysis of data and to create a better "match" of images for subtraction.

The post-processing scheme is shown in Figure 18:6. The method is useful in cases where patient motion has occurred. Therefore, it is not necessary to re-examine patients should motion present a problem during the examination.

Apart from subtraction and edge enhancement (the change of pixel values at the edge of an image), other post-processing techniques include image magnification (expansion), image rotation and image smoothing.

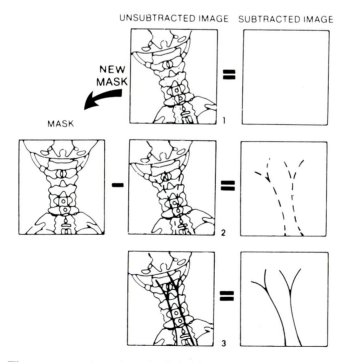

Figure 18:6. The post-processing scheme in digital fluoroscopy. See text for further explanation. (courtesy of Philips Medical Systems.)

Limitations of Temporal Subtraction

The primary limitation of temporal subtraction in digital radiography is related to patient motion. Motion usually occurs between the time when the mask image and post-contrast images are taken.

The mask is taken with the patient in a certain position. If the patient moves, then the post-contrast images are taken with the patient in a different position and images will not be in perfect alignment (misaligned or misregistered) with the mask image. This results in artifacts, since the vessels in the post-contrast images are not in alignment with those in the mask image.

To reduce motion artifacts in temporal subtraction digital angiography, another mask may be recorded just before the contrast arrives at the vessels of interest. This procedure is known as *remasking*.

Remasking, however, cannot eliminate the problem completely and therefore another method is needed. The method is based on superimposing images so that anatomical structures are in alignment. This is accomplished by an *image re-registration algorithm* which moves the information stored in memory (pixel values) to facilitate a successful subtraction.

Energy Subtraction

Another method of subtraction in digital radiography which is less susceptible to motion artifacts is *energy subtraction*. It is based on the the fact that x-ray attenuation is different for bone, soft tissues and contrast material, such as iodine, and depends on the energy of the x-ray beam.

When x-rays interact with matter, two main interactions occur. These are photoelectric absorption and Compton scattering (see any radiologic physics text). Soft tissues, for example, attenuate x-rays primarily by the Compton effect, iodine by the photoelectric effect, and bone by both the photoelectric and Compton interactions. It is clear then that since these interactions are related to the energy of the beam, acquiring images at different kVp values will permit successful energy subtraction to demonstrate a specific structure.

In energy subtraction, images are recorded at two different energies. Usually, one image is taken at a low energy (60-80 kVp) and the other at a somewhat higher energy level (120-140 kVp). The two images are then subtracted from each other, that is, the image taken at the low energy is subtracted from that taken at the higher energy. This method is typically referred to as *dual-energy subtraction* and usually only one material is cancelled out. Soft tissue and bone cannot be totally cancelled from the same image. Energy subtraction removes primarily soft tissues, since patient motion is most likely to occur is soft tissues.

The problems associated with energy subtraction are related to:

(a) Errors arising from the presence of scattered radiation.

(b) Beam hardening. Since the x-ray beam is polyenergetic (different wavelengths), attenuation in tissues is slightly different at different beam energies.

(c) Residual signals arising from non-contrast structures such as bone and soft tissues (with dual-energy imaging).

(d) The difficulty associated with developing an x-ray generator capable of switching kVp at the high rate of speed necessary.

The application of energy subtraction techniques ranges from non-vascular and vascular contrast studies to non-contrast studies such as in chest imaging. Table 18:1 gives a comparison between temporal and energy subtraction. In general, temporal subtraction techniques have found application in computed fluoroscopy (digital fluoroscopy), while energy subtraction is applied primarily to computed radiography or scanned projection radiography (to be discussed subsequently).

Table 18-1

A COMPARISON BETWEEN TEMPORAL AND ENERGY
SUBTRACTION METHODS

(From *Digital Radiography — An Assessment of its Potential Impact
on Radiological Practice.* General Electric. 1980.)

	TEMPORAL SUBTRACTION	DUAL-ENERGY SUBTRACTION
1. X-ray generator:	Dynamic kilovoltage switching is not required.	Dynamic kilovoltage switching is preferred.
2. X-ray spectrum filtration:	Static filtration is adequate.	Dynamic filter switching is preferred.
3. Control sensitivity:	Visualization of 1% contrasts for small objects is possible.	Comparable contrast sensitivity to temporal subtraction but at higher detected intensities.
4. Processing:	Simple subtraction between images.	Weighted subtraction between images. Higher order terms may be required to suppress beam hardening.
5. Misregistration artifacts:	Artifacts are a potential problem if the patient moves between both images.	Artifacts are not a severe problem since images can be acquired within milliseconds of each other.
6. Residual signals:	All structures common to both images are cancelled.	If two beams are used, then residual bone remains in tissue cancelled image and vice versa. 3-beam K-edge subtraction is required to give iodine isolation comparable to temporal subtraction.
7. Flexibility of subtraction:	With 2 initial images, one difference image is possible.	Various subtractions permitted; tissue or bone cancellation compromise bone-mimic-tissue, etc.

Hybrid Subtraction

Another form of subtraction which is based on both energy and temporal subtraction schemes is *hybrid subtraction*. In this technique, images are first obtained by the dual-energy method to eliminate soft tissue. The image taken before contrast arrives in the field of view (pre-contrast image) is then used as a mask image, and the other energy-subtracted images are temporally subtracted from the mask image (Figure 18:7).

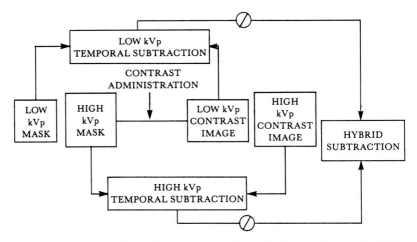

Figure 18:7. The concept of hybrid subtraction. (From Guthaner, D.; Brody, W.R. et al.: Clinical application of hybrid subtraction digital angiography: Preliminary results. *Cardiovascular Interventional Radiology.* 6: 1983.)

The advantage of this method of image subtraction is that soft tissue and motion arising from soft tissue are eliminated through energy subtraction. Bone, on the other hand, is eliminated by temporal subtraction.

EQUIPMENT AND TECHNOLOGY

Two schemes for digital radiography, energy and temporal subtraction, have been described so far. The equipment, therefore, falls into two broad categories, namely

    (a) Digital fluoroscopy (computed fluoroscopy)
    (b) Digital scanned projection radiography (computed radiography)

The essential elements and operational characteristics will now be described.

Digital Fluoroscopy

An overall diagrammatic representation of digital fluoroscopy equipment configuration is shown in Figure 18:2. It is clear from the figure that several of the imaging components are similar to a conventional intensified fluoroscopy scheme. With the point in mind, it is clear that conventional fluoroscopic equipment can easily be adapted to provide digital fluoroscopy.

A more detailed illustration of a digital fluoroscopic system is given in Figure 18:8. The main components of relevance to this chapter are: the x-ray generator and tube, the image intensifier, the lens and aperture system, the television camera tube, the logarithmic processor, the ADC, digital frame memories, the computer system and data storage.

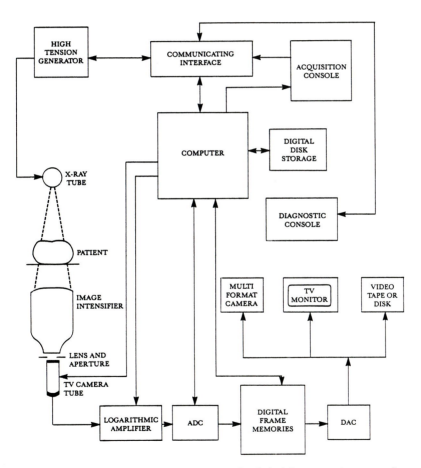

Figure 18:8. The basic equipment configuration of a digital fluoroscopic system. See text for further explanation.

A detailed description of each of these components is not within the scope of this text, however, a brief discussion and statement of their role in the total digital imaging scheme are in order.

The X-ray Tube and Generator

The application of digital fluoroscopy to digital subtraction angiography may involve intravenous and intraarterial injections. In intravenous digital subtraction angiography, there is a substantial dilution of contrast by the time it arrives at the arteries of concern. To image the diluted contrast successfully, an essential requirement is high radiation flux (low noise).

The x-ray tube should be of a high-speed rotation type and should feature a high anode heat-storage capacity. The focal spot should be large enough to generate a high photon flux, since it is not essential that a small focal spot be used (Kruger, 1982).

The generator should be flexible to accommodate the requirements of the various subtraction modes in digital subtraction angiography. For example, for successful cardiac imaging, at least 30 pulses per second are necessary. Another feature of the generator is that it should be computer controlled in order to determine accurate exposure factors. In general, an automatic exposure control system permits the generator to select appropriate kVp and mA values. Once this is accomplished, then a test exposure is made and the final exposure is computed accurately. If short exposure times are used in examinations, then generators featuring 1000 mA or more are needed.

The Image Intensifier

This is the detector in a digital fluoroscopy system. The principle of operation of image intensifiers is described in Chapter 12.

The light output from the intensifier is an important consideration in digital fluoroscopy, since the proper function of the television camera tube depends on a fixed amount of light.

The image intensifier characteristic to digital fluoroscopy is the cesium iodide (CsI) image intensifier. In general, large-format image intensifiers (36-cm input screen) are preferable, since they offer very high contrast resolution and a large field of view.

The Lens and Aperture

The light gain at the output screen of the image intensifier (CsI) is very high and is not suited for imaging at the high radiation levels needed in digital subtraction angiography.

The image intensifier is coupled to the television camera tube by an infinity-focused tandem lens system. Since the light level of the output screen is too high for the level required for proper operation of the television camera tube, it must be controlled or regulated to meet the requirements of the television camera tube. This control or scaling is done by the aperture or *video aperture,* as it is sometimes referred to.

The aperture is usually variable to facilitate a wide range of radiation exposures to the input screen of the image intensifier. This is necessary so that small apertures can be used for the high exposures needed in digital fluoroscopy and large apertures for conventional intensified fluoroscopy.

The Television Camera Tube

The television camera tube is a critical element in the digital imaging scheme, since it converts the light image at the output screen of the image intensifier into an output electrical signal (voltage waveform), which is then digitized for input into the computer.

Television camera tubes were described in Chapter 13. For digital subtraction angiography the Plumbicon® camera tube (lead oxide Vidicon) is generally used, since (a) it exhibits short image lag compared to the standard vidicon (antimony trisulfide), and (b) "the output video signal is linearly dependent on the incident x-ray flux" (Kruger, 1982). Lag causes image blurring, especially with fast-moving structures such as the heart.

The target of the television camera tube may be scanned in two different ways, namely, interlaced and progressive (Chapter 13).

In interlaced scanning, once the first line is read the electron beam moves onto the third line, then to the fifth and to the seventh and so on until it gets to the last line on the raster. In the total scanning of odd-numbered lines, (252 ½), 250 lines are read in one sixtieth sec. This is referred to as a *video field.* The scanning of even-numbered lines results in another video field, which when combined with the first field creates a *video frame.* The video frame consists of 525 lines scanned in one thirtieth sec.

In progressive scanning, each line is scanned sequentially and the 525 lines are read in one thirtieth sec.

In an interlaced scanning system, the x-ray exposure and the video signal occur at the same time, while in progressive scanning the video signal occurs just after the x-ray exposure. This has implications for digital fluoroscopy.

For cameras with interlaced scanning, the first set of video frames cannot be used in the production of a digital image, since the video signal is not stable at this point. Progressive scanning, on the other hand, makes use of all of the radiation to produce the digital image.

In summary, the scanning of the television camera raster is thus represented by a set of horizontal lines. Each line is then represented by an output video signal (voltage waveform) which is related to the image brightness through a direct proportionality. These voltage waveforms are then sent to a logarithmic amplifier before arriving at the analog-to-digital converter.

Another factor to be considered with respect to television cameras is the SNR. The SNR for camera tubes used in digital fluoroscopy should range from about 500:1 to 1000:1 (Kruger, 1981). The noise levels of the tube must also be low enough in order to demonstrate very small contrast differences. Noise may arise from the x-ray flux (quantum noise), the electrical components of the system (electrical noise) and digitization.

Logarithmic Processing

Patient thickness is not uniform and varies in different portions of the body. Such thickness will affect x-ray attenuation, in that more attenuation occurs in the thicker regions than in the thinner areas of the patient.

The opacification of vessels will also vary from point to point throughtout the part because the contrast is diluted as it flows further into the vessels. Because of this, opacification of vessels may not be uniform throughout the region of interest. This is illustrated in Figure 18:9.

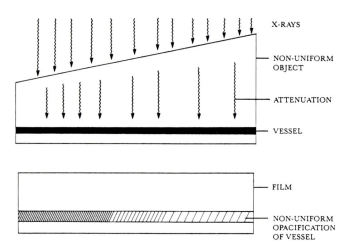

Figure 18:9. The non-uniform opacification of a vessel from a non-uniform object. This problem is eliminated through logarithmic processing.

To eliminate this problem in digital fluoroscopy, a *log amplifier* may be used to process data prior to subtraction, so that the digital image contrast does not change with changes in patient thickness. In some cases, another technique, called *linear amplification,* is used and this also results in a digital subtracted image which shows less perceptible noise and subtraction of those structures which are not opacified. It appears at present that logarithmic processing or amplification is the most widely used technique because it generates a uniform iodine signal despite the patient thickness and overlying structures.

Logarithmic amplication is usually done prior to analog-to-digital conversion and this requires an 8-bit ADC (to be discussed in the next subsection) for adequate gray-scale resolution.

In another method, the data is digitized before it is subject to logarithmic processing. In this case a table, called a digital look-up table, is used to do the logarithmic processing.

Analog-to-Digital Conversion

The ADC is based on integrated circuit technology which will not be discussed further in this text. The purpose of the ADC is to convert the video output signal (voltage waveform) from the television camera to digital data, by sampling the voltage waveform at certain time intervals. The sampling frequency is of importance, since it determines the number of samples for each horizontal television line and is related to spatial resolution.

Two parameters of the ADC which are of relevance to digital fluoroscopy are speed and accuracy. *Accuracy* refers to how close the digital data represents the analog signal or voltage waveform. The range of the waveform is divided into a number of parts (increments). The more parts to the waveform, the better the accuracy of the ADC.

In the ADC, the unit of the parts is the *bit* (contraction for *b*inary dig*it* — recall that the binary number system has a base 2). One bit can be either 0 or 1. A 1-bit ADC is represented as 2; which means that the range of the waveform is divided into 2 equal parts. A 2-bit ADC ($2^2 = 4$) will generate 4 equal parts, while a 6-bit ADC ($2^6 = 64$) will divide the range of the signal into 64 equal parts. Therefore, the higher the bits, the more accurate is the ADC.

The ADC also determines how many shades of gray will be represented in the image (gray-scale resolution). For example, after quantization (see Chapter 15), a 1-bit ADC will generate two integers (0 and 1) and these will be represented by two shades, usually black and white. A 2-bit ADC will generate a gray scale with 4 shades, a 6-bit ADC will generate 64 shades of gray, while an 8-bit ADC will generate 256 integers ranging from 0-255 and 256 (2^8 shades of gray. This concept is illustrated in Figure 18:10 for a 4-bit ADC.

The other parameter of the ADC is *speed*. The speed of the ADC refers to the time it takes to digitize the input analog signal. Speed and accuracy of an ADC are related in an inverse fashion, that is, the higher the accuracy of the ADC, the longer it takes to digitize the signal.

Frame Memories

The images acquired in a digital fluoroscopy system, once digitized, must be stored in some way before digital processing. For example, the mask image is digitized and stored before post-contrast images are obtained. These images are stored in memory referred to as *frame memories* (solid-state memories). This is necessary as a means of processing images very quickly, since the computer does not have external memory to subtract images from the mask image.

This memory is part of the computer system and is made of a printed circuit

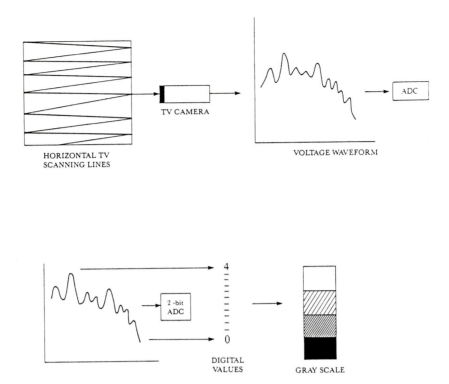

Figure 18:10. Analog-to-digital conversion. The television camera produces a voltage waveform from one horizontal line shown here. The waveform is converted into digital values (4) bit a 4-bit ADC, to generate an image with four shades of gray.

board consisting of an array of logic chips. Each chip may store as much as 64,000 bits (64K) of information, although some chips may be capable of storing more information.

Digital data represent a series of numbers arranged in a matrix fashion where each pixel in the matrix must be represented in the memory. The matrix size is related to the memory capacity through a direct proportionality, that is, a higher matrix demands a higher memory storage capacity. For example, a 256×256 (65,536 pixels) would require a 64K memory, while a 512×512 matrix (261,144 pixels) would require a 256K memory.

Computer Processing

Computer processing invovles input, processing, and output. Information must be fed into the computer (input) which then performs mathematical operations (subtraction and enhancement) on the data. The results of processing may either be stored in memory or displayed on suitable output devices for subsequent viewing and documentation.

Processing may be accomplished in two ways by:

(a) Hard-wired processing
(b) Minicomputer

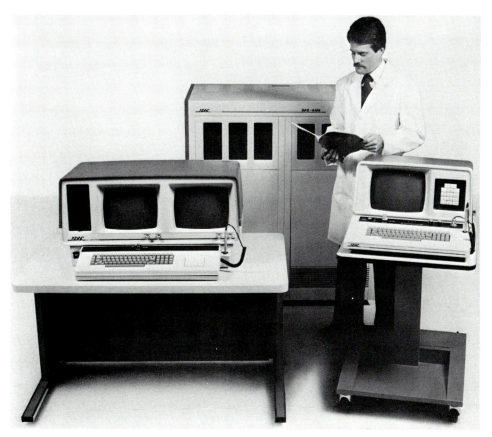

Figure 18:11. A digital radiography image processing system. Instead of a single general purpose computer, it utilizes many small, highly specialized computers. Each is dedicated to a specific set of tasks, operating both independently and in convert with others in the system. (courtesy of ADAC Laboratories.)

A *hard-wire processing* scheme was developed by Mistretta at the University of Wisconsin. It consists of fixed electrical circuits and does not permit programs to be changed (non-programmable subtraction circuits). It is relatively cheap and allows for real time fluoroscopy (high image acquisition rate).

The other processing concept which utilizes a *minicomputer* was developed at the University of Arizona. This concept makes use of programmable subtraction circuits and programs which are interchangeable to facilitate specific tasks, such as image enhancement. Although the minicomputer concept is limited in terms of image acquisition rates, it is more flexible with regards to software and other image processing capabilities. A digital image processing system is shown in Figure 18:11.

Data Storage

One form of data storage was mentioned earlier in the subsection dealing with frame memories. The data collected in digital fluoroscopy can be stored either in two ways: as analog images or digital images. These images may be stored on a short-term or long-term basis.

In short-term storage, images are stored from the time they are acquired to the time it is decided or agreed upon as to which images should be kept for archival storage. On the other hand, long-term storage refers to archival storage.

For short-term or long-term storage, data may be stored on analog or digital devices. Analog devices include video-disk recorders (which hold about 30 images per second) and magnetic tape recorders. However, there is some loss of image quality with these devices because of the noise arising from them.

Digital storage devices, such as digital disks, ensure a storage rate of about six 512×512 images per second (compared to analog storage devices) without loss of image quality.

In general, archival storage in digital fluoroscopy is done on film through the use of the multiformat camera. However, such storage may also be done on magnetic tape, either in analog or digital form.

Finally, images may be stored on laser disks in the near future.

Image Display and Viewing

Once images are proccessed, they are presented to the observer for viewing and recording. The images are displayed on a cathode ray tube (CRT) display device which generally consists of a control console. One such control and evaluation unit is shown in Figure 18:12.

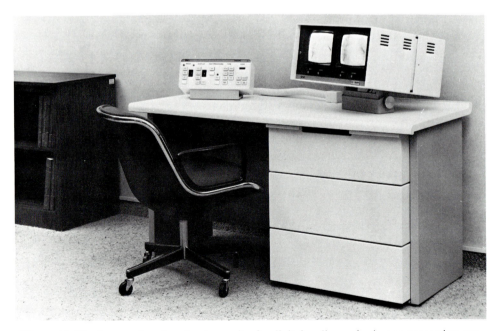

Figure 18:12. A control and evaluation unit of a digital radiography image processing system. (courtesy of Philips Medical Systems.)

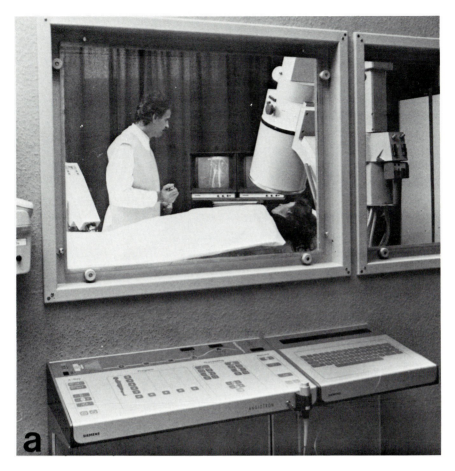

Figure 18:13. (a) The ANGIOTRON® (Siemens) digital fluoroscopy unit; (b) diagramic layout of the unit. The image signal from the image intensifier television chain is processed in real-time. The analog image signal first passes through a logarithmic amplifier to achieve a homogeneous vascular reproduction in the subtraction image independent of body thickness. The signal is subsequently digitized in a broadband analog-digital-converter (ADC). This is processed with the aid of a pipeline processor and three semi-conductor memories. In each case, a number of individual images are summarized to reduce noise. They are either summated or sliding weighted. Following subtraction, the image signals pass through a window amplifier, a lin/delogarithmic amplifier and a digital-analog converter (DAC), and are displayed at the subtraction monitor in analog form; (c) Real-time image processing "on-line" — after preparing the patient and determining the most favourable projection direction, the necessary function parameters are selected at the ANGIOTRON® console. After the contrast medium injection and shortly before the contrast medium bolus reaches the target area, the mask is set. With this, the subtraction process begins automatically and the image is displayed at the monitor in real time. Whenthe maximum contast medium concentration has been reached in the vascular region of interest, the subtraction is stopped by the examiner. (courtesy of the Siemens Corporation.)

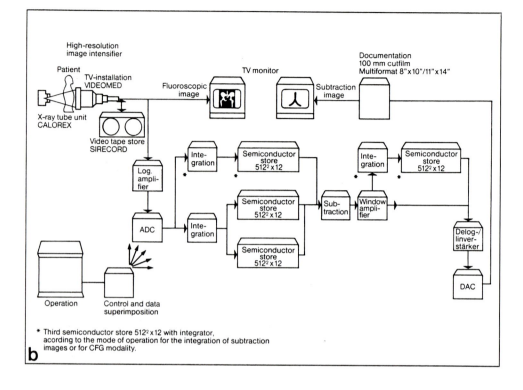

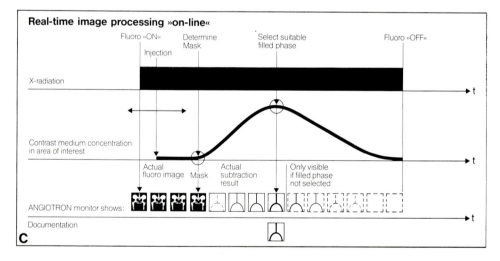

There are several controls on the console which are typical of digital fluoroscopic units. Some of these controls enable the operator to choose one of the four modes of temporal subtraction, record and store images, change contrast of images through windowing, image manipulation and so on.

Finally, one commercially available unit for digital fluoroscopy, the Angiotron® (Siemens Medical Systems), is shown in Figure 18:13. The control field and evaluation units are shown in Figures 18:14 and 18:15, respectively.

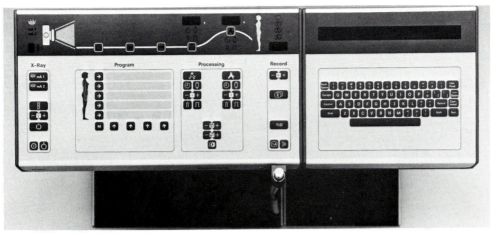

Figure 18:14. A close-up view of the control field of the ANGIOTRON® digital image acquisition and processing system for digital subtraction angiography. (courtesy of Siemens Corporation.)

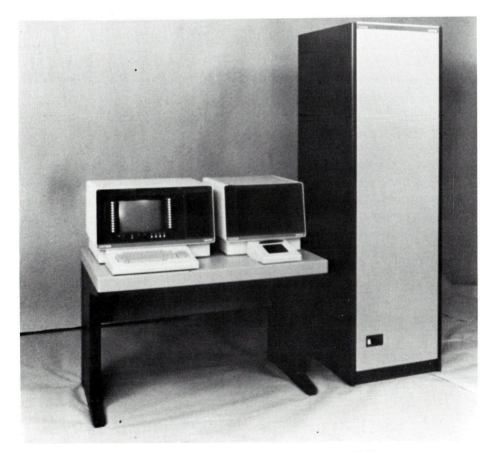

Figure 18:15. The control and evaluation unit of the DIGITRON® (Siemens) digital image acquisition and processing system for digital subtraction angiography. The text monitor with floppy disk drive and keyboard is seen on the left while the processor and memory cabinet is seen on the right. (courtesy of the Siemens Corporation.)

Digital Scanned Projection Radiography

Digital *scanned projection radiography* (SPR) or *computed radiography* (CR) is a technique which is used in computed tomography to provide precise localization of CT slices. Dr. Brody of Stanford University points out that "the term projection is used to indicate the 'non-tomographic' nature of the image to avoid confusion with computed tomography."

In the CT technique, the x-ray tube and detectors remain stationary while the patient moves through the gantry aperture during the exposure. The transmitted x-rays are collected and digitized for input into the computer.

The fundamental concept of SPR involves some form of scanning the patient through mechanical motion of the x-ray tube and detector using special collimation schemes. Two such approaches are available for SPR and they include (a) the line scanning approach using a single detector element (single detector method) and (b) the fan beam scanning approach using a linear array of detectors (line detector method).

Single Detector Approach

In this approach, the x-ray beam is highly collimated ("pencil beam") and the x-ray tube is coupled to a single detector. Together, the tube and detector scan the patient in a point-by-point manner to generate "line images." This technique has been referred to as the *"flying spot"* (pencil beam) technique.

A digital radiography unit based on the flying spot technique is shown in Figure 18:16. A pencil beam of radiation is produced by the collimator in conjunction with a rotating aperture wheel. The wheel rotates at a speed of about 1800 rpm and the beam scans the patient, since the tube, wheel, and detector move parallel to the long axis of the table.

The transmitted beam is detected by a single detector located above the patient. The detector is a sodium iodide (NaI) crystal coupled to a photomultiplier tube. The tube generates an output electrical signal which is digitized and fed into the computer for processing and storage. This is illustrated in Figure 18:17.

The time taken to generate a single image (512 × 480 pixel) is about 16 seconds.

The flying spot digital radiography concept is limited by "tube loading and mechanical scanning considerations. Tube limits restrict the dose delivered to the patient and throughput. Efficient dose utilization allows diagnostic imaging at 0-5 mR, and x-ray tubes with higher heat-storage capacity and higher dissipation will improve the throughput substantially. The requirement to scan mechanically will tend to keep exposure times in the order of seconds. This will prevent it being used for very high speed radiographs" (Bjorkholm, Annis and Frederick, 1982).

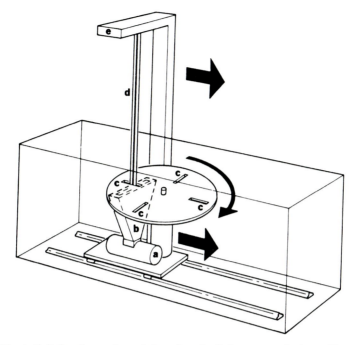

Figure 18:16. A digital radiography unit based on the flying-spot technique. Shown are (a) x-ray tube; (b) collimator; (c) rotating disk; (d) pencil x-ray beam; and (e) detector. (courtesy of American Science and Engineering, Inc.)

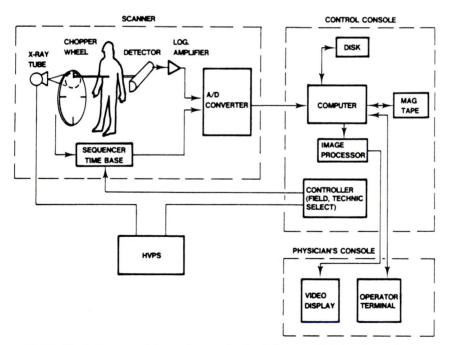

Figure 18:17. Block diagram of the equipment for the flyingspot digital radiography system. (courtesy of American Science and Engineering, Inc.)

Line Detector Approach

This approach to digital SPR has its origin from the CT concept which involves the localization of CT slices, as shown in Figure 18:18.

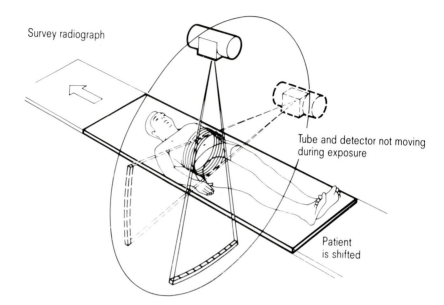

Figure 18:18. The line detector approach to digital scanned projection radiography. The x-ray tube and detector array remain stationary while the patient is moved through the gantry of the scanner. (From Rienmüller, R. and Sommer, B., et al.: The topogram in mediastinal computerized tomography. *Electromedica* 2: 1981.)

The line detector approach utilizes a linear array of detectors coupled to the x-ray tube. In producing a digital image, the x-ray tube and detectors remain stationary (positioned either for a lateral or frontal view), while the patient is moved through the gantry of the scanner.

Transmitted x-rays are collected by the detector array which converts x-ray photons into electrical signals. These signals are then digitized (AD conversion) before they are sent to the computer for processing, storage, and display.

The detectors may be either bismuth germanate (BGO) or sodium iodide crystals coupled to photomultiplier tubes or gas-ionization chambers (xenon). The x-ray beam is collimated in such a way to produce a fan beam which covers the detector array.

This method of digital radiography results in faster scan times and makes better use of x-ray sources compared to the point-by-point scanning of the single detector system.

Presently, a number of these fan beam digital units are being evaluated for use in chest (Mattson et al., 1981; Fraser et al., 1983) and other examinations such as intravenous angiography (Sashin et al., 1982).

It is interesting to note that patient motion is not displayed as a lack of sharpness in this type of scanning but rather displayed as distortion in the image.

Applications

Temporal and energy-subtraction approaches have been applied to digital scanned projection imaging. In intravenous angiography, for example, temporal subtraction may be used based on the acquisition of pre- and post-contrast scans. The post-contrast images will demonstate the vessels.

Another application of digital SPR is *digital tomosynthesis*, a digital imaging technique which is used to provide digital images of selected planes of the patient.

Other Methods of Digital Radiography

Imaging Plates

Apart from the specific schemes employed in digital fluoroscopy and digital scanned projection radiography, other approaches to digital radiography exist. These approaches are based on first acquiring information in analog form, followed by digital transformation and computer processing.

Acquiring the information is accomplished through the use of special radiographic imaging plates consisting of *photostimulable phosphor*. These plates are used in the same fashion as cassettes (screen/film) are used in conventional radiography.

The radiation beam falling on the plate stimulates the phosphor (stores the energy absorbed) to produce a latent image. When the plate is exposed to ultraviolet radiation, light is emitted. This phenomenon is known as *photostimulable luminescence*. The light emitted is detected by a photodetector which produces an output voltage. This voltage is subsequently amplified and digitized for input into the computer.

Another form of imaging plate stores the image as electrical charges. This is referred to as the *charged plate method*.

The plate is then read by an electrometer (device for detecting the amount of charge on various portions of the plate) which generates an electrical signal. This signal is amplified and digitized for processing by a digital computer.

IMAGE QUALITY CONSIDERATIONS

The fundamental parameters of image quality are spatial resolution, contrast resolution and noise. *Spatial resolution* is the ability of the imaging system to demonstrate small high-contrast objects. In general, it is related to the smallest object that can be demonstrated by the system. *Contrast resolution,* on the other hand, refers to the ability of a system to show small changes in tissue contrast.

Noise refers to unwanted signals which interfere with the faithful transfer and reproduction of information.

Digital Fluoroscopy

The factors influencing spatial resolution in digital fluoroscopy are focal spot size, exposure time, patient motion, magnification, the image intensifier and the television chain, the analog-to-digital converter and the size of the image matrix.

In this section, only at least three will be dealt with briefly since the student is already familiar with the influence of the other factors on resolution.

For a given field size (input screen diameter of the image intensifier tube), a 512 × 512 matrix generates higher spatial resolution than a 256 × 256 image matrix. That is, the larger the number of pixels, the smaller are the pixels and higher spatial resolution results. One should bear in mind that this resolution is ultimately related to the x-ray intensity and the inherent spatial resolution capability of the imaging system. For example, the 525 scan lines per television frame is related to the vertical resolution of the television chain. If the number of scan lines are increased, then the resolution can be increased.

For a given field size, the spatial resolution may range from about 2 line pairs per millimeter (for an 11-cm input screen) with a 512 × 512 matrix to about 1 line pair per millimeter with a 256 × 256 matrix for a field size of about 23 cm. Therefore, it should be clear that to maintain acceptable resolution with large-format image intensifiers, the matrix size must be increased.

Another point worth mentioning here is related to the field of view (input screen diameter of image intensifier tube) and the video line rate. As the field of view increases with increasing line rates, the resolution increases. For example, a 228-mm (9 inches) input screen in conjunction with a 525 line rate results in a 1.1 line pair/mm resolution compared to a 355-mm (14 inches) input screen in conjunction with a 2048 line rate which gives a resolution of almost 3 line pairs/mm (Vizy, 1983).

The line pairs/mm can be calculated through the use of the following relationship:

$$\text{Maximum Line Pairs/mm} = \frac{[\dfrac{\text{Line rate}}{2}] \; \text{LP}}{\text{input screen diameter}}$$

The ADC influences the contrast resolution in digital fluoroscopy in such a way that the higher the digitization capability of the ADC, the greater the contrast sensitivity. For example, a 2-bit ADC will generate only 4 (2^2) levels of gray which are observable on an image as opposed to a 10-bit ADC which will generate 1024 (2^{10}) levels of gray, thus providing a gain in contrast sensitivity and information.

Noise in digital fluoroscopy can be attributed to several sources, but the two most common are quantum noise and electronic noise.

If too few x-ray photons arrive at the image intensifier tube, then the image will show quantum mottle and lack detail. Therefore, in digital fluoroscopy, since the subtraction process has the effect of increasing noise in the system, it is mandatory to use high radiation levels to control the noise.

The other type of noise is referred to as electronic noise and it arises from the electronic components of the imaging system, for example, pre-amplifiers and amplifiers. One of the main sources of electronic noise is the television camera tube. The noise in this regard is important, since a high SNR of the camera tube is necessary to minimize the effect of noise on subtraction images (degrading). Such noise may be reduced by additional and more expensive electronics, however, in digital fluoroscopy, a technique referred to as *signal averaging* may be used.

In signal averaging, several television frames which have been collected sequentially are averaged together to generate an average signal. Mistretta (1981) has reported that signal averaging can result in an SNR of about 1200:1.

Computed Radiography

Image quality in computed radiography (SPR) is related to spatial resolution and contrast sensitivity. Since the beam is highly collimated, scatter is small and therefore contrast resolution is excellent. Other factors such as increased radiation dose and better detectors also influence contrast resolution.

Spatial resolution is related to several factors including magnification, scan speed, width of the x-ray beam, focal spot size, sample time, sample distance and, more importantly, the detector aperture.

The spacing of the detector cells influences the spatial resolution (lateral direction) in SPR. Smaller cells and closer spacing provide greater lateral resolution, but there must be a trade-off with respect to noise, quantum detection efficiency and the field of view.

The width of the beam influences the spatial resolution in the horizontal direction and hence depends on the collimation within a certain limit. Beyond this limit, the focal spot size affects this resolution.

For SPR, SNR may be increased by increasing photon flux, which demands an increase in x-ray tube output and increased detector efficiency.

The scan speed also plays a role in the spatial resolution in longitudinal direction, as well as contrast sensitivity. In general, an increase in speed tends to destroy both these parameters.

CLINICAL CONSIDERATIONS

Applications

Digital imaging techniques have been received with much enthusiasm and research continues to assess its true potential in clinical medicine.

Applications may be grouped into three areas:

(a) Intravascular contrast examinations
(b) Non-vascular contrast examinations
(c) Non-contrast procedures

Presently, digital imaging has found widespread applications in intravascular contrast examinations, especially with digital fluoroscopy.

Energy-subtraction techniques have been mostly suitable for studies involving non-vascular contrast procedures such as pyelography, cholangiography (both intravenous and oral) and imaging tumors. The removal of gas shadows in the area of the kidney and gallbladder is yet another application of energy-subtraction imaging.

Finally, for non-contrast studies, digital imaging has already been applied to various parts of the body, especially in examinations of the chest. In this application, digital techniques ensure contrast enhancement and selective tissue or bone subtraction as well as image manipulation.

Contrast Media and Injection Methods

Present clinical studies in digital subtraction angiography are based on the use of contrst media with a high level of iodine concentration and low toxicity and viscosity.

Ionic contrast media such as Renografin 76® and Conray 400 have been used, although non-ionic contrast such as Amipaque® (metrizamide) has also been used.

The amount of contrast and rate of injection may vary from institution to institution, but, in general, 30-40 cc per injection and a rate of about 10-12 cc per second is not uncommon.

Hand injection techniques are not used in digital subtraction angiography, since they do not opacify arteries satisfactorily; hence, pressure injectors are used.

Two catheterization approaches are used in digital subtraction angiography. The first is one in which the catheter is placed in an anti-cubital vein for peripheral venous injections. Sometimes, a femoral venous approach is also used. The second method is a central venous approach, in which the catheter tip is placed in the subclavian vein or the superior vena cava.

These intravenous injection techniques are used because of the improved contrast resolution provided by digital subtraction. It is also possible to use intra-arterial injections in digital subtraction angiography because of the improved contrast resolution. For example, injections into the subclavian artery in some cases have been successful in the study of vertebral artery circulation in older patients.

LIMITATIONS

Digital radiography is not a perfect system (no system is) and therefore it presents several limitations in imaging.

In general, patient motion poses a serious limitation since it causes problems in the subtraction process. However, complex computer programs are being developed to provide solutions to the problems imposed by motion.

Noise is also a limiting factor in digital imaging systems.

The amount of contrast media used in digital angiography is also among the list of limitations; since large amounts are used in intravenous digital angiography, there is an increase in the probability that vessels may be damaged.

The cost factor may also be a limitation. Although hardware costs are on the decline, the cost of software is significant.

In conclusion of this chapter, the following point is in order. As a new mode of imaging, digital radiography has provided solutions to many problems arising from conventional imaging in addition to generating more problems, both technical and clinical. Research in digital radiography continues to gain momentum, and the results so far appear to indicate that digital radiography is a very promising technique in diagnostic medicine.

DIGITAL IMAGE ARCHIVING AND COMMUNICATION

The previous chapters have described various methods of producing images. Static, dynamic and computer-reconstructed images are obtained in the imaging department on a daily basis. These images may be either analog or digital or both and they may be stored on film and magnetic tape or disks.

The technologist is already familar with the storage of film and in most cases the storage of magnetic tape and disks.

With the advent of digital image processing in imaging departments, there arises a need for other approaches to archiving and communication of digital images.

The following paper is reproduced in this chapter in its entirety, since it addresses and discusses digital image archiving and communication strategies for imaging departments with digital imaging equipment.

Filmless Picture Archiving and Communication in Diagnostic Radiology. Duerinckx, A.J., and Pisa, E.J. Society of Photo Optical Instrumentation Engineers, Vol. 318 (Part I), Picture Archiving and Communication Systems (PACS) for Medical Applications, 1982.

Abstract

"A survey is presented of recent changes in digital image acquisition for diagnostic radiology. New digital image archiving, communication and management strategies are proposed and discussed. A possible scenario for the development of digital Picture Archiving and Communication Systems ("digital PACS") in diagnostic radiology is presented, starting with a research/teaching environment and ending with a large-scale clinical environment. This scenario is presented as a sequence of five strategies with increasing levels of digital archiving and communication and requires five key concepts. We briefly discuss each key concept and present possible implementations, given today's technology. A preliminary evaluation of proposed image archiving strategies is made. The paper concludes that the development of a PACS that provides partial on-line digital storage is feasible today.

Introduction

"A Picture Archiving and Communication (PAC) system is part of every diagnostic radiology and nuclear medicine department. However, most of today's PACS consist of centralized analog film file rooms. The current film file room manages both the analog generated radiographic images and the the video raster film recordings used for imaging of digital diagnostic images. Several diagnostic image management strategies relying upon film file room type PACS are in use today.[1,2]

The purpose of this paper is to identify and discuss a '*digital PACS*' development scenario in diagnostic radiology suitable for the next few years. The scenario will assume today's technology and the need for digital storage to facilitate medical research and perhaps to improve the clinical usage of digitally acquired diagnostic images. We divide our scenario into a sequence of five "digital PAC" strategies with increasing amounts of digital archiving and communication. Different implementations of this scenario for the development of digital PACS are technically feasible today, and we attempt to give several examples of implementation of key concepts or components which will be discussed in this paper.

"This paper will focus on 'digital PACS'; i.e., PAC systems providing full digital storage of images. On-line digital storage precludes the use of analog film-based storage.' However, off-line digital storage can be realized by digitally encoding images on a strip of film. So, even though 'digital' does not necessarily imply 'filmless,' in this paper we will sometimes loosely refer to 'digital PACS' as 'filmless PACS.' 'Analog PACS' i.e., PAC systems providing analog storage of images (such as film file rooms,[1,2] microfilm systems[3] or analog video tapes/discs, will not be addressed.

"Today, departments of diagnostic radiology are using a greater percentage[4] of imaging systems that generate digital images. These systems include computed tomography scanners for head and body imaging, ultrasound scanners equipped with digital display memories, nuclear medicine gamma cameras and digital radiography imaging systems. Eventually other imaging systems, such as nuclear magnetic resonance scanners, will be added to the list. In the future these digital systems may also include systems that digitally acquire chest x-ray images (which are now generated in analog form) and other new imaging modalities.

"There are many reasons to examine 'digital PACS' and the consequent new image management strategies for diagnostic radiology. First, as stated above, more and more imaging systems produce images in digital form. Second, technological breakthroughs in digital storage[5] and broadband communication[6] make small-scale filmless digital PACS feasible today. Third, according to a study of a 600-bed hospital in Kansas City,[7] the cost of storing *digital* radiographic images in analog form on film, and the management of this archive, accounts for 75% of the total cost of digital image management. This fact indicates that a shift in archiving and management strategy away from analog video film recordings might induce a reduction in image archiving and management costs.

Current Procedures for PAC

"We will review and compare the ways in which digitally acquired diagnostic images are archived in both a clinical setting and a research/teaching setting. We emphasize that today only a fraction (approximately 30%) of all diagnostic radiographic images is acquired in digital form. This fraction will increase [11] to 50% during the next few years. Digitization of chest x-ray size images is not considered in this section. We will limit our comparison to x-ray CT, ultrasound and nuclear medicine imaging. Modalities such as digital fluorography, digital radiography and nuclear magnetic resonance imaging are not in sufficiently widespread use to be included.

"In a clinical environment, digitally acquired images are usually recorded on film using multiformat video raster gray-scale film recorders and then added to the film jacket, which is stored in a centralized film file room. In some hospitals, all digital CT images produced during one day are stored on a magnetic disc or tape which is purged at the end of each day. However, for most x-ray CT images the radiologist has a preferred CT window setting for each anatomical site, and the windowed digital image is recorded as an analog image on film. Nuclear medicine images require less storage than CT or ultrasound images, usually need to be processed (for dynamic studies), are stored on film or Polaroid and are not routinely archived in digital form for long periods of time. Most ultrasound scanners have digital scan converters and a digital image memory but only provide a video display output. There is usually no convenient interface to the digital image memory, and ultrasound images are stored on multiformat film, Polaroid or analog video tape/disc.

"The shortcomings of today's use of digital images in a clinical environment can be summarized as follows. Digitally acquired images are recorded in analog form with a video raster gray-scale film. Most of the advantages of "digital" access to the information and are therefore lost. However, today's use of an analog storage medium is a necessity. Diagnostic radiology departments have rooms equipped with 'light-boxes' to read film. Many physicians have small light-boxes in their offices. It would be very inconvenient to the average clinician if all diagnostic images could not be viewed in the same way. The majority of diagnostic images still consists of analog-generated large x-ray film and, therefore, dictates the choice of the viewing station.

"The factors dictating the choice of an analog viewing station in a clinical environment will become less important during the next few years for several reasons. First, more and more quantitative information, such as ultrasound tissue characterization and x-ray dual-energy analysis, is being used by clinicians for research and specialized exams. This type of information will soon be used in everyday clinical practice and wil require the use of digital viewing stations as a complement to the conventional (analog) light-box. Second, the fact that all pictures are now added to the patient film jacket, and stored in the film file room, increases the file room size needed for analog storage on film (more so than digital storage would require) and adds to the inconveniences of manual film retrieval. Third, today's utilization of available computation power, especially in nuclear medicine, is not optimal. If all computing were made available on a shared and distributed basis, the equipment would be used in a more efficient way.

"In a teaching/research environment, digitally acquired images are kept in digital form for as long as they are needed or for as long as it is physically possible to keep them given the size limitations of the archive. Both x-ray CT and nuclear medicine images are usually archived on magnetic tape or disc. Some ultrasound equipment images are usually archived on magnetic tape or disc. Some ultrasound equipment manufacturers now provide interfaces to the scanner's image memory and thus allow direct retrieval of the digital image informatin. In the case of x-ray CT and ultrasound images, one is limited in the total amount of images that can be stored (see Refs. 4 and 7 for data on memory size needed for different images).

"The shortcomings of today's use of digital images in a teaching/research environment can be summarized as follows. The only flexible, practical and widely used digital storage medium is magnetic tape. Clinical researchers want to be able to store any image in digital form. Because the volume of magnetic tapes required for such purposes increases very rapidly, and the image retrieval is slow and sequential, this type of data base cannot be used efficiently. To compound the problem, each imaging modality usually produces a different image format.

These restrictions somtimes force the researcher to use a viewing station connected to the instrument being used for clinical exams to view images and put the researcher and clinician in direct competition for access to clinical instruments.

"Without affecting the operation of today's clinical diagnostic department, research and/or teaching could drastically be improved and facilitated. In order to do so, a digital PAC sub-system needs to be developed within existing radiology departments[8] that provides one or a combination of the following capabilities. The first capability is an *image communication network*, which is a digital link between each imaging device and computing, archiving, and viewing stations. An image communication network allows any digital image to be archived at any time in a temporary archive. The second capability is a digital *image/ data base* that is sufficiently large to accommodate the volume of images needed for research/teaching during a number of days or weeks. The third capability is a system that allows *shared use* of computer power and viewing stations. If all three of these capabilities were available, researchers and teachers could have easy access to any diagnostic image with interesting pathological, clinical or technical features. The clinical radiologist would not be affected, because each digital image would still be recorded on film as usual. The radiologist's help would be needed, however, in selecting the clinically interesting images.

Proposed Image Archiving and Management Strategies

"As stated above, digital PAC sub-systems might be helpful for teaching/research and are not too difficult to develop. On the other hand, the development for clinical use of a full-scale digital PACS to replace today's centralized analog film file room will take many years of experimenting and research. A global digital and filmless PACS will have to be easy to use, be effective, provide fast access, be user friendly and cost effective to the average clinical diagnostic radiologist. We therefore do not foresee any major quantum jumps in the development and utilization of filmless PAC systems. Rather, we expect a slow, steady evolution in time. Cost may become a less important factor in the decision to switch to digital PACS, as routine clinical demand for quantitative parameters (such as tissue characterization or dual-energy radiography) may become major determinants in the decision to change. Technological breakthroughs will soon remove the last roadblocks to a totally digital PACS.

"We will now describe a possible 'digital PACS' development scenario, consisting of a sequence of five different strategies for images archiving and management, starting with a status quo strategy and ending with a full-scale digital PACS strategy. We foresee a 'digital PACS' development scenario where equipment manufacturers and the medical community join efforts to proceed from one strategy level to the next. Each strategy in our list brings us further from the analog film file room and closer to a filmless digital PACS. Each strategy is one step in a PACS development scenario for the coming years. For each strategy we give different ways to implement the general features of the strategy. While giving this step-by-step prediction of the evolution of PAC system development, we identify five key components or concepts needed for filmless PACS. These concepts are discussed in more detail in the next section.

Strategy #1

"This strategy is the starting point in our PACS development scenario and consists of leaving things the way they are today: a status quo. Archiving is done in centralized film file rooms. The image management strategy is a function of both the non-picture patient record filing system and the film file room organization. As mentioned earlier, some of the diagnostic images are stored digitally on tape or disc for special research or teaching purposes. Long-term archiving is sometimes achieved with movable shelf microfilm systems.[3]

Strategy #2

"This strategy is the second step in the 'digital PACS' development scenario and basically corresponds to what was suggested at the end of the previous section: provide researchers/teachers with easy access to the digital information, but in a way that is transparent to the clinician. His strategy does not affect the day-to-day operation of clinical diagnostic imaging procedures and does not interfere with the clinician's work.

"Strategy #2 calls for a digital PAC sub-system, consisting of a combination of any of the following four parts:

- A digital optical disc based archive, allowing on-line storage of several weeks' worth of research related images (see discussion of concept #1 in the next section).
- A fast access magnetic disc based archive, allowing storage of data acquired in real-time.
- An image communication network (see discussion of concept #2 in the next section) connecting nuclear medicine cameras, ultrasound scanners, x-ray CT scanners, a central computer and a small archive (see Ref. 8).
- High-resolution displays for parallel and sequential viewing of images (see discussion of concept #4 in the next section).

Strategy #3

"This strategy is the third step in the "digital PACS" development scenario/and it involves slightly more than strategy #2, in that it affects the way the technologist uses the imaging equipment and his/her interaction with the radiologist. Three examples of capabilities that would allow a partial implementation of strategy #3 are:

- Local on-line archives for each imaging modality (i.e., distributed data base), with each archive large enough to store several days' worth of images. This data base would take away the need to store images on film during the patient's examination (see discussion of concept #1 in the next section).
- Shared distributed computing and display resources in nuclear medicine.
- A flimless PAC sub-system for ultrasound. Such a PAC subsystem would interconnect all ultrasound examination rooms and scanners with one main viewing room, and also provide on-line archive capability of to 3 days' worth of images. The system would totally change the operation of ultrasound procedures: there would be no need to first make hard copies of the ultrasound images before the patient can be released. The radiologist can quickly check all the images prior to releasing the patient. No film is wasted.

Strategy #4

"This strategy is the fourth step in the "digital PACS" development scenario, and it will have a stronger effect on the operation of the clinical part of the radiology department than strategy #3. This strategy allows the clinician to use conventional light-boxes to view large-size x-ray images, but high-resolution video displays (see discussion of concept #4 in the next section) will be available to view digital images stored in digital form. Hard copy on film will only be provided for long-term archiving or outside consulting by another physician.

"Strategy #4 calls for on-line digital storage capability of all images produced in digital form over a period of time. Two implementation approaches can be taken: a centralized archive or a distributed archive (see concept #1).

"A first approach is the *centralized archive*, where all images are stored on a day-to-day basis and patient-by-patient basis. The time period over which the data base is maintained can be chosen in many different ways:

- a fixed time period; e.g., 3 days, 20 days or 2 months;
- the duration of the patient's stay in the hospital;
- the time needed for the course of therapy;
- the time needed to complete a clinical research project.

"A second approach is a *distributed archive* where a physical archive partition is provided for each imaging modality; i.e., each imaging modality will have its own archive. Because different imaging modalities produce different picture formats, a different amount of data will be archived for each imaging modality; for example: 3 days' worth of images for ultrasound, 40 days' worth for nuclear medicine, and 5 days' worth for x-ray CT.

"Another useful capability to be implemented at the level of strategy #4 is the sharing of image display, recall and processing resources.

Strategy #5

"This strategy represents the final step in the 'digital PACS' development scenario and brings us toward a fully digital, partially on-line PACS in diagnostic radiology and nuclear medicine. The strategy will, when implemented, drastically change the clinical operation of a radiology department. We distinguish, rather arbitrarily, three different ways to implement the strategy:

- Digital encoding of all diagnostic images on a patient-by-patient basis on an individual image 'credit card' for long-term archiving (the image 'credit card' is concept #3, to be discussed in the next section).
- Digital acquisition (also for x-ray; see discussion of concept #5 in the next section) and short-term (e.g., several days or weeks) on-line storage of all diagnostic images;
- Digital acquisition (also for x-ray) and long-term (e.g., several months or years) on-line storage of all diagnostic images, i.e., a digital radiology department.

"It should be noted that none of the above five strategies addresses the problem of management information systems (MIS) with computerized patient record keeping and patient file management. A standard way of encoding the final radiology consulting report has not been agreed upon yet. Therefore, we do not wish, in this paper, to dilute the main issue (i.e., a scenario for the development of 'digital PACS') by incorporating uncontrollable and unpredictable *human factors* into our discussion (see Refs. 1, 2 for such discussions). We want to make it very clear that a PACS, providing the physician with picture access and a patient name and date, is a viable concept with virtually none of the human interface problems and disagreements about a standard encoding method for computerized patient record keeping. It is beyond the scope of this paper to consider the combination of both MIS and PACS.

New Concepts Needed for PACS

"While presenting our PACS development scenario and discussing the above five strategies, we identified five key concepts needed to proceed from a film-based 'analog PACS' to a fully filmless, partially on-line "digital PACS." We will now detail these concepts, state their purpose and give possible implementations.

1. *The electronic picture archive*

"The purpose of the electronic picture archive is to provide on-line short-term or long-term digital image archiving, with fast retrieval of images. Short-term refers to several days or a few weeks. Long-term refs to many weeks or several months. Fast retrieval means: fast enough to allow user friendly parallel viewing of up to 30 images.

"An electronic picture archive could be implemented by using any one or a combination of:

- digital optical disc recorders;
- laser film encoders;
- magnetic tape/disc drives;
- solid-state memories.

"Such an electronic archive would allow both hard and soft copy production. Quantitative image informaiton extraction becomes possible. Also, savings in film otherwise wasted on poor pictures and repeat radiographs are to be expected.

2. *A picture communication network*

"The purpose of a picture communication network is to provide fast (broadband) digital communication between imaging devices, different on-line archives, and viewing stations.

"The picture communication network could be implemented using coax of fiber optic technology. The network configuration could be a local area network based on a single or double ring or a bus structure. The information exchange could be accomplished using a standard network communication protocol. Ethernet has been mentioned as a possible choice.[9]

"The picture communication network could be used for transfer of three types of information: control information (short 'packets' for status reporting); electronic mail (consultation reports, patient data, management data); and image records.

3. *An image "credit card"*

"The purpose of the image 'credit card' is to provide off-line long-term digital storage of images on a patient-by-patient basis. It might eventually replace the patient film jackets in use today. The term 'image credit card' is somewhat misleading because its implementation does not necessarily require a medium similar to a conventional (financial) credit card. However, it is called a 'credit card' to convey the message that its implementation will be significantly less bulky than today's film jacket.

"The image 'credit card' could be implemented by using an optical medium with digital encoding, such as a mini optical disc or a strip of film. Another approach would be to use a solid-state memory. VLSI technology will certainly open up new possibilities in the area of large memories. In order to be practical, the 'credit card' should be either updatable or cheap to replace and duplicate. Widespread use of such a digital archive will require the introduction of standard viewing stations in many locations within the hospital.

"The very real requirement for long-term storage (i.e., over a period of several years) should never be overlooked. The two most important reasons for keeping diagnostic image records over a long period of time are, first, for legal reasons and this requires storage for a period of several years. But even more important, the second reason is that many diagnoses depend on a comparison of an image acquired now with an image acquired last yeat, the year before, etc. A fairly significant number of diagnoses would be missed if previous images were not available for comparison, since small changes in pathology can only be recognized by comparison with previous images. Therefore, until an image 'credit card' medium becomes available, radiologists will have to rely on bulky and costly media (film or conventional digital storage) for long-term archiving.

4. *A high resolution display*

"The purpose of the high resolution display is the parallel (i.e., simultaneous) viewing up to 30 pictures and also the sequential viewing of dynamic studies.

"For its implementation, a special purpose image computer architecture seems most appropriate. Several manufacturers[12,13] provide partial solutions to this problem.

5. *A system for real-time digital acquisition of large x-ray images*

"The primary purpose of such a digitizer would be to complete the last step in making diagnostic radiology a fully digital operation. It will allow widespread use of digital radiogrpahy techniques.

"Several digitization methods for large x-ray film are presently being tested.[9,10] Knowledge gained in developing cheap and fast film digitizers could later lead to cheap systems that acquire large x-ray images directly in digital form.

Evaluations of Archiving Strategies

"The evaluation of archiving strategies requires criteria by which to predict the need for different PACS and PAC sub-systems in clinical diagnostic radiology. One can readily list three classes of criteria:

1. Technical factors, such as:
   - the daily volume of digital image data;
   - the speed required for image communication;
   - access protocols;
   - access speeds.
2. Cost-benefit factors, such as:
   - the archiving cost for each strategy;
   - the operating costs of different system configurations.
3. User interface factors, such as:
   - human acceptance of filmless operation.

"We will limit the criteria used in our preliminary evaluation to technical and cost-benefit factors. Unfortunately, few studies[7] are available that attempt to estimate the cost of conventional analog film file room based archiving. More studies are available[7,9] that give estimates of the daily volume of data produced and the data rates required for communication.

"We will use the results of a detailed study[7] at the University of Kansas Medical Center in 1981. The medical center is not necessarily representative of other hospitals or medical centers but is a good (and the only available) start for any future discussions on and evaluation of PACS. The University of Kansas Medical Center is a 614-bed teaching hospital where most imaging modalities commercially available today are in clinical use. The detailed list of the instrumentation used and the daily flow of patients for each imaging modality are given in Reference 7 and will not be repeated here. We will only restate two of the conclusions of the study:

(1) Use of imaging modalities such as x-ray, CT, ultrasound, nuclear medicine and (projected use of) digital radiography will generate between 254 and 502 megabytes of digital data daily. This number does not include analog-generated radiographic film.

(2) Seventy-five percent (75%) of the cost of archiving and managing these image data is due to the use of video raster multi-format film recording.

"It is also worthwhile to look at data available from European medical centers[10] and the New York University Medical Center.[9] These studies not only consider imaging modalities that produce digital images but include digitization stations for analog-generated radiographs. Maquire[9] envisions a 10-year transition period during which all old film is digitized each time it is recalled, and new film is immediately digitized. This transition period (toward an era where all images are acquired in digital form) will put heavy demands on a broadband communications system. Maquire estimates that about 5,500 megabytes of image data would have to be stored daily during that transition period.

"The conclusions of the above studies are that we need to store a lot of digital image data, and that we need a 'very broadband' communication network. When one surveys today's available storage media, nothing comes close to being able to provide more than several days' worth of on-line digital image storage capacity. Even the non-erasable digital optical disc recorder only allows the recording of up to 1,000 MBytes on each side of a disc.[5] A typical 2,400-foot magnetic tape reel, at a 1,600 byte/inch recording rate, only stores about 42 MBytes of data. Thus for short-term archiving more clever on-line archiving strategies will have to be developed to match both the clinical needs for immediate recall of part of the diagnostic images and the availability of storage hardware that is not overly complex or costly. For long-term archiving, an image 'credit card' type medium will have to be developed.

"The cost estimates[7,9] for image archiving and management available so far are only a portion of the total cost. Difficult to include are cost factors such as: hidden personnel cost, cost of infrequently used modalities (real-time archiving, etc.), and the hidden cost of software development and maintenance. The number of beds, hospital size, and whether or not all imaging modalities are available are factors that heavily influence cost estimates.

"Cost may be less important[14] than patient care delivery and access to new technology. If digital PACS drastically improves short-term access to diagnostic images, it will most certainly replace analog film recordings for short-term archiving.

Conclusions: The Future of Filmless PACS

"The future of digital PAC subsystems looks very promising. After the first introduction of PAC subsystems, the usage of film will, initially, not decrease significantly, but the access to diagnostic information will improve. Even after full-scale 'digital PACS' will become an integral part of diagnostic radiology departments, a moderate amount of hardcopy on film will still be needed because of its convenience and portability.

Acknowledgements

"We would like to thank Samuel J. Dwyer III (University of Kansas Medical Center), Carla Marceau (NCR Corporation), Fritz Arink (Philips Medical Systems Division), Dietrich Myer-Ebrecht (Philips Research Lab, Hamburg) and Norman Baily (University of California, San Diego) for their helpful comments on a preliminary draft of this paper. We thank the participants in the 1982 PACS Conference for providing valuable information of the topic of digital PACS. We also thank Paul Brown, managing editor of *Diagnostic Imaging,* for providing Figure 1 (see Ref. 15). Finally, we thank Alma Faught who typed the manuscript on a Philips MICOM word processor."

References

1. Arenson, R.L., Morton, D., London, J., *Comprehensive Radiology Management System Without PACS.* Proceedings of the First International Conference and Workshop on Picture Archiving and Communication Systems (PACS) for Medical Applications (Abbreviated: Proceedings of the 1982 PACS Conference), Edited by Andre J. Deurinckx, SPIE Vol 318-61, January 18-21, 1982, Newport Beach, CA.

2. Quintin, J., Simborg, D., *The University of California at San Francisco Automated Radiology Department Without PACS,* Proceedings of 1982 PACS Conference, SPIE Vol 318-62, January 18-21, 1982, Newport Beach, CA.

3. *Medical Records Round Up: Part II:* Radiology/Nuclear Medicine Magazine, Vol. III, No. 5, pp. 63-67, October 1981.

4. Robinson, R.G., *The Use of Medical Images in Today's Hospital,* Proceedings of the 1982 PACS Conference, SPIE Vol 318-01, January 18-21, 1982, Newport Beach, CA.

5. Nadan, J., Blom, G., Chandra, S., Kenny, G., McFarlane, R., *Recent Advances in Digital Optical Recording*, Proceedings of the 1982 PACS Conference, SPIE Vol 318-07, January 18-21, 1982, Newport Beach, CA.

6. Kreutzer, H.W., Hermes, T., *Fiber Optic Broadband Communication Systems — Design and Realizations*, Proceedings of the 1982 PACS Conference, SPIE Vol 318-16, January 18-21, 1982, Newport Beach, CA.

7. Dwyer III, S.J., Templeton, A.W., *The Cost of Managing Digital Radiographic Images*, Proceedings of the 1982 PACS Conference, SPIE Vol 318-02, January 18-21, 1982, Newport Beach, CA.

8. Dwyer III, S.J., Templeton, A.W., Anderson, W.B., Tarlton, M.A., *A Distributed Diagnostic Image Information System*, Proceedings of the 1982 PACS Conference, SPIE Vol 318-33, January 18-21, 1982, Newport Beach, CA.

9. Maquire, Jr., G.O., Zeleznik, M.P., Horii, S.C., Schimpf, J.H., Noz, M.E., *Image Processing Requirements in Hospitals and an Integrated Systems Approach*, Proceedings of the 1982 PACS Conference, SPIE Vol 318-35, January 18-21, 1982, Newport Beach, CA.

10. D. Meyer-Ebrecht (private communication)

11. G.J. Arink (private communication); the 50% fraction refers to the share of images produced with x-ray equipment.

12. La Jeunesse, R.P., *A New System Architecture for Medical Image Processing*, Proceedings of the 1982 PACS Conference, SPIE Vol 318-42, January 18-21, 1982, Newport Beach, CA.

13. Clouthier, R., *Digital Storage and Fast Communication Links for Medical Image Analysis*, Proceedings of the 1982 PACS Conference, SPIE Vol 318-43, January 18-21, 1982, Newport Beach, CA.

14. Vanden Brink J.A., *Present Practice and Perceived Needs — the Medical Imaging Market*, Proceedings of the 1982 PACS Conference, SPIE Vol 318-74, January 18-21, 1982, Newport Beach, CA.

15. Deurinckx, A.D., Dwyer III, S.J., Pisa, E.J., *Digital Image Archiving and Management*, Diagnostic Imaging, November 1981 (pp. 62-63), a Miller-Freeman Publication.

SUMMARY

1. Digital radiography is a technique in which data (analog) collected from the patient is converted into digital form so that it is suitable for processing by a digital computer.

2. Several terms are used to describe digital radiography and these have been identified as digital fluoroscopy, digital subtraction angiography, digital vascular imaging, computerized fluoroscopy, digital video angiography and digital scanned projection radiography, to mention only a few.

3. This chapter uses the term digital radiography to impress upon the student that the technique is based on non-tomographic principles and to distinguish it from computed tomography.

4. The limitations of radiography, fluoroscopy and computed tomography are removed by digital radiography. Such limitations include the problem of superimposition, inflexible display of images, poor demonstration of

low contrast structures and so on.

5. One of the main advantages of digital radiography is its improved detectability of low contrast structures. Other advantages include quantitative analysis, data storage, image enhancement and manipulation, image transmission and so on.

6. The development of digital imaging in medicine is based on previous works done in several areas such as in astronomy.

7. The fundamental concept of digital radiography involves digitization of the analog data collected from the patient and subsequent processing by a digital computer. Since the concept also involves projection imaging in a non-tomographic fashion, the problem of superimposition also exists. This problem is eliminated through some form of subtraction technique.

8. Three forms of subtraction are used in digital radiography: temporal, energy and hybrid subtraction.

9. In temporal subtraction images are subtracted in time. Usually a pre-contrast image (mask image) is recorded and post-contrast images are then subtracted from it. Several modes of temporal subtraction are discussed.

10. Energy subtraction involves subtraction of images based on the energy level at which they are recorded. Energy subtraction is less susceptible to motion artifacts, a shortening of temporal subtraction.

11. Hybrid subtraction uses both temporal- and energy-subtraction schemes in producing images.

12. Equipment for digital radiography can be divided into two main classes: digital fluoroscopy and digital scanned projection radiography, or computed radiography as it has often been referred to.

13. Digital fluoroscopy makes use of almost the same equipment components as in conventional fluoroscopy except for a few differences. Digital fluoroscopy consists of an image intensifier-television chain, a logarithmic processor, an analog-to-digital converter, digital frame memories, a computer and data storage equipment.

14. The image from the image intensifier is picked up by the television camera tube. The voltage output from the camera tube is digitized by the analog-to-digital converter and the information may then be stored in the frame memories. The computer system then uses this data for processing and storage.

15. The data (processed) may then be displayed on suitable devices (television screen) for viewing and recording.

16. A brief description of each of the components in a digital fluoroscopy scheme is presented.

17. The fundamental concept of digital scanned projection imaging involves some form of scanning the patient through mechanical motion of the x-ray tube and detectors.

18. Two approaches, the line scanning approach which uses a single detector

element, and the fan beam scanning approach, which uses a linear array of detectors are used to collect data from the patient. The transmitted x-ray photons are detected and are converted into electrical signals which are subsequently digitized for processing a digital computer.

19. Temporal subtraction has found its main application in intravenous angiography, while energy subtraction has been applied to scanned projection imaging.

20. Other methods of digital radiography involve the use of special imaging plates. These plates are either photostimulable phosphors or electrically charged plates. The signals arising from the plates are digitized for processing by the computer.

21. Image quality was discussed for both digital fluoroscopy and digital scanned projection imaging, in terms of spatial and contrast resolution and noise. Factors influencing resolution were also identified.

22. Digital radiography has found applications in three areas, namely, intravascular contrast studies, non-vascular contrast studies, and non-contrast precedures.

23. While the contrast media used in digital-subtraction angiography must be of low toxicity and viscosity, it must also have a high level of iodine concentration. Pressure injectors are also used in digital angiography. Other characteristic features in clinical imaging involves catheterization through a peripheral venous and central venous approaches.

24. Digital radiography is limited with respect to patient motion, noise, the amount of contrast media used and cost.

Part C

QUALITY ASSURANCE

Section E

QUALITY-ASSURANCE OVERVIEW

CHAPTER 19

QUALITY-ASSURANCE CONCEPTS

THE end product in diagnostic imaging is an image from which a diagnosis is made. If the image is poor, the extraction of useful information becomes a problem and the image may be discarded for a better quality image. This process involves the use of more films to produce such images and additional radiation exposures to the patient.

One of the fundamental goals of an imaging department is to provide the best possible image with minimal radiation doses and at minimal cost to the patient and institution. To establish, and most of all maintain, the production of high-quality images, it is essential that a quality-assurance program be developed and implemented.

DEFINITION OF QUALITY ASSURANCE

The idea and concepts of *quality assurance* (QA) are becoming increasingly important and commonplace in imaging departments.

According to the Food and Drug Adminstration (FDA, 1979), United States Department of Health, Education and Welfare (USHEW), quality assurance is defined as "the planned and systematic actions that provide adequate confidence that a diagnostic x-ray facility will produce consistently high-quality images with minimum exposure of the patients and healing-arts personnel. The determination of what constitutes high quality will be made by the facility producing the images. Quality-assurance actions include both 'quality control' techniques and 'quality administration' procedures."

The definition focuses attention on several concepts, including (a) the concept of minimal exposure doses to patients and personnel, (b) the concept of image quality standards, (c) quality control, and (d) quality administration.

Quality control (QC) and *quality administration* are two terms that require further clarification. In this regard the FDA (1979) points out that:

1. "Quality control techniques are those techniques used in monitoring (or testing) and maintenance of the components of an x-ray system. The quality control techniques thus are concerned directly with the equipment."
2. "Quality administration procedures are those management actions intended to guarantee that monitoring techniques are properly performed and evaluated and that necessary corrective measures are taken in response to monitoring results. These procedures provide the organizational framework for the quality-assurance program."

In other words, quality administration ensures that a QC program is developed, implemented and maintained on a regular basis, that the results of monitoring procedures are examined carefully, and that corrective and preventive actions be taken if necessary. It also takes into account other considerations such as delegating responsibility for carrying out QC tests, training staff to perform QC tests, determination of image quality standards and so on.

HISTORICAL BACKGROUND

The history of quality assurance in x-ray imaging may be traced back to the early 1970s based on the experiences of the National Institute for Occupational Safety and Health (NIOSH), in which coal miners were provided with periodic chest x-rays to check for the presence and extent of pneumoconiosis. In this project, the radiologists interpreting the films were faced with the problem of poor film quality, in that about 30 percent of these films were unacceptable (Felson et al., 1973). The radiologists attributed the poor quality to poor processing technique, poor beam geometry, overexposure and underexposure. In other words, the *reject rate* (rate at which unacceptable films are discarded) was very high.

Around the same period the Bureau of Radiological Health (BRH) examined the reject rate and used it as an index of radiographic quality. Later, in another study (Burnett et al., 1975), retake rates were reported as being significant in British and American hospitals.

In 1974, these experiences prompted the BRH to develop instructional materials on quality assurance (Federal Register — FDA, 1979). At that time also, other groups such as Dupont, Agfa-Gavaert, Eastman Kodak Company, Radiation Measurements Incorporated and the American College of Radiology (ACR) joined in the effort to promote the idea of quality assurance. They offered seminars and workshops and developed educational materials on quality assurance.

Today, quality assurance is an acceptable program in most radiology departments. The literature is replete with articles on quality-assurance concepts, and recently several textbooks on quality control (for example, Gray et al., 1983) have appeared. Quality-assurance courses are becoming commonplace in educational institutions and are provided on a regular basis by several film manufacturers and other groups such as the American Association of Physicists in Medicine (AAPM).

A QUALITY-ASSURANCE SCHEME — DEFINING RESPONSIBILITIES

It is important to establish and define responsibilities to maintain a successful quality-assurance program, since there are a number of elements in the total scheme.

A typical quality-assurance scheme in terms of responsibilities is illustrated in Figure 19:1. The scheme can be discussed in terms of primary and secondary responsibilities.

Primary Responsibility

The FDA (1979), the BRH (1980) and the Joint Committee on the Accreditation of Hospitals (JCAH — 1980) identify the radiologist in charge of the imaging department as the individual responsible for the entire scheme and for implementation and maintenance of the program.

Secondary Responsibility

Although the radiologist assumes the full responsibility for the program, this responsibility is (in general and in practice) shifted to either the medical

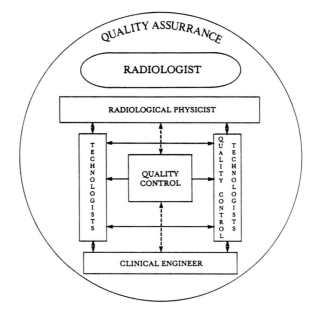

Figure 19:1. A quality control scheme, showing responsibilities and interaction among different individuals. The radiologist is seen as being responsible for the entire scheme. See text for further explanation.

physicist, clinical engineer or the technologist.

The responsibility of quality control rests upon all technical staff in the department, the interrelationships of which are shown in Figure 19:1. In some departments the responsibility is that of the physicist who works in conjunction with staff technologists to ensure an effective program. Since physicists are trained at a higher level, it is beneficial to the program if they assume the role of developing tests and educating staff technologists in carrying out test procedures and interpreting tests results. In this regard, the physicist may also assume the role of a consultant. On the other hand, the clinical engineer's role is to make necessary repairs and to adjust and calibrate the equipment.

In other departments, the idea of a quality-control technologist is appealing and quality control becomes the prime function of this individual. The quality-control technologist is seen as the individual who performs the test procedures, documents, and in some cases interprets and makes recommendations for corrective action, especially in small-scale institutions.

In summary, there must be an interaction among a number of people to implement and maintain an effective quality-assurance program.

FUNDAMENTAL PRINCIPLES OF QUALITY ASSURANCE

Quality-assurance principles must be organized and executed in a specific and defined manner. Since quality-control tests involve a definite set of rules

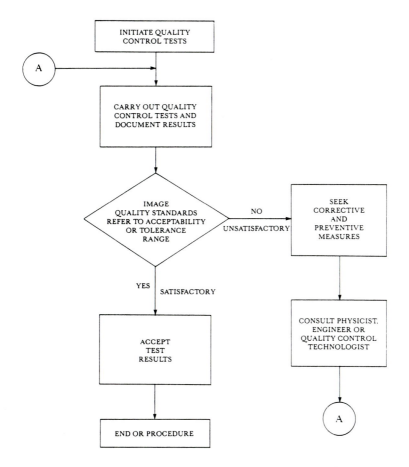

Figure 19:2. A flowchart, illustrating the fundamental principles of quality control.

and procedures, perhaps an *algorithmic approach* (use of algorithms, a defined set of rules for solving a problem) may best describe the fundamental principles. Such an algorithm is shown in Figure 19:2 in the form of a flowchart.

The flowchart consists of a starting point and a finishing point with a number of definite steps in between. The steps are:

(a) carry out the test procedure.
(b) document the results.
(c) interpret the results.
(d) accept the results if image quality standards are met.
(e) reject results if image quality standards are not met.
(f) seek corrective and preventive measures.
(g) consult physicist, engineer, QC technologist and/or other appropriate resources.
(h) having consulted, repeat the test until satisfactory results are obtained.

PARAMETERS FOR QC MONITORING

This text is concerned with x-ray imaging equipment, and hence the material described in the previous chapters deal with three aspects of x-ray imaging instrumentation, namely: radiographic, fluoroscopic and computer-aided imaging such as computed tomography and digital radiography.

The parameters to be monitored in a quality-assurance program are therefore related to these three categories of equipment. There are five key components (FDA, 1979) that require monitoring:

(a) cassettes and grids.
(b) processing room.
(c) processing of film (processor).
(d) view boxes or illuminators.
(e) basic characteristics of the x-ray unit.

In Tables 19:1, 19:2, 19:3, and 19:4, the essential parameters to be monitored in a QC program are summarized. It is not within the scope of this chapter to describe how these parameters are monitored.

In item (e) above, the x-ray unit refers to radiographic, fluoroscopic, image intensified units and automatic exposure control. Other units which must be considered include conventional tomographic and computed tomography units.

QC TEST PROCEDURES

Once the QA program is established and responsibilities have been delegated, the next phase involves the actual test procedures. The test procedure should be in a clearly defined format, and in this regard the BRH (1979) outlines the following format for these tests:

(a) *Objective of the test.* This is a statement of the purpose of the test. It should indicate what will be accomplished at the end of the test procedure.

(b) *Equipment to carry out the test.* This includes all necessary equipment for the test procedure. In some cases, diagrams and/or photographs are useful to demonstrate the actual set up of the equipment. Figure 19:3 shows a quality-control kit for radiography and fluoroscopy which contains several pieces of equipment used for various test procedures. These include a Wisconsin kVp test cassette, a focal spot test tool, a half-value layer attenuator set, a timing and mAs test tool, a high and low contrast resolution test tool, a screen-film contact test tool, a beam-alignment test tool, a low-energy dosimeter and a dosimeter charger.

(c) *Testing frequency.* This indicates how often the test should be carried out. For example, collimator accuracy, timer accuracy, kVp measurement, grid alignment and film/screen contact should be checked

Table 19-1

PARAMETERS TO BE MONITORED FOR FILM PROCESSING

(Adapted from the *Federal Register*, Volume 44,
Number 239, 1979.)

FILM PROCESSING PARAMETERS

— Index of speed.

— Index of contrast.

— Base plus fog.

— Solution temperature.

— Film artifact identification.

Table 19-2

PARAMETERS TO BE MONITORED FOR THE BASIC PERFORMANCE CHARACTERISTICS OF
THE X-RAY UNIT

(Adapted from the *Federal Register*, Volume 44, Number 239, 1979.)

PERFORMANCE CHARACTERISTICS OF THE X-RAY UNIT			
RADIOGRAPHY	FLUOROSCOPY	IMAGE INTENSIFIED SYSTEMS	AUTOMATIC EXPOSURE CONTROL
— Reproducibility of x-ray output.	Table top exposure rates.	Resolution.	Reproducibility.
— Linearity and re-producibility of mA stations.	Centering alignment.	Focussing. Distortion.	kVp compensation. Field sensitivity matching.
— Reproducibility and accuracy of timer stations.	Collimation. kVp accuracy and re-producibility.	Glare. Low contrast performance.	Minimum response time.
— Reproducibility and accuracy of kVp stations.	mA accuracy and re-producibility.	Physical alignment of cam-era and collimating lens.	Back-up timer varification.
— Accuracy of source-to-film distance.	Exposure time ac-curacy and reproduci-bility.		
— Light/x-ray field congruence.	Reproducibility of x-ray output.		
— Half value layer.	Focal spot size consis-tency.		
— Focal spot size consistency.	Half value layer.		
— Representative entrance skin ex-posures.	Representative en-trance skin exposure.		

Table 19-3

PARAMETERS TO BE MONITORED FOR CASSETTES, GRIDS AND
VIEW BOXES

(Adapted from the *Federal Register,* Volume 44, Number 239, 1979.)

CASSETTES	GRIDS	VIEW BOXES
Film/screen contact. Screen condition. Light leaks. Artifact identification.	Alignment and focal distance. Artifact identification.	Consistency of light output with time. Consistency of light output from one box to another. View box surface conditions.

Table 19-4

PARAMETERS TO BE MONITORED FOR SPECIALIZED EQUIPMENT

(Adapted from the *Federal Register,* Volume 44, Number 239, 1979.)

CONVENTIONAL TOMOGRAPHY	COMPUTED TOMOGRAPHY
Accuracy of depth and cut indicator. Thickness of cut plane. Exposure angle. Completeness of tomographic motion. Flatness of tomographic field. Resolution. Continuity of exposure. Flatness of cassette. Representative entrance skin exposures.	Precision (noise). Contrast scale. High and low contrast resolution. Alignment. Representative entrance skin exposures.

every 2 months, 6 months, 3 months, 6 months, and 6 months, respectively (BRH, 1979).

(d) *Test procedure.* This phase of a test procedure format outlines the steps of the test and demonstrates how the equipment is utilized. It should be described step by step and written in an itemized format.

(e) *Documentation of test results.* This refers to the documentation (recording) of all the data obtained during the test procedure. The data must be recorded on special forms (data forms) so that the results can be compared with the acceptance test data (acceptance criteria) in order to determine satisfactory equipment performance and also to be used for consultation purposes. Four such forms are shown in Tables 19:5, 19:6, 19:7, and 19:8.

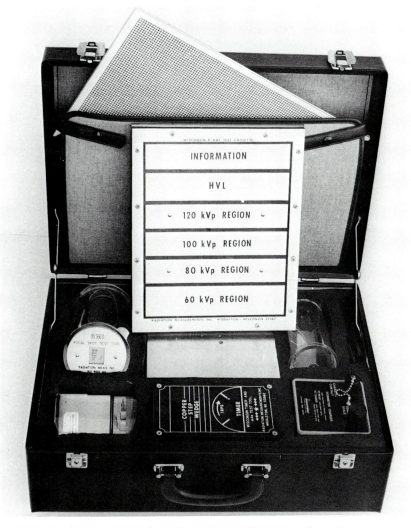

Figure 19:3. A quality control kit for radiography and fluoroscopy. Several test instruments are shown. (courtesy of Radiation Measurements, Inc.)

(f) *Interpretation of results.* The results of the test procedure must be checked and should match the acceptance criteria or standards for acceptable image quality.

(g) *Action limits and corrective actions.* These are measures taken to rectify unsatisfactory results. The test may be done again to verify the previous results.

(h) *Test procedure limitations.* These limitations in general relate to the problems encountered with the test procedure.

(i) *Alternate test procedure.* This is the final phase of the format and it refers to other techniques and methods that can be used for the same objective of the QC test.

Table 19-5

AN EXAMPLE OF A DATA FORM FOR DOCUMENTATION OF QC
TEST RESULTS ON RADIOGRAPHIC UNITS

(Courtesy of Radiation Measurements, Inc., 1977.)

Room _____   Tube _____   Date _____   Surveyor _____

1. kVp	Generator Kvp	Match Step	Measured kVp	Variance kVp	% Variance	Acceptable Yes	No
Set mA____							

2. HVL	Set true 60 kVp	mAs 1φ____ 3 φ	Match Step		Estimated HVL mm AL	Acceptable Yes	No

3. Timer	Generator Set Time	Angle Measured Time	Time Variance	% Variance	Acceptable Yes	No

4. mAs Reciprocity	Generator mA	Generator Time	Total mAs	Is there a Step Variance	% Variance	Acceptable Yes	No

5. Collimator	F.F.D. (SID)	Long Axis	Short Axis	Measured Variance	% Variance	Acceptable Yes	No
	40" Standard						
	Other						

6. Beam Alignment	Focal Film Distance (SID)	Is the Screw Shadow within the Washer	Acceptable Yes	No

7. mR output	kVp	mAs	F.F.D. (SID)	mR	mR/mAs	Acceptable Yes	No

8. Focal Spot Size	Tube Focal Size	Technique Used	Smallest Group Resolved	Measured Focal Spot Sized	% Variance	Acceptable Yes	No
Tube 1 Large							
Small							
Tube 2 Large							
Small							

Table 19-6

AN EXAMPLE OF A DATA FORM FOR DOCUMENTATION OF
QC TEST RESULTS ON FLUOROSCOPIC UNITS

(Courtesy of Radiation Measurements, Inc., 1977.)

Room: _____ Tube: _____ II Tube: _____ Date _____ Surveyor _____

kVp		Generator kVp Set	MA Time	Match Step	Measured kVp	kVP Variance	% Variance	Acceptable Yes	No
Spot Film Mode	A								
	B								
	C								
	D								
Fluoro Mode	A								
	B								
	C								
	D								

HVL	Set 60 kVp	mAs 1φ_____ 3φ	Match Step	Estimated HVL mmAl	Acceptable Yes	No

Maximum Output	Dosimeter between tube and phantom	kVp_____ mA	Exposure_____ Time	R/Min_____	Acceptable Yes	No

Focal Spot	Specified Spot Size	SID (24")	Technique Used	Smallest Group Resolve	Measured Focal Spot Size	% Variance	Acceptable Yes	No
Large								
Small								

Automatic Brightness Control		kVp (80 if constant)	mA	Image Brightness Change	No Change	Acceptable Yes	No
	1/32"						
Phantom 3/4"							
	1-1/2"						
1-1/2" and lead							

High Contrast Resolution	kVp	mA	Smallest Mesh Resolved				Acceptable Yes	No
			Direct View		Television			
			Center	Edge	Center	Edge		
6"								
9"								
mag.								

Low Contrast Resolution	kVp	mA	4% Contrast		2% Contrast		Acceptable Yes	No
			No. of Holes Resolved		No. of Holes Resolved			
			Direct View	Tele-vision	Direct View	Tele-vision		
6"								
9"								
mag.								

Phototimer	kVp (Constant)	mA	Phantom Thickness	Spot Film Density No change	Change ΔD	Acceptable Yes	No
1							
2							
3							

Table 19-7

AN EXAMPLE OF A DATA FORM FOR DOCUMENTATION OF QC TEST RESULTS ON TOMO-
GRAPHIC UNITS

(Courtesy of Radiation Measurements, Inc., 1977.)

Room: _____   Date: _____   Surveyor: _____

1. Location of Fulcrum	Machine Set CM.	Measured CM.	CM. Variance	% Variance	Acceptable Yes	No

2. Thickness of Plane		Type of Motion	Amplitude or Angle	Measured Thickness	Acceptable Yes	No
	1.					
	2.					
	3.					

3. Resolution		Type of Motion	Amplitude or Angle	Smallest Mesh Resolution	Acceptable Yes	No
	1.					
	2.					
	3.					

4. Exposure Uniformity Beam Path		Type of Motion	Amplitude or Angle	Visual Path of Motion Complete	Incomplete Overlap	Visual Density Uniformity	Acceptable Yes	No
	1.							
	2.							
	3.							
	4.							
	5.							
	6.							

Table 19-8

AN EXAMPLE OF A DATA FORM FOR DOCUMENTATION OF QC TEST RESULTS
ON FILM PROCESSOR UNITS

(Courtesy of Radiation Measurement, Inc., 1977.)

Processor: _____ Month: _____ 19 _____

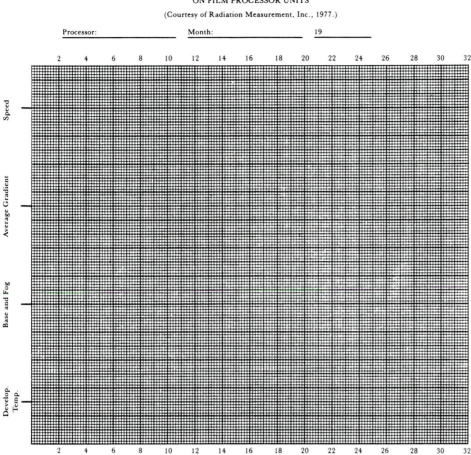

MONTHLY SERVICE AND INFORMATION RECORD
(cleaning, chemical change, adjustments)

| DATE | Replenishment | | DATE | SERVICE |
	Developer	Fixer		

IMAGE QUALITY STANDARDS

In any quality-assurance program there must be standards for image quality which determine whether the results of a test procedure are acceptable or not acceptable. In establishing these standards, it may be beneficial to set up *acceptance criteria* or "certain defined limits" (FDA, 1979). If the results of the test procedure fall within these limits, the acceptance criteria would have been met and the equipment performance is rated as being acceptable.

In establishing image quality standards, both subjective and objective standards are the focus of concern. The FDA (1979) recommends that standards should be objective, for example, "acceptability limits for the variations of parameter values." If the standards are based on "the opinions of professional personnel," then they are classed as subjective. Objective standards, on the other hand, are based on the results of research studies. As more and more research studies provide substantial and definitive expressions of image quality, objective standards will prevail.

OTHER CONSIDERATIONS

Maintaining a Quality-Assurance Program

Once a QA program is developed and implemented, it must be maintained to ensure its total effectiveness. It would be beneficial if the maintenance aspect of the program features *preventive* as well as *corrective maintenance.*

The ultimate objective of preventive maintenance is to prevent "breakdowns due to equipment failing without warning signs detectable by monitoring." Such maintenance procedures would entail, for example, a visual check of the equipment for unusual occurrences such as a crack i the insulation of the high tension cables, smooth motion of the x-ray tube on its support and tracks, and so on.

Corrective maintenance, on the other hand, implies that measures must be introduced in the QA program to deal with "potential problems" which must be removed "before they cause a major impact on patient care" (FDA, 1979).

Record Keeping

Documentation of test procedure results is especially important to the total effectiveness of the QA program. Record keeping is therefore recommended in order to maintain the overall quality of the program.

Education and Resources

A QA program must include some allotment of time for the education of staff with respect to all aspects of the QC portion of the program. This is particularly important for staff technologists who may have to carry out the actual QC test procedures and interpret the results.

Continuing education is of vital importance, especially as more research studies indicate acceptance criteria for objective image quality standards. The introduction and development of new techniques in imaging, particularly computer-assisted imaging techniques, demand that the QA program keep up with new concepts.

Resource material such as books, articles from research journals and manufacturer's literature on quality assurance should be made available. In cases where quality-assurance or quality-control courses are available at educational institutions, staff should be encouraged to participate in these classes. In-service lectures by either the charge QC technologist, the radiologist, the physicist and/or the clinical engineer or the manufacturers' representative should be encouraged.

Policy and Procedural Manual

Since a QA program involves a large number of parameters, it is beneficial to develop a policy and procedural manual, a document that is somewhat analogous to the department's policy and procedural manuals.

A manual promotes and maintains coherence to a QA program since it defines what protocols are used in executing the program.

In developing a manual, the FDA suggests a specific format which includes a number of items that should be included. In Table 19:9, a format for preparing a QA manual is given and it includes those items suggested by the FDA, as well as additional items.

Table 19-9

PERTINENT ITEMS THAT MAY BE INCLUDED IN THE DEVELOPMENT
OF A QUALITY ASSURANCE MANUAL

- Introduction.
- Objectives of the QA program.
- Individual responsibility protocol.
- Parameters to be monitored.
- Frequency of testing.
- Image quality standards.
- Test equipment available.
- Description of each test procedure.
- Photographs and/or diagrams illustrating the equipment set up procedure.
- Record keeping protocol.
- Protocol for reporting problems.
- References.
- Additional educative materials including audiovisual aids.
- An appendix which includes all data recording forms.

CONCLUSION

Quality-assurance concepts are becoming increasingly important, and, in the future, these concepts may become mandatory in all imaging departments.

Benefits of a QA Program

The development and implementation of an effective QA program ensures the acquisition of the overall objectives of the imaging department. Such acquisition reflects the benefits of the program:

    (a) improvement and maintenance of image quality standards
    (b) reduction of radiation exposures to both patients and staff
    (c) reduction of costs to the patient and to the imaging department.

In addition to these, other tangible benefits include the provision of a motivational factor in providing staff with the need to generate the best possible image and take pride in their work, as well as to encourage active participation in the learning process.

Evaluation

The process of quality assurance dictates a close interrelationship among all the elements involved. In summary, these elements include the objectives of the program, equipment needed to carry out the tests, test procedures, documentation, consultation, imge quality standards, frequency of testing, maintenance, development of a QA manual and education.

A determination of the interrelationships and overall effectiveness of the QA program can only be assessed by an evaluation scheme. Such a scheme may ensure that the test results meet the acceptance criteria for image quality, that minimal doses are used to provide the best possible image, and that costs are kept to a minimum. In other words, evaluation of the QA program is essential to determine whether the objectives have been met.

The evaluation process may differ from institution to institution and is not within the scope of this text.

SUMMARY

1. The fundamental goal of the imaging department is to provide the best possible image using minimal radiation doses at minimal cost to the patient and institution.
2. Quality assurance (QA) is a concept which ensures that high-quality images are produced consistently with minimal radiation exposure. It includes both quality-control techniques and quality administration procedures.

3. Quality control (QC) deals with monitoring and maintenance of the components of the x-ray imaging system and focuses directly on the equipment.

4. Quality administration refers to the management aspects which guarantee that quality-control tests ae implemented and maintained and that corrctive measures are taken if necessary.

5. The history of quality assurance goes back to the early 1970s based on experiences of NIOSH. In these experiences, radiologists were faced with images of very poor quality, which were attributed to poor processing, poor beam geometry and poor exposure factors.

6. Today, quality assurance has become an integral part of x-ray imaging, in that a variety of activities are available to assist departments in setting up quality-assurance programs.

7. The primary responsibility of quality assurance rests upon the radiologist in charge of the imaging department.

8. This responsibility is, in general, usually shifted to a radiological physicist, a clinical engineer or a senior technologist. In some cases, all three work together to maintain an effective quality-assurance program.

9. The fundamental principles of quality assurance follow a definite set of rules which allow for effective implementation and maintenance.

10. The parameters to be monitored relate to five key components, including cassettes and grids, processing room, processing film, view boxes or illuminators and the basic characteristics of the x-ray unit.

11. The test procedure in a quality-assurance program must be clearly stated in a defined format. Such format includes the objective of the test, equipment needed, testing frequency, test procedure, documentation, interpretation, limits and corrective measures, test procedure limitations and alternative test procedure.

12. In determining whether the results of the test procedures are acceptable or unacceptable, it is essential to establish acceptance criteria.

13. Acceptance criteria may be based on both objective and subjective standards. As more and more research studies provide substantial and definitive expressions of image quality, objective standards will prevail.

14. Quality-assurance programs must feature preventive as well as corrective maintenance. While preventive maintenance prevents equipment breakdowns, corrective maintenance ensures that certain measures must be introduced to deal with potential problems before they pose a serious impact on patients.

15. It is essential to document and keep records for the total effectiveness of a quality-assurance program.

16. Personnel must also be kept informed about quality assurance

through the availability of courses and library materials, including audiovisual aids and so on.

17. A policy manual for quality-assurance programs ensures coherence and defines protocols.

18. The benefits of a quality-assurance program include improvement and maintenance of image quality standards, reduction of radiation doses and costs, as well as other benefits.

19. Finally, it is mandatory to evaluate the quality-assurance program to determine whether the objectives have been met.

APPENDICES

APPENDIX A

SYMBOLS DEPICTED ON X-RAY IMAGING EQUIPMENT
(Internationally adopted codes)

SYMBOL	MEANING
	AC mains supply line.
	Mains power 'on'.
	Mains power 'off'.
	Tilting table.
	Movement of the Bucky.
	Movement of table top.
	Varying source-to-image distance.
	Spot film control indicator. Diaphragms fully closed.

SYMBOL	MEANING
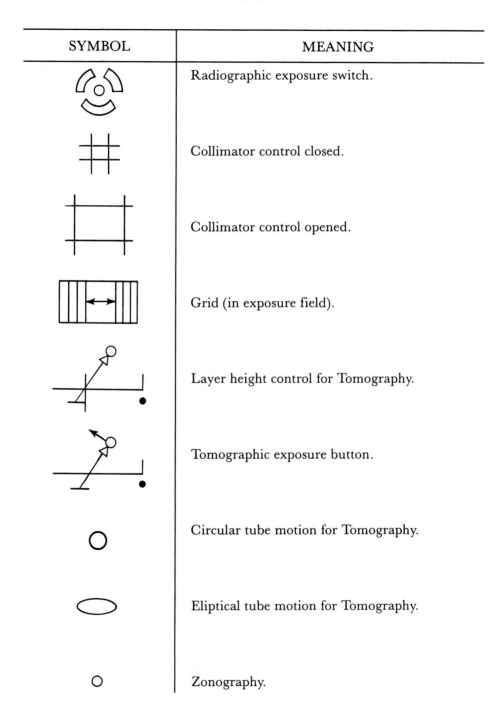	Radiographic exposure switch.
	Collimator control closed.
	Collimator control opened.
	Grid (in exposure field).
	Layer height control for Tomography.
	Tomographic exposure button.
	Circular tube motion for Tomography.
	Eliptical tube motion for Tomography.
	Zonography.

SYMBOL	MEANING
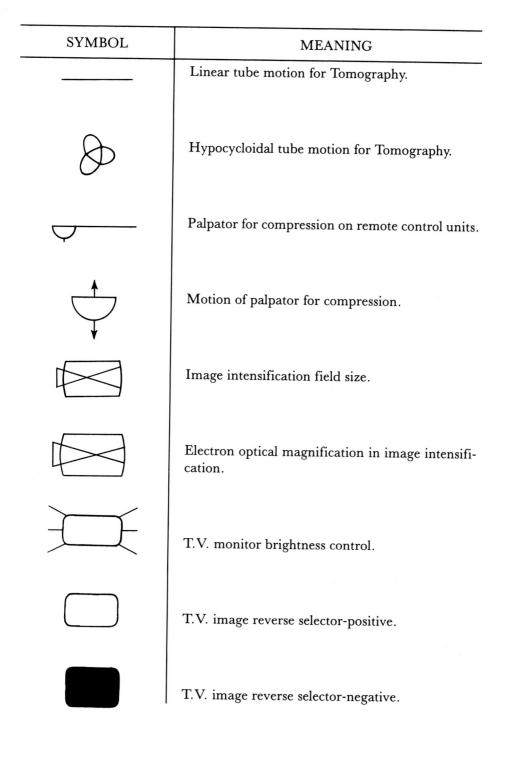	Linear tube motion for Tomography.
	Hypocycloidal tube motion for Tomography.
	Palpator for compression on remote control units.
	Motion of palpator for compression.
	Image intensification field size.
	Electron optical magnification in image intensification.
	T.V. monitor brightness control.
	T.V. image reverse selector-positive.
	T.V. image reverse selector-negative.

SYMBOL	MEANING
	T.V. image reserve selector — left.
	T.V. image reverse selector — right.
	T.V. image reverse selector — head-up.
	T. V. image reverse selector — head-down.
	Large focal spot.
	Small focal spot.

APPENDIX B

FIELD SELECTION GUIDELINE
(Courtesy of Picker International)

THREE-FIELD UNIVERSAL BUCKY

ANATOMICAL AREA	THREE-FIELD SELECTION AND RADIOGRAPHIC VIEW	REASON FOR SELECTION
	PA & AP ■■ □	Senses an area to include a portion of both lungs and mediastinum
Thorax	PA or AP ■□ □■ □ □	Senses an area of right or left lung and mediastinum
Chest for lungs and heart	*RAO or rt. □■ lateral ■	Senses superimposition of heart and lungs and portion of upper mediastinum with right side of chest nearest film plane
	†LAO or lt. ■□ lateral ■	Senses similar areas with left side of chest nearest film plane
	Collimated beam senses □□ cardiac area or lung field ■ ■■ ■	Senses fields collimated to 8 × 10 inch [18 × 24 cm] lengthwise or smaller Senses field collimated to 10 × 12 inch [24 × 30 cm] or larger for large heart
Thorax — Bony rib cage Ribs above diaphragm	See selection for lungs	To optimize radiography above and below the diagphragm, use appropriate density settings. Example — auxiliary line — use –1 density Ribs through cardiac shadow +1 density Area of diaphragm — Inspiration and expiration
Ribs below diaphragm	See selection for abdomen	
Small anatomical parts hip, shoulder girdle, sternum, knee, scapula & clavicle	All views □□ ■	Area of interest is sensed — PA obl. sternum, lat. sternum head of humerus, scapula & clavicle
	■■ ■	Survey of entire shoulder girdle 10 × 12-inch [24 × 30 cm] film size or larger

Note: Darkened block represents field selection.

*Reverse for RPO.

†Reverse for LPO.

THREE-FIELD UNIVERSAL BUCKY

ANATOMICAL AREA	THREE-FIELD SELECTION AND RADIOGRAPHIC VIEW	REASON FOR SELECTION
Renal area	AP ■■ / □	Right and left kidney and portion of vertebral column
	AP ■□ □■ / □ □	Sense area of left or right kidney
Caution: If positioned too high may sense lung area above diaph.	Obl. or collimated view ■■ / ■	Sense area of right or left kidney (Obl.) Sense any area collimated to 8″ × 10″ [18 × 24 cm] size or smaller
	Collimated view ■■ / ■	Sense large area right or left kidney
Cholecystogram (Gallbladder)	All views □□ / ■	Sense area of gallbladder 8 × 10 inch [18 × 24 cm] portal coverage or smaller. If gallbladder is very dense, use −1 density selection
	■■ / ■	Collimated to 10 × 12-inch [24 × 30 cm] field size
Abdomen	All views ■■ / ■	Survey of abdomen — soft tissue and vertebral column 10 × 12-inch to 14 × 17-inch [24 × 30 cm to 35 × 43 cm] portal size coverage
	■■ / □	Sense area of liver, spleen, kidneys and diaphragm
	■□ □■ / □ □	Sense soft tissue right or left area
	□□ / ■	Sense collimated area of abdomen 8 × 10-inch [18 × 24 cm] film size or smaller
Head — skull, sinuses facial bones	All views □□ / ■	Sense mid area of all anatomical positions for collimated views which are very dense, use −1 density selection
	All views ■□ □■ / ■ ■	Sense two (2) areas of extremely different densities for average film density. Employ collimation for 8 × 10 [18 × 24 cm] widthwise or 10 × 12-inch [24 × 30 cm] area

THREE-FIELD UNIVERSAL BUCKY

ANATOMICAL AREA	THREE-FIELD SELECTION AND RADIOGRAPHIC VIEW	REASON FOR SELECTION
GI & BE	All views ■■ ■ Caution — If centered too high, upper pickups may sense lung area just above diaphragm instead of upper abdomen (liver area)	Sense areas of barium filled GI tract, abdomen, organs and other soft-tissue structures as well as vertebral column
Trunk of body— (Vertebral Column)	All views □□ ■	Senses vertebral column area of primary interest All film sizes
	□■ ■□ ■ ■	In extreme cases of kyphosis, lordosis and scoliosis 10″ × 12″ film or larger. Selections that follow the spinal curvature may be employed
Pelvic girdle	All views ■■ ■	Survey films
	AP ■■ □	Right and left iliac area
	AP □■ ■□ □ □	Iliac area right or left
	Obl. & lat. □■ ■□ ■ ■	Right or left pelvic area Sense area of sacrum and coccyx as well as area of ilium overlap

Note: Routinely use center field pickup only when collimation is 8 × 10-inch [18 × 24 cm] size or smaller. Also, use only the center field when the selected x-ray tube angulation exceeds 20°-25°.

THREE-FIELD UNIVERSAL BUCKY

ANATOMICAL AREA	THREE-FIELD SELECTION AND RADIOGRAPHIC VIEW	REASON FOR SELECTION
Thorax (Bucky)	PA & AP ■	Senses an area to include a portion of both lungs and mediastinum
	PA or AP ■	Senses an area of right or left lung and mediastinum
Chest for lungs and heart	RPO, RAO, or Rt. Lateral ■	Senses superimposition of heart and lungs and portion of upper mediastinum with the right side of chest nearest the film plane
Small anatomical parts	LPO, LAO or Lt. Lateral ■	Senses similar areas with left side of chest nearest the film plane
hip, shoulder girdle, sternum, knee, scapula & clavicle	Collimated beam covers the cardiac area or lung field ■	Senses collimated fields
Thorax — bony rib cage Ribs above diaphragm	See selection for lungs	To optimize radiography above and below the diaphragm, use appropriate density settings. Example — auxiliary line — use –1 density Ribs through cardiac shadow +1 density Area of diaphragm — Inspiration and expiration
Ribs below diaphragm	See selection for abdomen	
	All views ■	Area of interest is sensed — PA obl. sternum, lat. sternum head of humerus, scapula, clavicle and survey of entire shoulder girdle

THREE-FIELD UNIVERSAL BUCKY

ANATOMICAL AREA	THREE-FIELD SELECTION AND RADIOGRAPHIC VIEW	REASON FOR SELECTION
Renal area	AP ■	Right and left kidney and portion of vertebral column Use −1 or −2 density selection
Caution — If positioned too high, may sense lung area above diaphragm	AP ■ Obl. or collimated view ■	Sense area of left or right kidney (area of interest centered) Sense area of right or left kidney AP or obl. Sense any area collimated. Depending upon the structure of interest (soft tissue), employ density variation
Cholecystogram (Gallbladder)	All views ■	Sense area of gallbladder 8 × 10-inch [18 × 24 cm] portal coverage or smaller. If gallbladder is very dense, use −1 density selection
Abdomen	All Views ■ ■	Survey of abdomen — Soft tissue and vertebral column Sense area of liver, spleen, kidneys and diaphragm Sense soft tissue right or left (area of interest centered)
Head — skull, sinuses facial bones	All views ■	Sense area of anatomical position for views

THREE-FIELD UNIVERSAL BUCKY

ANATOMICAL AREA	THREE-FIELD SELECTION AND RADIOGRAPHIC VIEW	REASON FOR SELECTION
GI & BE series (Overtable)	All views ■ Caution — If centered too high, pickup may sense lung area just above diaphragm instead of upper abdomen (liver area)	Sense areas of barium filled GI tract, abdomen, organs and other soft-tissue structures as well as vertebral column
Trunk of body — (vertebral column)	All views ■	Senses vertebral column area of primary interest All film sizes
Pelvic girdle	All views ■	Survey films
	AP ■ Obl. & lat. ■ also Collimated areas	Iliac area right or left (anatomical area centered) Right or left pelvic area Sense area of sacrum and coccyx as well as area of ilium (anatomical area centered)

Note: Routinely use small (■) field pickup only when collimating small areas. Also, use only the small field when performing radiography requiring x-ray tube angulation.

APPENDIX C

STUDY QUESTIONS

THE purpose of these study questions is to provide a quick and comprehensive review of the essential elements of the text. These questions will also assist you to identify areas of weaknesses, which should be reviewed in preparation for the final examination in x-ray imaging equipment.

For each of the following multiple-choice questions, circle the correct answer.

Chapter 1

1. Which of the following supplies high voltage (kV) to the x-ray tube?
   (a) the control unit.
   (b) the high tension generator.
   (c) the detector system.
   (d) the mains voltage supply.
2. The input information to the image processing system in an x-ray imaging scheme is derived from:
   (a) the control unit.
   (b) the imaging object.
   (c) the x-ray tube.
   (d) the high tension generator.
3. Which component in the imaging scheme renders the latent image visible?
   (a) the image processor.
   (b) the image detector.
   (c) the recording medium.
   (d) the x-ray tube.
4. The main source of x-rays is:
   (a) the filament.
   (b) the target.
   (c) the step-up transformer.
   (d) the rectifier.
5. The requirements for the production of x-rays include the following *except*:
   (a) the x-ray exposure timer.
   (b) a source of a electrons.
   (c) a source of high voltage.
   (d) a target for electron bombardment.

Chapter 2

6. The main purpose of the x-ray control console is to:

    (a) control the high voltage to the x-ray tube.

    (b) allow the technologist to select the appropriate mA for the examination.

    (c) allow the technologist to select other parameters influencing the production of the x-rays.

    (d) all of the above.

7. A device which converts a low voltage to a high voltage is the:

    (a) autotransformer.

    (b) step-up transformer.

    (c) line voltage compensator.

    (d) step-down transformer.

8. The purpose of a rectification circuit is to:

    (a) decrease the voltage to the x-ray tube.

    (b) increase the voltage to the x-ray tube.

    (c) control the input voltage to the autotransformer.

    (d) change alternating current to direct current.

9. The x-ray tube filament is subjected to about:

    (a) 50 volts.

    (b) 50 kilovolts.

    (c) 10 kilovolts.

    (d) 10 volts.

10. The filament current in the x-ray tube is used to:

    (a) produce x-rays.

    (b) produce electrons.

    (c) produce heat in the anode.

    (d) heat the entire x-ray tube.

11. Which is used to measure the x-ray tube current?

    (a) the x-ray exposure timer.

    (b) the voltmeters

    (c) the milliammeter.

    (d) the line voltage compensator.

12. Which of the following is *not* used to prevent electrical overloads in the x-ray machine?

    (a) fuses.

    (b) circuit breakers.

    (c) insulators.

13. Which of the following is of primary concern in protecting the operator from radiation during an examination?

    (a) collimation.

    (b) filtration.

    (c) good operational practices.

    (d) shielding the patient's gonads with lead.

Chapter 3

14. Which type of table is characteristic of the spotfilm device?
    (a) radiographic.
    (b) radiographic-fluoroscopic.
    (c) tomographic.
    (d) urological.
15. Which type of table is most likely to have a floating tabletop?
    (a) radiographic-fluoroscopic.
    (b) radiographic.
    (c) tabletop for a dedicated skull unit.
    (d) all of the above.
16. The function of the spotfilm device is to:
    (a) produce high-quality radiographs.
    (b) allow the radiologist to make instantaneous recordings of the anatomy under study.
    (c) allow the radiologist to choose films of different sizes.
    (d) allow the radiologist to palpate the patient's abdomen during an upper gastrointestinal examination.
17. The most efficient tube support system is the:
    (a) ceiling-suspended.
    (b) ceiling-floor.
    (c) floor stand.
    (d) parallelogram type.
18. The Bucky mechanism characteristic to most radiographic, radiographic-fluoroscopic and tomographic tables consists of:
    (a) a tray to hold the cassette.
    (b) a device called a grid.
    (c) an electronic circuitry to move the grid.
    (d) all of the above.

Chapter 4

19. The basis of an electronic timer is:
    (a) charging a capacitor through a variable resistor.
    (b) ionization of a volume of gas.
    (c) the use of a thyratron tube to start the x-ray exposure.
    (d) determining the capacitance of a capacitor.
20. The time taken for a capacitor to charge up to a certain critical value is proportional to the product of the resistance (R) and the capacitance (C) of a capacitor. The product RC is called the:
    (a) time constraint.
    (b) time constant.

(c) resistance curve.

(d) time control.

21. Grid-controlled switching is used for very short exposure times needed in angiography because:

(a) of the time needed for high-voltage cables to lose their charge.

(b) of hysteresis current in the high-voltage transformer.

(c) the primary contactor is limited in time to 0.002 second.

(d) all of the above.

22. Which of the following timer integrates the tube current into a capacitor?

(a) the clockwork timer.

(b) the mAs timer.

(c) the automatic timer.

(d) all of the above.

23. Which of the following techniques allow the phototimer of three-phase generators (x-ray units) to terminate the exposure more accurately?

(a) forced extinction.

(b) ionization.

(c) the minimum exposure concept.

(d) the minimum response time.

24. When using automatic timers, the primary structure of interest to be x-rayed is referred to as the:

(a) dominant.

(b) target.

(c) measuring field.

(d) detector field.

25. The minimum response time of an automatic exposure timer is the:

(a) upper time limit of the timer.

(b) back-up time.

(c) back-up mAs.

(d) lower time limit of the timer.

26. Which of the following is common to both electronic and automatic exposure timers?

(a) a capacitor.

(b) a phototube.

(c) an ionization chamber.

(d) only one measuring field.

27. In the ionization-type automatic exposure timer, the chamber is generally positioned:

(a) between the patient and x-ray tube.

(b) between the patient and the grid.

(c) between the grid and cassette.

(d) behind the cassette.

28. A spinning top test is carried out on a full-wave rectified unit operating on single-phase power. If the number of dots on the film is 10, what is the exposure time used to check the accuracy of the timer?
    (a) 1/12 second.
    (b) 1/6 second.
    (c) 12 seconds.
    (d) 6 seconds.

Chapter 5

29. The main source of x-rays in an x-ray tube is the:
    (a) copper rod.
    (b) tungsten filament.
    (c) tungsten target.
    (d) all of the above.
30. The main source of electrons in an x-ray tube is:
    (a) tungsten target.
    (b) the tungsten filament.
    (c) the vacuum.
    (d) the copper rod.
31. In the stationary anode x-ray tube, tungsten is embedded in a copper rod, the purpose of the copper is to:
    (a) conduct heat away from the filament.
    (b) conduct heat away from the tungsten target.
    (c) to make the tube heavy and stable.
    (d) to increase the quality of the x-ray beam.
32. Rotating anode x-ray tubes offer the following:
    (a) increase tube ratings.
    (b) increase in the heat-storage capacity of the tube.
    (c) permit the use of higher mA and shorter exposure times.
    (d) all of the above.
33. The force of rotation of the anode disk is brought about by:
    (a) the stator.
    (b) the rotor.
    (c) the steel ball bearings.
    (d) the speed at which the electrons strike the target.
34. A new target material is used today in rotating anode disks, in combination with other materials. A typical combination is given to be:
    (a) tungsten and lead.
    (b) rhenium and molybdenum.
    (c) 10% rhenium and 90% tungsten.
    (d) 10% tungsten and 90% rhenium.
35. Anode disks which are made of more than one material are referred to as:

(a) simple anode disks.
(b) complex anode disks.
(c) compound anode disks.
(d) conventional anode disks.

36. Other materials used in the construction of the type of disk in the question above are:
    (a) titanium.
    (b) graphite.
    (c) zirconium.
    (d) all of the above.

37. The ratings of x-ray tubes can be discussed in terms of:
    (a) fluoroscopic ratings.
    (b) radiographic ratings.
    (c) thermal ratings.
    (d) all of the above.
    (e) only a and b of the above.

38. Two factors which affect radiographic ratings are:
    (a) the nature of the anode construction and the nature of the circuit providing the voltage to the tube.
    (b) focal spot size and the length of the tube.
    (c) the amount of kVp and mA used.
    (d) focal spot size and the nature of the circuit providing the high voltage to the tube.

39. The speed of rotation of the anode disk can be increased by:
    (a) increasing the frequency of the mains supply to the stator.
    (b) decreasing the frequency of the mains supply to the induction motor.
    (c) using silver ball bearings.
    (d) increasing the acceleration of the electrons.

40. Erosion (or pitting) of an x-ray tube target results in:
    (a) unsharpness of the image.
    (b) no change in image sharpness.
    (c) reduction of the intensity of the beam towards the anode site.
    (d) a and c of the above.

41. The curve which describes the anode thermal characteristics is generally referred to as:
    (a) a thermal curve.
    (b) a cooling curve.
    (c) an anode curve.
    (d) a radiographic curve.

42. Which of the following insulates the x-ray tube?
    (a) oil.

    (b) tungsten.

    (c) the tube housing.

    (d) the lead lining of the housing.

43. The abbreviation RTM refers to:

    (a) rotating-target-material.

    (b) rhenium-tungsten-molybdenum.

    (c) rhenium-tungsten-material.

    (d) rhenium-transfer-mechanism.

44. The principle of inclining the anode face at a small angle is referred to as the:

    (a) angle of inclination effect.

    (b) Roentgen principle.

    (c) line focus principle.

    (d) the bevelled effect.

45. Heat dissipation in the x-ray tube is accomplished by:

    (a) convention.

    (b) conduction.

    (c) radiation.

    (d) all of the above.

46. Which of the following will *not* extend the life of the x-ray tube?

    (a) reduction in the filament preparation time.

    (b) use of lower tube currents when possible.

    (c) use of repeated exposures for a tomographic series.

    (d) use of high-speed anode rotation only when desired.

47. Which of the following is characteristic of the metal-ceramic x-ray tube?

    (a) the metal envelope.

    (b) ceramic insulation.

    (c) double-bearing axle and large disk.

    (d) all of the above.

48. Failure of the stator to turn the rotor will result in:

    (a) cracking of the anode disk.

    (b) a poor vacuum.

    (c) a reduction of the insulating property of the glass.

    (d) wobbling of the disk.

49. The formation of a reflecting surface on the glass envelope due to heavy exposures which may cause vaporization of the metal parts of the tube will:

    (a) reduce the cooling capability of the tube.

    (b) reduce the speed of electrons.

    (c) decrease the speed of rotation of the anode disk.

    (d) reduce the insulating properties of the glass envelope.

Chapter 6

50. Which of the following is the *main* source of scattered rays in an x-ray room?
    (a) the patient.
    (b) the cassette.
    (c) the grid.
    (d) the tabletop.

51. A decrease in the kilovoltage for a particular examination will result in:
    (a) a decrease in the production of scattered rays and an improvement in image contrast.
    (b) a decrease in image contrast.
    (c) an increase in scattered rays.
    (d) a reduced number of x-ray photons.

52. Compression as an anti-scattered technique ensures a:
    (a) decrease in the amount of scattered rays arriving at the image receptor.
    (b) more uniform exposure at the image plane.
    (c) sharper image than that obtained without compression.
    (d) all of the above.

53. Which of the following ensures that a space is left between the image receptor and the object for the purpose of eliminating scattered rays?
    (a) the compression technique.
    (b) the collimation of the primary beam.
    (c) the use of a grid.
    (d) the air gap technique.

54. Collimation of the primary beam is primarily intended for:
    (a) improved density of the image.
    (b) protection of the patient.
    (c) protection of the operator.
    (d) improved image contrast.

55. The reduction of scattered rays by restriction of the primary beam is not accomplished by:
    (a) filters.
    (b) collimators.
    (c) cones.
    (d) diaphragms.

56. Which is the most widely used anti-scatter technique?
    (a) The scattered radiation grid concept.
    (b) The air gap technique.
    (c) The collimation method.
    (d) The compression technique.

57. The main purpose of a scattered radiation grid is to:
    (a) improve contrast.
    (b) reduce the density on the film.
    (c) reduce scattered rays reaching the patient.
    (d) reduce scattered rays reaching the operator.

58. The primary purpose of a focussed grid is to:
    (a) minimize grid cutoff.
    (b) improve image contrast.
    (c) improve image sharpness.
    (d) use higher kVp values.

59. Exposure factors are usually increased when a grid is used because:
    (a) the grid is thick.
    (b) the lead strips are thick.
    (c) a significant amount of scattered rays is absorbed by the grid.
    (d) a significant fraction of the primary beam is absorbed by the grid.

60. The performance of a grid is related to the:
    (a) Bucky factor and relative patient exposure.
    (b) grid ratio and grid frequency.
    (c) contrast improvement factor.
    (d) all of the above.

61. The ability of a grid to improve contrast is specified by the:
    (a) grid ratio.
    (b) width of the grid.
    (c) grid frequency.
    (d) contrast improvement factor.

62. The idea of moving the grid during the exposure was conceived by:
    (a) Roentgen.
    (b) Bucky.
    (c) Potter.
    (d) Hollis.

63. The ability of a grid to remove scattered radiation is referred to as the:
    (a) grid efficiency or cleanup efficiency.
    (b) grid ratio.
    (c) grid cutoff.
    (d) grid radius.

64. The absorption of a fraction of the primary beam, by a grid during normal usage is called:
    (a) grid efficiency.
    (b) grid cutoff.
    (c) grid lag.
    (d) the improvement factor.

65. The grid frequency is defined as:
    (a) the number of grid strips per inch or per centimeter.
    (b) the number of grid strips plus the number of interspace strips.
    (c) 110 lines per inch.
    (d) the distance between two lead strips.
66. The selectivity of a grid is the:
    (a) ratio of the contrast with a grid to the contrast without a grid.
    (b) ratio of the transmitted scattered rays to the transmitted primary rays.
    (c) ratio of the height of a lead strip to the distance between the strips.
    (d) ratio of transmitted primary rays to the transmitted scattered rays.
67. The use of a grid is necessary when exposing a patient to higher peak kilovoltages because:
    (a) more back-scattered radiation reaches the film.
    (b) the contribution of unmodified scattering to beam attenuation becomes significant.
    (c) a greater fraction of the scattered rays reaches the film along with the primary beam.
    (d) much more of the primary radiation is scattered in bone.
68. The purpose of moving the grid is to:
    (a) get rid of grid lines.
    (b) increase the kVp.
    (c) decrease the exposure time.
    (d) absorb more scattered rays.
69. In which type of grid motion does the grid move back and forth several times during the x-ray exposure?
    (a) single stroke motion.
    (b) reciprocating.
    (c) oscillating.
70. In which type of grid motion does the grid move in a circular fashion, just as the exposure is made?
    (a) reciprocating.
    (b) single stroke.
    (c) oscillating.
71. The effect which produces the presence of pronounced grid lines, when the grid motion and x-ray pulsations are not synchronized, is referred to as:
    (a) the pulsation effect.
    (b) the stroboscopic effect.
    (c) the oscillating effect.
    (d) the stationary effect.
72. What is the effect produced on the film when the central ray is not

positioned in the center of a focussed grid?

(a) Partial grid cutoff over the entire film (hence the film lacks the correct density over its entire surface area).

(b) Only the center of the film receives the radiation and is therefore black.

(c) The two sides of the film are black.

(d) There is one dark band down the center of the grid.

73. What effect is produced on the film when a 72-inch parallel grid is used at 40-inch source-to-image receptor distance?

(a) The two sides of the film are black.

(b) A dark band is produced down the center of the film.

(c) Only the right side of the film is blackened.

(d) Only the left side of the film is blackened by the radiation.

74. What effect is produced on the film if a 40-inch focussed grid is placed on top of a 72-inch parallel grid? This combination is used at a 40-inch source-to-image receptor distance.

(a) the two sides of the film are black.

(b) a dark band is produced down the center of the film.

(c) only the right side of the film is blackened by the radation.

75. One major disadvantage that accompanies the use of grids is the increased patient dose required. Use of a moving grid instead of a stationary grid with similar physical characteristics results in approximately:

(a) 30% more radiation to the patient.

(b) 20% more radiation to the patient.

(c) 15% more radiation to the patient.

(d) 5% more radiation to the patient.

76. Which of the following factors must be remembered when selecting a grid?

(a) Patient dose increases with increasing grid ratio.

(b) High-ratio grids are usually employed for high kVp examinations.

(c) Patient dose at high kVp is less than at low kVp.

(d) All of the above.

77. The main limitation of an anti-scatter grid is that it:

(a) requires an increase in exposure factors.

(b) does not absorb all the scattered rays.

(c) requires a circuit to move the grid.

(d) does not transmit the primary beam efficiently.

Chapter 7

78. The waveforms in three-phase AC power supplies are out of phase by:

(a) 60°.

(b) 30°.

(c) 180°.

(d) 120°.

79. Solid-state rectifiers are made of semi-conducting material such as:

(a) germanium.

(b) silicon.

(c) lead telluride.

(d) all of the above.

80. Solid-state rectifiers:

(a) exhibit very low heat loss.

(b) have a longer life span than valve tubes.

(c) produce a more consistent radiographic output.

(d) all of the above.

81. In which type of rectification is the bridge or Graetz circuit used?

(a) self-rectification.

(b) half-wave rectification.

(c) full-wave rectification.

(d) all of the above.

82. Which type of generator would be best suited in terms of providing the shortest possible exposure time during automatic exposure control?

(a) constant potential generator.

(b) falling load generator.

(c) single-phase single-pulse generator.

(d) two-pulse single-phase generator.

83. Which of the following generator types exhibit minimum ripple?

(a) twelve-pulse, three-phase.

(b) six-pulse, three-phase.

(c) two-pulse, single-phase.

(d) single-pulse, single-phase.

84. Which of the following is located in the primary circuit of the auto-transformer?

(a) on-off switch on the control panel.

(b) autotransformer.

(c) expsoure switch.

(d) the kVp meter.

85. The following are located in the primary circuit of the high tension transformer except the:

(a) autotransformer.

(b) kVp selector.

(c) exposure switch.

(d) mains switch.

86. Which of the following is located in the secondary circuit of the high tension transformer?
    (a) the anode of the x-ray tube.
    (b) the exposure timer.
    (c) the exposure switch.
    (d) the kVp selector.
87. The following are located in the filament heating circuit of the x-ray tube except the:
    (a) step-down transformer.
    (b) rectifiers.
    (c) space charge compensator.
    (d) mA selector.
88. The mA meter is located in the:
    (a) primary circuit of the autotransformer.
    (b) primary circuit of the high tension transformer.
    (c) secondary circuit of the high tension transformer.
    (d) filament heating circuit of the x-ray tube.

Chapter 8

89. The simplest motion in geometric tomography is:
    (a) circular.
    (b) spiral.
    (c) hypocycloidal.
    (d) linear.
90. The most complex motion in geometric tomography is:
    (a) hypocycloidal.
    (b) circular.
    (c) linear.
    (d) elliptical.
91. The amplitude in geometric tomography is related to the:
    (a) angle of tube swing.
    (b) angle of the tomographic x-ray tube disk.
    (c) angle at which the slice is oriented to the film.
    (d) speed at which the tube travels.
92. Which of the following motion gives the most highly effective blurring?
    (a) circular.
    (b) elliptical.
    (c) hypocycloidal.
    (d) linear.
93. In geometric tomography, the fulcrum corresponds to this:
    (a) surface of the object.
    (b) layer of the anatomy under study.

    (c) thickness of the object layer.

    (d) angle of the tube swing.

94. In geometric tomography, zonography refers to:

    (a) narrow-angle tomography.

    (b) wide-angle tomography.

    (c) an angle of 30.̈

    (d) a very thin layer.

95. Zonography is primarily used for:

    (a) examination of thick layers.

    (b) examination of very thin layers.

    (c) longer tube travel.

    (d) longer exposure times.

96. The fundamental objective of multi-directional movements in geometric tomography is to:

    (a) increase the contrast resolution.

    (b) decrease exposure times.

    (c) improve the definition of structures by examining thin layers.

    (d) use higher kVp values.

97. Which of the following is used to describe a technique which can manipulate the tomographic image by electronic means?

    (a) body-section radiography.

    (b) stratigraphy.

    (c) tomography.

    (d) tomosynthesis.

98. Which of the following methods of tomosynthesis involves a recording step followed by a reconstruction step?

    (a) televised electronic tomography.

    (b) flashing tomosynthesis.

    (c) cinetomosynthesis.

    (d) tomoscopy.

99. In which of the following techniques are sixteen x-ray tubes used in conjunction with sixteen magnetic deflector coils to produce a tomographic section?

    (a) flashing tomosynthesis.

    (b) televised electronic tomography.

    (c) cinetomosynthesis.

    (d) tomoscopy.

100. In tomoscopy, the tomographic angle and the thickness of cut (layer height) are determined by the:

    (a) radius of the circle traced by the focal spots of all x-ray tubes.

    (b) image intensifier imaging ratio.

    (c) distance between the x-ray tube and the image intensifier.

    (d) all of the above.

Chapter 9

101. The following classes of mobile x-ray units exist based on the total radiographic output:
    (a) low- and medium-powered units.
    (b) low- and high-powered units.
    (c) medium- and high-powered units.
    (d) low-, medium- and high-powered units.

102. In some mobile x-ray units, the filament transformer, the high tension transformer and the x-ray tube are all encased in a special unit referred to as:
    (a) the tube head.
    (b) the collimator box.
    (c) the insulator unit.
    (d) the tube tank.

103. In a mobile capacitor discharge x-ray unit, x-rays are produced:
    (a) when the capacitor is being charged.
    (b) after the film has been properly positioned.
    (c) during the period when the capacitor is being discharged.
    (d) when the capacitor reaches a certain value.

104. Mobile x-ray units operate only through:
    (a) self-rectification.
    (b) half-wave rectification.
    (c) full-wave rectification.
    (d) all of the above.

105. The term "cordless mobile" implies that the unit:
    (a) does not have an exposure cord.
    (b) does not have high tension cables.
    (c) operates on battery power ad hence requires no power from the AC mains supply.
    (d) requires the technologist to use an electrical cord to recharge the batteries.

106. The primary purpose of a capacitor discharge mobile x-ray unit is to:
    (a) give high x-ray output on the low power mains supply.
    (b) protect the operator.
    (c) protect the patient.
    (d) offer the best possible image to the radiologist.

107. In which of the following dental units does the x-ray tube and film move around the patient?
    (a) intra-oral unit.
    (b) panoral unit.
    (c) craniostat.
    (d) conventional dental unit.

Chapter 10

108. The imaging requirements for mammography include the following except:
    (a) the use of lower kVp values in the 25 to 40 range.
    (b) the use of the x-ray tubes with molybdenum targets.
    (c) the use of high voltages (80-100 kVp) to provide the best possible image of soft tissues.
    (d) modification of the transformer circuitry to operate at low kilovoltages.

109. The geometric blurring in mammography is attributed to the following except:
    (a) size of the focal spot.
    (b) source-to-image receptor distance.
    (c) object-to-image receptor distance.
    (d) motion of the object.

110. Electrostatic imaging refers to a process whereby:
    (a) x-rays are converted into a latent charged image.
    (b) x-rays are converted to light.
    (c) charges are converted to x-rays.
    (d) light photons are converted into a charge pattern.

111. Which of the following is a gas-discharge imaging process?
    (a) conventional radiography.
    (b) xeromammography.
    (c) xeroradiography.
    (d) electron radiography.

112. Which of the following is a dry non-silver electrostatic imaging process?
    (a) conventional radiography.
    (b) electron radiography.
    (c) xeroradiography.
    (d) ionography.

113. In remote-controlled radiography and fluoroscopy, the television monitor should be positioned:
    (a) at a point along the direction in which the radiologist views the patient.
    (b) to the right of the observer.
    (c) to the left of the observer and behind the patient.
    (d) close to the ceiling.

114. The scattered radiation levels in overhead fluoroscopy is:
    (a) greater than undercouch fluoroscopy.
    (b) less than in mobile fluoroscopy.
    (c) the same as in undercouch fluoroscopy.
    (d) less than in undercouch fluoroscopy.

115. High-voltage radiography is defined as:
    (a) The use of voltages higher than 100 kVp.
    (b) the use of long source-to-image receptor distances.
    (c) the use of the air gap technique.
    (d) the use of high-ratio grids.
116. The concept of field emission radiography is based on the:
    (a) hot cathode x-ray tube.
    (b) high-speed anode rotation.
    (c) cold cathode x-ray tube.
    (d) photoemission principle.
117. In field emission radiography, electrons are emitted from the x-ray tube by:
    (a) thermionic emission.
    (b) the Compton effect.
    (c) the presence of a strong electric field at the surface of the emitter.
    (d) photoemission.
118. Photofluorography is:
    (a) a magnetic recording process.
    (b) photography of a fluorescent screen.
    (c) an intensifying mechanism.
    (d) photography of the radiographic image.
119. The purpose of a filter in radiography is to:
    (a) protect the patient.
    (b) protect the radiologist during fluoroscopy since higher kVp's are used.
    (c) protect the technologist.
    (d) produce high-contrast films.
120. The thickness of a filter increases as the:
    (a) exposure time increases.
    (b) mA increases.
    (c) kVp increases.
    (d) kVp decreases.
121. A filter is used to:
    (a) absorb preferentially low-energy waves in the primary beam.
    (b) absorb the short-wavelength x-rays.
    (c) absorb scattered rays arising from the patient.
    (d) generate "soft" x-rays.
122. The material most commonly used as a primary filter in diagnostic radiography is:
    (a) tin.
    (b) aluminum.
    (c) copper.
    (d) lead.

123. Filtration results in the following except:
    (a) beam hardening.
    (b) reduced patient dose.
    (c) improved image quality.
    (d) low energy x-rays (soft beam).
124. If a patient is to be held for an x-ray examination the most likely person to restrain him/her should be the:
    (a) technologist.
    (b) radiologist.
    (c) parents or relatives.
    (d) darkroom technologist.
125. An example of a mechanical immobilizer is the:
    (a) compression band.
    (b) balsa wood.
    (c) sponges.
    (d) masking tape.

Chapter 11

126. The phosphor used in the conventional fluoroscopic screen is:
    (a) calcium tungstate.
    (b) barium lead sulphate.
    (c) zinc cadmium sulphide.
    (d) cesium iodide.
127. The conventional fluoroscopic image is inferior to the radiographic image with respect to:
    (a) contrast.
    (b) detail.
    (c) brightness.
    (d) all of the above.
128. In conventional fluoroscopy, the radiologist is protected from radiation by:
    (a) lead glass in front of the fluoroscopic screen.
    (b) lead apron hanging from the spotfilm device.
    (c) lead apron which he wears.
    (d) all of the above.
129. In conventional fluoroscopy, which of the following is used to protect the patient?
    (a) collimation of the primary bean.
    (b) filtration added to the x-ray tube.
    (c) the use of a cumulative fluoroscopic timer.
    (d) all of the above.

Chapter 12

130. Visual acuity increases as:
    (a) light intensity decreases.
    (b) light itensity increases.
    (c) light is reflected by a mirror.
    (d) the x-ray photons increase.

131. Image intensification is:
    (a) the brightening of the radiograhic image.
    (b) an increase in the illumination at the photocathode.
    (c) increase in brightening of the fluoroscopic image.
    (d) creating an image at the output phosphor which lacks detail, contrast and brightness.

132. Brightness gain refers to:
    (a) an increase in intensity at the input phosphor.
    (b) increase in intensity at the output phosphor.
    (c) decrease in kV across the tube.
    (d) increase in electrons at the photocathode.

133. In an x-ray image intensifier tube, which is an emitter of electrons?
    (a) input phosphor.
    (b) output phosphor.
    (c) photocathode.
    (d) electron lens.

134. What is the approximate potential difference across the image intensifier tube?
    (a) 10-15 kVp.
    (b) 80-100 volts.
    (c) 25-30 kVp.
    (d) 50-60 kVp.

135. What is meant by stating that an image intensifier tube is 9 inches?
    (a) the length of the tube is 9 inches.
    (b) the diameter of the output screen is 9 inches.
    (c) the diameter of the input screen is 9 inches.
    (d) the radius of the input screen is 9 inches.

136. The term *brightness gain* has been superseded by the term:
    (a) conversion factor.
    (b) conversion coefficient.
    (c) resolution gain.
    (d) conversion process.

137. If the diameter of the output screen of an image intensifier tube is 0.5 cm, what is the radius of the input screen?
    (a) 5.0 cm.

    (b) 0.005 cm.
    (c) 25 cm.
    (d) 2.5 cm.
138. Contrast in image intensification refers to:
    (a) brightness gain.
    (b) conversion factor.
    (c) the brightness ratio of the periphery to the center of the ouptut screen.
    (d) the ratio of the brightness at the input screen to the brightness at the output screen.
139. The loss of brightness at the periphery of the image in x-ray image intensification is:
    (a) vignetting.
    (b) quantum noise.
    (c) resolution.
    (d) contrast.
140. The conversion factor of an image intensifier tube is the:
    (a) ratio of the luminance at the output screen to the exposure rate at he input screen.
    (b) ratio of the exposure rate at the input screen to the diameter of the output screen.
    (c) ratio of the flux gain to the minification gain.
    (d) ratio of the square of the diameter of the input phosphor to the square of the diameter of the output screen.

Chapter 13

141. Which of the following consists of a set of hollow glass cylinders closely packed together?
    (a) the image intensifier tube.
    (b) a microchannel plate.
    (c) a panel electron tube.
    (d) the solid-state image intensifier.
142. A television camera tube is a photoelectric tube which:
    (a) is used only in x-ray image intensification.
    (b) is capable of converting visual information to electrical information.
    (c) is capable of converting x-rays into light.
    (d) acts as an image intensifier.
143. The largest of the camera tubes for television is the:
    (a) isocon.
    (b) image orthicon.
    (c) Plumbicon.
    (d) vidicon.
144. The vidicon television camera tube works on the principle of:

(a) phosphorescence.
(b) electroconductivity.
(c) photoconductivity.
(d) thermionic emission.

145. Lead oxide is used in which of the following?
(a) the image orthicon.
(b) the vidicon.
(c) the Plumbicon.
(d) the isocon.

146. Which of the following television camera tubes is most suitable for a hip-pinning procedure?
(a) the vidicon.
(b) the image orthicon.
(c) the isocon.
(d) the Plumbicon.

147. The area scanned by the electron beam in a television camera tube is referred to as a:
(a) kinescope.
(b) scanning target.
(c) a lined area.
(d) raster.

148. The purpose of a shadow mask in a color television monitor is to:
(a) ensure that each electron beam excites its respective color dot within a dot trio.
(b) brighten the colors.
(c) improve the image contrast.
(d) ensures that each electron beam excites all three dots in the dot trio.

149. One of the functions of the cathode ray tube (TV monitor) and its associated circuitry is to:
(a) accelerate electron in an air-filled space.
(b) convert visual information into electrical information.
(c) convert x-ray photon into visible pattern.
(d) convert electrical information into visual information.

150. The range of frequencies that can be transmitted by a television system is referred to as the:
(a) bandwidth.
(b) contrast.
(c) aspect ratio.
(d) brightness.

151. In the television principle, the ratio of the width to the height of the picture frame is referred to as the:
(a) aspect ratio.

      (b) conversion factor.

      (c) contrast improvement.

      (d) resolution.

152. The proper viewing distance for television images is given to be:

      (a) six meters.

      (b) two to four times the picture height.

      (c) four to eight times the picture height.

      (d) four to eight times the picture width.

153. Improvements in the transmission properties of a high resolution x-ray television chain have been made to the:

      (a) lens, which provides better resolution and a more uniform image field.

      (b) magnetic deflection and focussing for the electron beam.

      (c) video amplifier, to facilitate a wider bandwidth.

      (d) all of the above.

154. Compared to 13 million bits of information which can be transmitted by conventional x-ray television systems, a high resolution x-ray television system can transmit up to:

      (a) four million bits of information.

      (b) two million bits of information.

      (c) four billion bits of information.

      (d) two billion bits of information.

Chapter 14

155. Which of the following is not a dynamic recording process?

      (a) spotfilm single-exposure technique.

      (b) spotfilm series exposure.

      (c) cinefluorography.

      (d) videotape recording.

156. Videotape recording of the intensified image is:

      (a) an electrostatic image recording process.

      (b) a magnetic recording process.

      (c) a photographic recording process.

      (d) an ionization process.

157. Which of the following is true for videotape storage?

      (a) tape should be stored on its edge and shielded from magnetic fields.

      (b) tape must be stored under the proper temperature and humidity conditions.

      (c) tape must be stored in an environment free of dust.

      (d) all of the above.

158. Laser videodisk recording is:

      (a) a magnetic recording process.

      (b) a photographic recording process.

    (c) non-magnetic recording process.

    (d) an ionization process.

159. The image distributor ensures that the film camera receives about:

    (a)   90$\hat{}$of the light from the image intensifier.

    (b)   10$\hat{}$of the light from the intensifier.

    (c) 100$\hat{}$of the light from the intensifier.

    (d)   70$\hat{}$of the light from the intensifier.

160. In cine fluorography, as the aperature is covered by the shutter of the camera:

    (a) the film is exposed to x-rays.

    (b) the film is held firmly by the pressure plate and does not move.

    (c) the film is pulled down by the "teeth-like" mechanism which fits into the perforations on the film.

161. In which of the following is the diameter of the fluoroscopic field larger than the width of the frame in cine fluorography?

    (a) overframing.

    (b) underframing.

    (c) exact framing.

    (d) satisfactory framing.

162. Orthochromatic cine film is sensitive to the following except:

    (a) green light.

    (b) yellow light.

    (c) blue light.

    (d) red light.

163. Pulsed cine radiography refers to:

    (a) the x-ray tube being continuously energized during filming.

    (b) the x-ray tube is only heated when the mains supply switch is activated.

    (c) filming the anatomy of interest using the patient's pulse as a reference point.

    (d) the x-ray tube is not continuously energised during cine but passes current only during periods when the camera shutter is opened.

164. Which of the following is considered the most important factor in terms of dose in cine fluorography?

    (a) synchronization.

    (b) framing frequency.

    (c) f-number.

    (d) all of the above.

165. Large-field serial radiography is achieved by:

    (a) short source-to-image receptor distances.

    (b) long source-to-image receptor distances.

    (c) moving the tabletop.

    (d) compensating filters.

Chapter 15

166. Images of objects can be represented only as:
    (a) pictures.
    (b) optical images.
    (c) mathematical functions.
    (d) all of the above.
167. Subjecting numerical representations of objects to a series of operations using the computer to produce a devised result is referred to as:
    (a) digital image processing.
    (b) pattern recognition.,
    (c) analog-to-digital conversion.
    (d) digital-to-analog conversion.
168. The logical steps in digitizing an image are:
    (a) sampling, scanning and quantization.
    (b) scanning, sampling and quantization.
    (c) scanning, quantization and sampling.
    (d) quantization, scanning, and sampling.
169. Which is a measure of the brightness level at each pixel location in digital image processing?
    (a) scanning.
    (b) quantization.
    (c) pixelization.
    (d) sampling.
170. Which of the following involves dividing up a picture into elements called pixels?
    (a) sampling.
    (b) scanning.
    (c) quantization.
    (d) pixelization.
171. Which is a measure of the brightness level at each pixel location in digital image processing?
    (a) sampling.
    (b) scanning.
    (c) brightness detection.
    (d) quantization.
172. The process of representing a brightness level measured at each pixel location by an integer is referred to as:
    (a) integration.
    (b) scanning.
    (c) sampling.
    (d) quantization.
173. In digital image processing theory, a pixel is:
    (a) a device which converts electricity into digits.

(b) a shade of gray.

(c) an integer.

(d) a picture element.

174. An analog-to-digital converter:

(a) is an output device.

(b) converts voltage into binary digits.

(c) converts binary digits into a graphic display.

(d) converts binary digits into voltage.

175. A digital-to-analog converter:

(a) is an output device.

(b) converts binary digits into voltage.

(c) converts binary digits into a "numerical picture."

(d) converts voltage into binary representation.

Chapter 16

176. The logical steps in computer processing are:

(a) programming, output and processing.

(b) input, output and processing.

(c) input, processing and output.

(d) input, programming and output.

177. In which of the following are problems solved by using arithmetic and logical operations through a set of instructions?

(a) a computer.

(b) an analog-to-digital converter.

(c) a quantizer.

(d) an algorithm.

178. The binary representation 1011 is equivalent to the decimal number:

(a) 9.

(b) 10.

(c) 11.

(d) 12.

179. The decimal number 12 is equivalent to the binary number:

(a) 0101.

(b) 1100.

(c) 1110.

(d) 1111.

180. Computer hardware refers to:

(a) a program.

(b) an algorithm

(c) a flowchart.

(d) a central processing unit.

181. Computer software refers to:

(a) the arithmetic/logic unit.

   (b) the line printer.
   (c) the computer program.
   (d) the cathode ray tube.
182. The central processing unit constitutes the following except the:
   (a) arithmetic/logic unit.
   (b) memory unit.
   (c) control unit.
   (d) cathode ray tube.
183. All activities of the computer are coordinated by the:
   (a) control unit.
   (b) memory.
   (c) input device.
   (d) output device.
184. The component of primary storage is:
   (a) magnetic disks.
   (b) magnetic drums.
   (c) magnetic cores.
   (d) magnetic tapes.
185. The storage capacity of a computer is expressed as:
   (a) a group of binary digits.
   (b) the number of addressable locations.
   (c) the number of input/output devices.
   (d) the number of secondary-storage devices in a computer system.

Chapter 17

186. Which of the following reflects the limitations of geometric tomography?
   (a) poor contrast resolution.
   (b) persistence of image blur.
   (c) phantom images.
   (d) all of the above.
187. A voxel is:
   (a) the attenuation coefficient in tissue.
   (b) a matrix.
   (c) a picture element.
   (d) a volume of tissue in the patient.
188. The number of pixels in a 160 × 160 matrix is:
   (a)   320.
   (b)   160.
   (c) 16,000.
   (d) 25,600.
189. The decrease in scan time in CT is:
   (a) inversely proportional to the number of x-ray beams.

(b) inversely proportional to the number of detectors.

(c) directly proportional to the number of detectors.

(d) not related to the detectors.

190. The linear attenuation coefficients for bone and water are 0.380 and 0.190, respectively, and the scaling factor of the scanner is 1000. The CT number for air is:

(a) +1000.

(b) –1000.

(c) +380.

(d) +190.

191. Which of the following scanner is based on the translate/rotate principle using one or two x-ray beams?

(a) first generation.

(b) second generation.

(c) third generation.

(d) fourth generation.

192. Fourth-generation scanners are based on:

(a) five minutes to complete one scan.

(b) fan radiation beam coupled to an array of detectors which rotate synchronously.

(c) stationary circular detector array with a rotating fan beam of x-rays.

(d) multiple x-ray sources.

193. Which of the following determines the thickness of the section in CT?

(a) the collimation of the x-ray beam.

(b) the computer program.

(c) the speed of rotation of the x-ray tube.

(d) the technologist.

194. The problem of afterglow is characteristic of:

(a) sodium iodide detectors.

(b) bismuth germanate detectors.

(c) xenon detectors.

(d) calcium fluoride detectors.

195. Which of the following describes a set of rules for solving a problem using a specified number of steps?

(a) algorithm.

(b) logarithm.

(c) fourier transform.

(d) back projection.

196. The window width and window level settings on a scanner are 200 and 0, respectively. This means that:

(a) all CT numbers between +100 and –100 will spread through the gray scale.

(b) all CT numbers between ⅔ 200 and ffl200 will appear white.

(c) only those structures above 200 will appear white.

(d) all structures between 0 and ⅔ 200 will appear black.

197. The floppy disk in CT is:

(a) an example of a secondary-storage device.

(b) an example of primary storage.

(c) an example of an output device.

(d) designed to record images off the multiformat camera.

198. Image quality in CT is influenced by:

(a) the slice thickness.

(b) detector noise

(c) motion of the patient.

(d) all of the above.

199. Which is an example of a high-speed CT scanner?

(a) first-generation EMI machines.

(b) second-generation GE machines.

(c) fourth-generation CT scanners.

(d) the cine CT machine developed by Imatron Inc.

Chapter 18

200. Digital radiography involves:

(a) conversion of x-ray data collected from the patient to digital form
for processing by a computer.

(b) manipulation of x-ray images collected from an image intensifier
by an analog-to-digital converter.

(c) dividing the x-ray image into small regions called pixels.

(d) storage of all analog images in digital form.

201. Radiography and fluoroscopy are limited in the following ways.

(a) superimposition of structures.

(b) poor demonstration of low-contrast structures.

(c) inflexible display of images.

(d) all of the above.

202. The *main advantage* of digital radiography is:

(a) the improved detectability of low-contrast structures compared to
conventional radiography and fluoroscopy.

(b) the ability to perform quantitative analysis.

(c) the ability to transfer images via the telephone or by microwaves.

(d) the ability to store images on magnetic tapes and disks.

203. In digital radiography the problem of superimposition of structures is
eliminated through the use of:

(a) temporal-subtraction techniques.

(b) energy-subtraction techniques.

(c) hybrid-subtraction techniques.

(d) all of the above.

204. Temporal-subtraction digital radiography is a process which is based on:
    (a) subtraction of images which are separated only in time.
    (b) subtraction of images based on two different kilovoltages.
    (c) subtraction of images in both time and energy.
    (d) all of the above.

205. In which of the following subtraction techniques is a mask first obtained, then a difference or subtracted image is created from two images recorded while contrast is distributed in the vessels?
    (a) serial mask mode.
    (b) continuous mode.
    (c) time interval difference.
    (d) post processing.

206. A technique which is used to reduce motion artifacts in digital fluoroscopy, by recording another mask image just before the contrast arrives at the vessels of interest, is:
    (a) remasking.
    (b) windowing.
    (c) quantitative analysis.
    (d) energy subtraction.

207. Which of the following serves as the image detector in digital fluoroscopy?
    (a) The image intensifier tube.
    (b) The television camera tube.
    (c) The magnetic disk.
    (d) The television monitor.

208. The light output from the image intensifier tube is controlled by the:
    (a) lens in front of the television camera tube.
    (b) video aperture.
    (c) phosphor characteristics of the image intensifier tube.
    (d) kVp technique used.

209. In digital fluoroscopy, accuracy refers to:
    (a) the type of television scanning.
    (b) the number of scan lines which make up the picture.
    (c) how close the digital data represents the analog data collected from the patient.
    (d) the time required to digitize the input analog data.

210. A 6-bit analog-to-digital converter will divide a signal into the following equal parts:
    (a) 64.
    (b) 6.
    (c) 12.
    (d) 36.

211. Which of the following determines how many shades of gray are represented in an image?
    (a) the video aperture.
    (b) the type of television camera tube.
    (c) the analog-to-digital converter.
    (d) the logarithmic processor.
212. How many shades of gray are generated by a 6-bit analog-to-digital converter?
    (a) 64.
    (b) 256.
    (c) 12.
    (d)   6.
213. Digital scanned projection radiography is:
    (a) a non-tomographic digital radiographic imaging process.
    (b) a tomographic method of digital imaging.
    (c) not used in computed tomography.
    (d) not useful in evaluating chest problems.
214. The contrast resolution in digital fluoroscopy depends on:
    (a) the field size.
    (b) the number of television scan lines.
    (c) the matrix size.
    (d) the analog-to-digital converter.
215. Which of the following influences spatial resolution in computed radiography?
    (a) the width of the x-ray beam.
    (b) the focal spot size.
    (c) the scan speed.
    (d) all of the above.
216. Which of the following is related to the limitations of digital imaging systems?
    (a) noise.
    (b) patient motion.
    (c) the amount of contrast used.
    (d) all of the above.

Chapter 19

217. Quality control technique are concerned directly with:
    (a) equipment testing and maintenance.
    (b) mangement concepts.
    (c) film quality.
    (d) organizational features of a department.
218. According to the FDA, the BRH and the JCAH, the primary responsibility of a quality-assurance program rests upon the:

(a) radiologist in charge of the department.

(b) chief technologist.

(c) hospital administrator.

(d) quality control technologist.

219. In general, the responsibility of quality control rests upon:

(a) all x-ray technologists in the imaging department.

(b) the medical physicist.

(c) the biomedical engineering technologist.

(d) all of the above.

220. Components of an x-ray imaging scheme which require monitoring are:

(a) cassettes and grids.

(b) processing components and viewboxes.

(c) the x-ray unit.

(d) all of the above.

221. The benefits of a quality-assurance program include:

(a) cost control to patient and hospital.

(b) radiation protection to both patient and personnel.

(c) maintainance and improvement of image quality standards.

(d) all of the above.

222. The acceptance criteria in a quality-assurance program are based on:

(a) objective data.

(b) subjective data.

(c) the results of research studies.

(d) all of the above.

ANSWERS TO STUDY QUESTIONS

1. b	42. a	83. a	124. c
2. b	43. b	84. a	125. a
3. a	44. c	85. d	126. c
4. b	45. d	86. a	127. d
5. a	46. c	87. b	128. d
6. d	47. d	88. c	129. d
7. b	48. a	89. d	130. b
8. d	49. d	90. a	131. c
9. d	50. a	91. a	132. b
10. b	51. a	92. c	133. c
11. c	52. d	93. b	134. c
12. c	53. d	94. a	135. c
13. c	54. b	95. a	136. a
14. b	55. a	96. c	137. d
15. a	56. a	97. d	138. c
16. b	57. a	98. b	139. a
17. a	58. a	99. d	140. a
18. d	59. d	100. d	141. b
19. a	60. d	101. d	142. b
20. b	61. d	102. a	143. a
21. d	62. c	103. c	144. c
22. b	63. a	104. d	145. c
23. a	64. b	105. c	146. a
24. a	65. a	106. a	147. d
25. d	66. d	107. b	148. a
26. a	67. c	108. c	149. d
27. c	68. a	109. d	150. a
28. a	69. b	110. a	151. a
29. c	70. c	111. d	152. c
30. b	71. b	112. c	153. d
31. b	72. a	113. a	154. a
32. d	73. b	114. a	155. a
33. a	74. b	115. a	156. b
34. c	75. c	116. c	157. d
35. c	76. d	117. c	158. c
36. d	77. d	118. b	159. a
37. d	78. d	119. a	160. c
38. d	79. d	120. c	161. a
39. a	80. d	121. a	162. d
40. d	81. c	122. b	163. d
41. b	82. b	123. d	164. d

165. b	180. d	195. a	210. a
166. d	181. c	196. a	211. c
167. a	182. d	197. a	212. a
168. b	183. a	198. d	213. a
169. d	184. c	199. d	214. d
170. b	185. b	200. a	215. d
171. a	186. d	201. d	216. d
172. d	187. d	202. a	217. a
173. d	188. d	203. d	218. a
174. b	189. b	204. a	219. d
175. b	190. a	205. b	220. d
176. c	191. a	206. a	221. d
177. a	192. c	207. a	222. d
178. c	193. a	208. b	
179. b	194. a	209. c	

BIBLIOGRAPHY

THE references included in this section include those works which have been cited in the text, together with several others which have not been cited.

The student is encouraged to refer to these original works, particularly when a further insight into a specific topic is required.

1. Accreditation Manual for Hospitals. Chicago, Joint Commission for Accreditation of hospitals, 155, 1976.
2. Alvarez, R.E., Lehmann, L.A., Macovski, A., and Brody, W.R.: Limitations of accuracy in dual-energy digital fluoroscopy. Proceedings of the Society of Photo-Optical Instrumentation Engineers 314: 1196, 1981.
3. Amisano, P.: La stratigrafia toracicia a strato a strato trasverso. Radiol. Med. (Torino), 32: 418, 1946.
4. Andrews, J.R.: Planigraphy. American Journal of Roentgenology, 36: 575, 1936.
5. Andrews, J.R., and Stava, R.J.: Planigraphy. American Journal of Roentgenology, 38: 145, 1937.
6. Arnold, B.A., Eisenberg, H., Borger, D., and Metherel, A.: Digital Radiography — an overview. Proceedings of the Society of Photo-Optical Instrumentation Engineers, 273: 215, 1981.
7. Atkins, H.A., Fairchild, R.G., Robertson, J.S. et al.: Effect of absorption edge filters in diagnostic x-ray spectra. Radiology, 115: 431, 1975.
8. Ardran, G.M., and Crooks, H.E.: Field emission 350 kVp chest x-ray system. Radiography, 40: 227, 1974.
9. Baert, A.L., Marchal, G., Wilms, G., Haendle, J., Maass, W., and Wolf, H.D.: Computer angiography — intravenous arteriography. Electromedica, 2: 122, 1981.
10. Bailar, J.C., III: Mammography: A contrary view. Am. Intern. Med., 84: 77, 1976.
11. Bailar, J.C.: Screening for early breast cancer: Pros and cons. Cancer, 39: 2783, 1977.
12. Balter, S., Laughlin, J.S., Rothenberg R.L., Thomas, N.C., and Zandmanis, J.: A microchannel plate x-ray converter and intensifier tube. Radiology, 110: 673, 1974.
13. Banks, G.B.: Television pick-up tubes for x-ray screen intensification. British Journal of Radiology, 3: 319, 1958.
14. Barella, J.M., and Genefas, J.A.E.: A new video recorder for use in radiodiagnostics. Medicamundi, 14(2): 103, 1969.
15. Barnes, G.T., and Brezovich, I.A.: The design and performance of a scanning multiple slit assembly. Medical Physics, 6: 197, 1979.
16. Barnes, G.T.: Characteristics of scatter. In Logan, W.W. and Muntz, E.P. (Eds.): Reduced Dose Mammography. New York, Mason Publishing U.S.A. Inc., 1979.
17. Barnes, G.T., and Brezovich, I.A.: The intensity of scattered radiation in mammography. Radiology, 126: 243, 1978.
18. Barnes, G.T., Brezovich, I.A., and Witten, D.M.: Scanning multiple slit assembly: A

547

practical and efficient device to reduce scatter. American Journal of Roentgenology, 129: 497, 1977.

19. Barnhard, H.J., and Lane, G.B.: The computerized diagnostic radiology department: Update 1982. Radiology, 145: 551, 1982.

20. Barnhard, H.J.: The bedside examination: A time for analysis and appropriate action. Radiology, 129: 539, 1978.

21. Bartolotta, A., Calenda, E., Calicchia, A., and Indovina, P.: Dental orthopantomography: Survey of patient dose. Radiology, 146: 821, 1983.

22. Bednarek, D.R., Rudin, S., and Wong, R.: Artifacts produced by moving grids. Radiology, 147: 255, 1983.

23. Beekmans, A.A.G.: Image quality aspects of x-ray image intensifiers. Medicamundi, 27: 25, 1982.

24. Berci, G., and Seyler, A.J.: An x-ray television image storage apparatus. American Journal of Roentgenology, 90: 1290, 1963.

25. Birken, H., and Franken, A.A.J.: Use of the single-image store in general and preoperative x-ray diagnostics. Medicamundi, 20: 108, 1975.

26. Birken, H., and Heise, T.: An x-ray television chain with integrated exposure rate control. Medicamundi, 14: 107, 1969.

27. Birken, H., and Bejczy, C.I.: A new generation of x-ray image intensifiers — characteristics and results. Medicamundi, 18: 120, 1973.

28. Birken, H. and Heise, I.: An x-ray TV-chain with integrated exposure rate control. Medicamundi, 14(2): 97, 1969.

29. Bjorkholm, P.J., Annis, M., Frederick, E.E.: *Digital Radiography*. American Science and Engineering, Inc., Massachusetts, 1982.

30. Bloom, W.L.: *Image Intensification and Recording Principles*. Milwaukee, General Electric Company, 1962.

31. Bloom, W., Hollenbach, J., and Morgan, J.: *Medical Radiographic Technic*. Springfield, Thomas, 1965.

32. Bocage, A.E.M.: Method of, and apparatus for, radiography on a moving plate. French Patent No. 536464, 1922.

33. Botden, P.J.M., Feddema, J., Vijverberg, G.P.M.: First results with an experimental integrated image intensifier television system. Medicamundi, 14: 155, 1969.

34. Breed, T.: An x-ray system for paediatric examinations. Medicamundi, 18: No. 3, 128, 1973.

35. Brezovich, I.A., and Barnes, G.T.: A new type of grid. Medical Physics, 4(5):451, 1977.

36. Brody, W.R., and Macovski, A.: Dual-energy digital radiography. Diagnostic Imaging, 3: 18, 1981.

37. Brody W.R.: Scanned projection radiography (computed radiography): In Newton, T.H., and Potts, D.G.: *Modern Neuroradiology, Vol. 2: Advanced Imaging Techniques*. San Francisco, Clava Press, 1982.

38. Brooks, R.A. and Dichiro, G.: Principles of computer assisted tomography (CAT) in radiographic and radioisotopic imaging. Physics in Medicine and Biology, 21: 689, 1976.

39. Brody, W.R., Macovski, A., Lehmann, L.: Intravenous arteriography using scanned protection radiography — preliminary investigation of a new method. Investigative Radiology, 15: 220, 1980.

40. Brody, W.R.: Digital radiography. In Moss, A., Goldberg, H., and Norman, D. (Eds): *Interventional Radiologic Techniques: Computed Tomography and Ultrasonography*. New York, Academic Press, Inc., 1979.

41. Buchignani, J.S., Wagner, W.W., and Howley, J.R.: Radiation dosimetry in full chest tomography. Radiology, 99: 175, 1971.

42. Buchmann, F.: The principles of the dental tomography. Medicamundi, 20(1): 43, 1975.

43. Bull, K.W., Curry III, T.S., Dowdey, J.E., and Christensen, E.E.: The cut-off characteristics of rotating girds. Radiology, 114: 453, 1975.

44. Burnett, B.M., Massaferro, R.J., and Church, W.W.: A study of retakes in radiology departments of two large hospitals. New publication (FDA) 76-8016. Washington, D.C., 1975.

45. Bureau of Radiological Health: Regulations for the administration and enforcement of the radiation control for health and safety act of 1968. H.H.S. Publication No. (FDA) 80-8035. Bureau of Radiological Health, U.S. Department of Health and Human Services, Washington, D.C., 1980.

46. Burgess, A.E.: Contrast effects of a gadolinium filter. Medical Physics, 8(2): 203, 1981.

47. Burgess, A.E., and Pate, G.: Voltage energy and material dependence of secondary radiation. Medical Physics, 8(1): 33, 1981.

48. Bushong, S.C.: *Radiological Science for Technologists.* Missouri, The C.V. Mosby Company, 1980.

49. Cabansag, E.M.: Immobilization in pediatric and radiography. Radiologic Technology, 48(3): 269, 1976.

50. Cannon, T.M., and Hunt, B.R.: Image processing by computer. Scientific American, 1981.

51. Capp, M.P.: Radiological imaging — 2000 A.D. Radiology, 138: 541, 1981.

52. Chaney, E.L., Hendee, W.R., and Hare, D.L.: Performance evaluation of phototimers. Radiology, 118: 715, 1976.

53. Chamberlain, W.E.: Fluoroscopes and fluoroscopy. Radiology, 28: 383, 1942.

54. Chan, H.P., and Doi, K.: Physical characteristics of scattered radiation and performance of antiscatter grids in diagnostic radiology. Radiographics, 2: 378, 1982.

55. Chaney, E.L., Hendee, W.R., and Hare, D.L.: Performance evaluation of phototimers. Radiology, 118: 715, 1976.

56. Chang, C.H.: Specific value of computed tomographic breast scanner (CT/M) in diagnosis of breast diseases. Radiology, 132: 647, 1979.

57. Chesneys, D.N., and Chesneys, M.O.: *X-ray Equipment for Student Radiographers.* Oxford, Blackwell Scientific. 1971.

58. Chin, F.K., Anderson, W.B., and Gilbertson, J.D.: Radiation dose to critical organs during petrous tomography. Radiology, 94: 624, 1970.

59. Christensen, E.E., Curry, T.S. and Dowdey, J.E.: *An Introduction to the Physics of Diagnostic Radiology,* 2nd Edition. Philadelphia, Lea and Febiger, 1978.

60. De Marre, D.A., Kantrowitz, P., Zucker, L., and Simmons, D.: *Applied Biomedical Electronics for Technicians.* New York, Marcel Dekker, Inc., 1979.

61. Dennison, E.W.: Memory systems for signal generating photoelectric image detectors. NASA — C.R. — 140669 N75 — 10408 Hale Observatories, Pasadena, California, U.S.A., Nov. 14, 1974.

62. *Digital Radiography: An Assessment of its Potential Impact on Radiological Practice.* General Electric. 1980.

63. Doi, K., Frank, P.H., Chan, H.P., Vyborny, C.J., Makino, S., Iida, N., and Carlin, M.: Physical and clinical evaluaiton of new high-strip-density radiographic grids. Radiology, 147: 575, 1983.

64. Dome, R.B.: *Television Principles.* New York, McGraw-Hill, Inc., 1951.

65. Droege, R.T.: A quality assurance protocol for CT scanners. Radiology, 146: 244, 1983.

66. Dümmling, E.: Ein neues Verfahren zum Mehrfachschichten mit Hilfe von Fernschbildspeichern. Radiologie, 9(2): 37, 1968.

67. Dyke, W.P.: Advances in field emission. Scientific American, Jan. 1964.

68. Dyke, W.P., and Dolan, W.W.: Field emission. In Marton, L. (Ed.): *Advances in Electronics and Electron Physics.* New York, Adademic Press, 1956.

69. Dyke, W.P., Barbour, J.P., and Charbonnier, F.M.: Physical basis for 350 kV chest radiography. Oregon, Hewlett-Packard, 1975.

70. Editorial: New industrial contributions to medical instrumentation. Medicamundi, 22(2): 1, 1977.

71. Edholm, P.: The tomogram: Its formation and content. Acta Radiologica, 193: 1, 1960.

72. Edholm, P.R., and Jacobson, B.: Primary x-ray dodging. Dodger T Brochure. Sweden, Saab-Scania, 1972.

73. Euler, F.J.: Synchronization in cinefluorography. In Ramsey G.H., Watson, J.S., Tristan, T.A., Weinberg, S., and Cornwell, W.S.: (Ed.): *Cinefluorography.* Springfield, Thomas, 1960.

74. Feddema, J.: Considerations on x-ray examinations carried out by remote control. Medicamundi, 14: 74, 1969.

75. Feddema-Gorissen, A. and Staring, A.: Practical experiences with a new mobile condenser discharge unit. Medicamundi, 18(1): 44, 1973.

76. Felson, B. Morgan, W.K.C., Bristol, L.J., Pendergrass, E.P., Dessen, E.L., Linton, O.W., and Reger, R.B.: Observations on the results of multiple readings of chest films in coal miners pneumoconiosis. Radiology, 109: 19, 1973.

77. Field Emission Corporation: 300 kV x-rays. Technical Bulletin, 26: 1, 1972.

78. Field Emission Corporation: Field emission medical radiography. Oregon, 1973.

79. Fink, D.G., and Lutyens, D.M.: *The Physics of Television.* New York, Anchor Books, 1960.

80. Friedel, R., and Haberrecker, K.: Increased output of rotating-anode x-ray tubes. Electromedica, 4-5: 198, 1973.

81. Frost, M.M., Fisher, H.D., Nudelman, S. and Rolhrig, H.: A digital video acquisition system for extraction of subvisual information in diagnostic medical imaging. SPIE. Vol. 127. Optical Instrumentation in Medicine VI, 1977.

82. Gebauer, A., Lissner, J., and Schott, O.: *Roentgen Television.* New York, Grune and Stratton, 1967.

83. Geldner, E.: Electrical, thermal and load characteristics of rotating-anode x-ray tubes. Electromedica, 1: 14, 1981.

84. Gershon-Cohen, J., Hermel, M.B., and Birsner, J.W.: Advances in mammograhic technique. American Journal of Roentgenology, 108: 424, 1970.

85. Gilbert, M.A., and Cartlton, W.H.: Performance evaluations for diagnostic x-ray equipment. Radiologic Technology, 50(3): 243, 1978.

86. Gisvold, J.J., Karsell, P.R., and Reese, D.F.: Computerized tomographic mammography. In Logan, W.W. (Ed): *Breast Carcinoma.* New York, John Wiley, Inc., 1977.

87. Goldman, L, Vucich, J.J., Beech, S., and Murphy, W.L.: Automatic processing quality assurance program: Impact on a radiology department. Radiology, 125: 591, 1977.

88. Goodenough, D.J., Weaver, K.E., and Davis, D.O.: Comparative image aspects of radiography and computed tomography. Investigative Radiology, 17: 510, 1982.

89. Gordon, R., Herman, G.T., and Johnson, S.A.: Image reconstruction from projections. Scientific American, 233: 56, 1975.

90. Gould, R.G., Judy, P.F., and Bjarngard, B.E.: Image resolution of a microchannel plate x-ray image intensifier. Medical Physics, 5(1): 27, 1978.

91. Gray, Joel E., Winkler, Norlin T., Stears, John and Frank, Eugene: *Quality Control in Diagnostic Imaging.* Baltimore, University Park Press, 1983.

92. Grob, B.: *Basic Television.* New York, McGraw-Hill, 1964.

93. Gudden, F.: Imaging systems today and tomorrow. Electromedica, 2: 64, 1981.

94. Guthaner, D.F., Brody, W.R., Lewis, B.D. Keyes, G.S., Belanger, B.F.: Clinical application of hybrid subtraction digital angiography: Preliminary results. Cardiovascular and Interventional Radiology, 6: 290, 1983.

95. Haendle, J., Wenz, W., Sklebitz, H., Dietz, K., and Meinel, F.: A new electronic tomographic system. Electromedica, 2: 106, 1981.

96. Haendle, J., Horbaschek, H., and Alexandrescu, M.: High-resolution x-ray television and the high-resolution video recorder. Electromedica, 3-4: 83, 1977.

97. Hammerstein, G.R., Miller, D.W., White, D.R., Masterson, M.E., Woodward, H.Q., and Laughlin, J.S.: Absorbed radiation dose in mammography. Radiology, 130: 485, 1979.

98. Hancken, G., Dietrich, L.P., and Birken, H.: First clinical experience with a 14 in. image intensifier. Medicamundi, 22: 11, 1977.

99. Hartl, W.: A new type of x-ray tube: the suger rotalix ceramic. Medicamundi, 25: 17, 1980.

100. Haus, A.G.: Choice of image recording system in mammography, tomography, cerebral angiography in terms of system speed, resolution and noise. Journal of Applied Photographic Engineering, 4(2): 35, 1978.

101. Haus, A.G., Paulus, D.D., Dodd, G.D., Cowart, R.W., and Bencomo, J.: Magnification mammography: Evaluation of screen-film and xeroradiographic techniques. Radiology, 133: 223, 1979.

102. Haus, A.G.: Physical principles and radiation dose in mammography. Medical Radiography and Photography, W.58: No. 3, 70, 1982.

103. Hay, G., and Huges, D.: *First-Year Physics for Radiographers.* London, Bailliére Tindall, 1978.

104. Heintzen, Ph. Malerczyk, V., Pilarczy, J.O.: On-line processing of video image for left ventricular volume determination. Comp. Biomed. Res., 474, 1971.

105. Hellekamp, J.C., and Recourt, A.: A short history of tomography. Medicamundi, 16(1): 45, 1971.

106. Hendee, W.R.: *Medical Radiation Physics.* Chicago, Year Book Medical Publishers, 1970.

107. Hendee, W.R., Chaney, E.C., and Rossi, R.P.: *Radiologic Physics Equipment and Quality Control.* Chicago, Year Book Medical Publishers, Inc., 1977.

108. Henny, G.C., and Chamberlain, W.E.: Roentgenography: Fluoroscopy. In Glasser, O. (Ed.): *Medical Physics.* Chicago, Year Book, 1944.

109. Henny, G.: Dose aspects of cinefluorography. In Janower, M. (Ed): *Technical Needs for Reduction of Patient Dosage in Diagnostic Radiology.* Springfield, Thomas, 1963.

110. Hewlett-Packard. 350 kV chest x-ray technique. Technical Bullentin B-27. Oregon. 1974.

111. Hill, D.R.: *Principles of Diagnostic X-ray Apparatus.* London, MacMillan Press, 1977.

112. Hofmann, F.W: Image transfer from the x-ray image intensifier to subsequent systems. Electromedica, 4: 131, 1972.

113. Hohne, K.H., Nicolae, G.C., Pfeiffer, G., Bohm, M., Erbe, W., and Sonne, B.: Functional imaging — A new tool for x-ray functional diagnostics. Desy DV 78/01, 1978.

114. Holm, T., and Moseley, R.: The conversion factor for image intensification. Radiology, 82: 898, 1964.

115. Holmes, R.B., and Wright, D.J.: Image orthicon fluoroscopy of a 12-inch field and direct recording of the monitor image. Radiology, 79: 740, 1962.

116. Hollingdale, S.H., and Tootill, G.C.: *Electronic Computers.* New York, Penguin, 1971.

117. I.C.R.P. Report 15. *Protection Against Radiation from External Sources.* New York, Pergamon Press, 1969.

118. I.C.R.P. Report 3. *Protection Against X-ray up to Energies of 3MeV and Beta and Gamma Rays from Sealed Sources.* Nw York, Pergamon Press, 1960.

119. Jaffe, C., and Webster, E.W.: Radiographic contrast improvement by means of slit radiography. Radiology, 116: 631, 1975.

120. Jaundrell-Thompson, F., and Ashworth, W.J.: *X-ray Physics and Equipment.* Oxford,

Blackwell Scientific, 1965.

121. Jelaso, D.V., Southworth, G., and Purcell, L.H.: Telephone transmission of radiographic images. Radiology, 127: 147, 1978.

122. Johns, H.E., and Cunningham, J.R.: *The Physics of Radiology.* Springfield, Thomas, 1969.

123. Kazan, B.: A solid-state amplifying fluoroscopic screen. American Journal of Roentgenology, 79: 709, 1958.

124. Kieffer, J.: Analysis of laminographic motions and their values. Radiology, 33: 560, 1939.

125. King, M.A., Barnes, G.T., and Yester, M.V.: A mammographic scanning multiple slit assembly. Design considerations and preliminary results. Preceedings of the Conference on Reduced Dose Mammography. Buffalo, N.Y., October, 1978.

126. Kiver, M.S.: *Color Television Fundamentals.* New York, McGraw-Hill, 1959.

127. Kollath., Birken, H., and Jotten, G.: Image quality in image intensifier fluorography in relation to patient dose and exposure at the image device. Medicamundi, 23:   ,   .

128. Krohmer, J.S.: Patient dose distributions during hypocycloidal tomography. Radiology, 103: 447, 1972.

129. Kruger, R.A., Mistretta, C.A., Lancaster, J. et al.: A digital video image processor for real-time x-ray subtraction imaging. Optical Engineering, 17: 652, 1978.

130. Kruger, R.A., Mistretta, C.A., Houk, T.L. et al.: Computerized fluoroscopy in real time for noninvasive visualization of the cardiovascular system. Preliminary studies. Radiology 130: 49, 1979.

131. Kruger, R.A.: A method for time domain filtering using computerized flurorscopy. Medical Physics, 8: 466, 1981.

132. Kruger, R.A.: Basic physics of computerized fluoroscopy difference imaging. In Mistretta, C.A., Crummy, A.B., Strother, C.M. and Sackett, J.F. (Eds): *Digital Subtraction Arteriography: An Application of Computerized Fluoroscopy.* Chicago, Year Book Medical, 1982.

133. Kruger, R.A., Sorenson, J.A., and Niklason, L.T.: Effectiveness of antiscatter grids in digital subtraction angiography. Investigative Radiology, 18: 293, 1983.

134. Kuhn, H.: Optimization of the radiographic conditions in mammography. Electromedica, 2: 32, 1977.

135. Kuhn, H.: Reducing the patient dose by prefiltration. Electromedica, 2: 41, 1982.

136. Kyser, K., Mohr, H., and Reiber, K.: Improvements in radiographic imaging obtained with the Super Rotalix Ceramic x-ray tube. Medicamundi, 25(3): 118, 1980.

137. Lawrence, D.J.: A simple method of processor control. Medical Radiography and Photography, 49(1): 2, 1973.

138. Leeming, B.W.A., Hames, O.S., Gould, R.G., and Locke, E.: A comparison of fluoroscopically controlled patient positioning and conventional positioning, including comparative dosimetry. Radiology, 124: 231, 1977.

139. Lenk, J.D.: *Manual For Integrated Circuit Users.* Reston, Virginia, Reston, 1973.

140. Liebel-Flarsheim Company: Characteistics and application of x-ray grids. Ohio, Liebel-Flarsheim Co., 1968.

141. Lindblom, K.: Rotation tomography at small angles. Acta Radiologica, 43: 30, 1955.

142. Machlett Laboratories, Inc.: "Trade-Offs." A guide to the selection of diagnostic x-ray tubes. Connecticut, Raytheon Company, 1977.

143. Machlett Laboratories, Inc.: Guidelines for the proper use of rotating-anode tubes. Connecticut, Raytheon Company, 1982.

144. Maravilla, K.R., and Pastel, M.S.: Technical aspects of CT scanning Computerized Tomography, 2: 137, 1978.

145. McClenahan, J.: The uses of fluoroscopy. Radiology, 75: 64, 1960.

146. McCullough, E.C., and Coulam, C.M.: Physical and dosimetric aspects of diagnostic

geometrical and computer assisted tomographic procedures. Radiologic Clinics of North America, XIV(1):   Philadelphia, Saunders Co., 1976.

147. Mistretta, C.A., Crummy, A.B., and Strother, C.M.: Digital angiography: A perspective. Radiology, 139: 273, 1981.

148. Moore, R., Korbuly, D., and Kurt, A.: Removal of scattered radiation by moving-slot radiography. Applied Radiology, Nov. - Dec., 10: 85, 1981.

149. Moore, R., and Amplatz, K.: Rotational scanography. Electromedica, 1: 34, 1981.

150. Muntz, E.P. Meyers, H., Wilkinson, E., and Jacobson, G.: Preliminary studies using electron radiography for mammography. Radiology, 125: 517, 1977.

151. Nadjmi, M., Weiss, H., Klotz, E., and Linde, R.: Flashing tomogsynthesis — a new tomographic method. Neuroradiology, 19: 113, 1980.

152. N.C.R.P. Report 66: Mammography. Washington. National Council on Radiation Protection and Measurements. 1980.

153. N.C.R.P. Report 35: Dental X-ray Protection. Washington. National Council on Radiation Protection and Measurements. 1972.

154. N.C.R.P. R. Report 33: Medical X-ray and Gamma-ray Protection for Energies up to 10MeV. Washington. National Council on Radiation Protection and Meausrements. 1971.

155. Niklason, C.T., Sorenson, J.A., and Nelson, J.A.: Scattered radiation in chest radiography. Medical Physics 8(5): 677, 1981.

156. Oosterkamp, I.W.: Monochromatic x-rays for medical fluoroscopy and radiography? Medicamundi, 7: 68, 1961.

157. Ovitt, T.W., Capp, M.P., Fisher H.D., et al.: The development of a digital video subtraction system for intravenous angiography. In Miller, H.A., Schmidt, E.V., and Harrison, P.C. (Eds.): *Noninvasive Cardiovascular Measurements.* Society of Photo-Optical Instrumentation Engineers, 57: 61, 1978.

158. Ovitt, T.W., Capp, M.P., Christenson, P. et al.: Development of a digital video subtraction system for intravenous angiogrpahy. Society of Photo-Optical Instrumentation Engineers, 206: 73, 1979.

159. Ovitt, T.W., Christenson, P.C., Fisher, H.D. et al.: Intravenous angiography using digital video subtraction: x-ray imaging system. American Journal of Neuroradiology, 1: 387, 1980.

160. Pasche, O.: Uber eine neue blendenvorrichtung in der Rontgentechnik. Deutche Med Wocheuschr, 29: 266, 1903.

161. Peschmann, K.R., Couch, J.L., and Parker, D.L.: New developments in digital x-ray detection. Proceedings of the Society of Photo-Optical Instrumentation Engineers, 314: 50, 1981.

162. Pfeiler, M., and Marhoff, P.: Technical aspects of digitization x-ray image processing, especially digital subtraction angiography. Electromedica, 51: 1, 1983.

163. Potter, H.E.: The Bucky diaphragm principle applied to roentgenograhy. American Journal of Roentgenology, 7: 292, 1920.

164. Proto, A.V., and Lane, E.J.; 350 kVp chest radiography review and comparison with 120 kVp. American Journal of Roentgenology, 130: 859, 1978.

165. Quality assurance programs for diagnostic radiology facilities; Final recommendation. Federal Register: 44(239), 1979.

166. Quality assurance: An idea whose time has come: Editorial. American Journal of Roentgenology, 133: 989, 1979.

167. Radiation Measurements Incorporated: Middleton, Wisconsin, 1983.

168. Raithel, H.J., Stahnke, I., and Valentin, H.: Initial experience with a new large-screen x-ray image intensifier in the diagnosis of asbestosis and silicosis. Electromedica, 51(2): 73, 1983.

169. Richards, A.G., Barbour, G.L., and Badder, J.D.: Samarian filters for dental radiography. Oral Surgery, 29: 704, 1970.

170. Riemann, H.E., and Marhoff, P.: The clinical value of high-resolution x-ray television with a high number of scanning lines. Electromedica, 1: 18, 1981.

171. Rossi, R.P., Wesenberg, R.L., and Hendee, W.R.: A variable aperture fluoroscopic unit for reduced patient exposure. Radiology, 129: 799, 1978.

172. Rothenberg, L.N., Kirch, R.L.A., and Snyder, R.E.: Patient exposures from film and xeroradiographic mammographic techniques. Radiology, 117: 701, 1975.

173. Rücker, H.C., and Jalloul, M.K.: A modern universal angiography installation with a 14 in. image intensifier. Medicamundi, 27: 111, 1982.

174. Rudin, S.: Fore-and-aft rotating aperture wheel (RAW) device for improving radiographic contrast. Application of Optical Instrumentation in Medicine VII. Society of Photo-Optical Instrumentation Engineers, 173: 98, 1979.

175. Schmitmann, H., and Ammann, E.: Pandoros optimatic — an x-ray generator with new possibilities. Electromedica, 4-5: 177, 1973.

176. Schreiber, P.: New anode disk technology in Super Rotalix tubes. Medicamundi, 20(2): 87, 1975.

177. Schut, T.H.G., and Oosterkamp, W.J.: The application of electronic memories in radiology. Medicamundi, 5(2/3): 85, 1959.

178. Seeram, E.: *Computed Tomography Technology.* Philadelphia, Saunders Co. 1982.

179. Seeram, E.: The computer and its applications in diagnostic radiology. Canadian Journal of Radiography, Radiotherapy and Nuclear Medicine, VII: 238, 1976.

180. Seppanen, S., Lehtinen, E., and Holli, H.: Radiation dose in hysterosalpingography: Modern 100 mm fluorography vs. full-scale radiography. Radiology, 127: 377, 1978.

181. Shinozima, M., Kohirazawa, H., Kukota, K., and Tokui, M.: Tomorex (curved rotational tomography apparatus) in experimental and clinical practice. Oral Surgery, 53: 94, 1982.

182. Shrivastava, P.N.: Radiation dose in mammography: An energy balance approach. Radiology, 149: 483, 1981.

183. Siddon, R.L.: Scatter transmission through an ideal grid. Medical Physics, 8(6): 905, 1981.

184. Sklebitz, H., and Haendle, J.: Tomoscopy: Dynamic layer imaging without mechanical movements. American Journal of Roentgenology, 140: 1247, 1983.

185. Skucas, J., and Gorski, J.W.: Comparison of the image quality of 105-mm film with conventional film. Radiology, 118: 433, 1976.

186. Sorenson, J.A., Niklason, L.T., Jacobsen, S.C., Knutti, D.F., and Johnson, T.C.: Tantalum air-interspace crossed grid: Design and performance characteristics. Radiology 145: 485, 1982.

187. Spiegler, P., and Moler, C.L.: The effective exposure angle for spiral and hypocycloidal motion in tomography. Radiology, 108: 173, 1973.

188. Sprawls, P.: *The Physical Principles of Diagnostic Radiology.* Baltimore, University Park Press, 1977.

189. Stevels, A.L.N.: New phosphors for intensifying screens. Medicamundi, 20: 12, 1975.

190. Strum, R., and Morgan, R.: Screen intensification systems and their limitations. American Journal of Roentgenology, 62: 617, 1959.

191. Strum, R.E., and Morgan, R.H.: Screen intensification systems and their limitations. American Journal of Roentgenology, 62: 617, 1949.

192. Strother, C.M., Sackett, J.F., Crummy, A.B. et al.: Clinical applications of computerized fluoroscopy: The extracranial carotid artery. Radiology, 136: 781, 1980.

193. Ter-Pogossian, M.: *The Physical Aspects of Diagnostic Radiology.* New York, Harper and ROw, 1967.

194. Tristan, T.A., and Quick, R.S.: Radiation dose in image intensifier cinefluorography.

In Ramsey, G.H., Watson, J.S., Tristan, T.A., Weinberg, S., and Cornwell, W.S.: *Cinefluorography.* Springfield, Thomas, 1960.

195. Trout, E.D., Jacobson, G., Moore, R.T., and Shoub, E.P.: Analysis of the rejection rate of chest radiographs obtained during the coal miners' black lung program. Radiology, 109: 25, 1973.

196. Trout, D.E., and Kelly, J.P.: The deterioration of x-ray fluoroscopic screens. Radiology, 110: 103, 1974.

197. Vallebona, A.: Trattats di Stratigrafia. Italy, Vallardi, 1952.

198. Vallebona, A.: Una modalita di tecnica per la dissociazione radiografica della ombre applicata allo studio del cranio. Radiology in Medicine, 17: 1090, 1930.

199. Van der platts, G.J.: *Medical X-ray Technique.* Eindhoven, Centrex, 1969.

200. Villagran, J.E., Hobbs, B.B., and Taylor, K.N.: Reduction of patient exposures by use of heavy elements as radiation filters in diagnostic radiology. Radiology, 127: 249, 1978.

201. Vizy, K.N.: An overview of digital radiography systems. Cardiovascular and Interventional Radiology, 6: 296, 1983.

202. Wahl, F.A.: Beitrag zur verbesserung der bildqualitat in der Rontgen-technik. Rontgenpraxis, 3: 855, 1931.

203. Wang, S.P., Robbins, C.D., and Bates, C.W.: A novel proximity x-ray image intensifier tube. Optical Instrumentation in Medicine. Society of Photo-Optical Instrumentation Engineers, 127: 188, 1977.

204. Watson, W.: Differential radiography I. Radiography, 5: 81, 1939.

205. Watson, W., Differential radiography II. Radiography, 6: 161, 1940.

206. Watson, W.: Differential radiography III. Bodysection radiography in practice. Radiography, 9: 33, 1943.

207. Weaver, K.E., Barone, G.J., and Fewell, T.R.: Selection of technique factors for mobile capacitor energy storage x-ray equipment. Radiology, 128: 223, 1978.

208. Webber, M.M., Wilk, S., and Pirruccello, R., et al.: Telecommunication of images in the practice of diagnostic radiology. Radiology, 109: 71, 1973.

209. Webster, E.W., and Smith, L.C.: A system for stereoscopic fluoroscopy involving electronic storage. Radiology, 78: 117, 1962.

210. Weiss, J.: Large field cineradiography and image intensification utilizing the TVX system. Radiology, 76: 264, 1961.

211. Weiss, H.: Three-dimensional x-ray information retrieving by optical filtering. In *International Optical Computing Conference.* New York, Institute of Electrical and Electronics Engineers, 1974.

212. Wipfelder, R., Pendergrass, H., and Webster, E.: High definition versus standard television fluoroscopy. Radiology, 88: 355, 1967.

213. Woelke, H., Hanrath, P., Schlueter, M., Bleifeld, W., Klotz, E., Weiss, H., Waller, D., and von Weltzien, J.: Work in progress. Flashing tomosynthesis: A tomographic technique for quantitative coronary angiography. Radiology, 145: 357, 1982.

214. Wolf, M., Stargardt, A., and Angerstein, W.: Evaluation of image quality in tomographic imaging. Physics in Medicine and Biology, 22(5): 900, 1977.

215. Walter, I.: Loadix, a system for thermal monitoring of x-ray tubes. Electromedica, 2: 73, 1977.

216. Xonics, Inc.: Application of xonics electron radiography to mammography. Xonics Inc., Van Nuys, California, 1978.

217. Zatz, L.M., Finston, R.A., and Jones, H.H.: Reduced radiation exposure in the operating room with video disk radiography. Radiology, 110: 475, 1974.

218. Zeman, G.H., Osterman, F.A., Rao, G., Kirk, B.G., James E.A.: Xeromammograhic automatic exposure termination. Radiology, 126: 117, 1978.

219. Ziedes des Plantes, B.G.: *Subtraction.* Stuttgart, Georg Thieme, 1961.

220. Zworykin-Morton.: *Television.* New York, John Wiley and Sons, Inc., 1954.

NAME INDEX

557

SUBJECT INDEX

A

Air gap anti-scatter technique
 basis of, 112
 considerations, 113
 principle, 113, 138
  schematic representation, 113
 study question, 518
Alternating current
 advantages of, 142-143, 159
 definition, 141
 frequency of
  definition, 141, 159
  expression of, 141, 142, 159
 power to hospitals, 141, 159
 rectification of (*see* Rectification of alternating
   current)
 rectifiers, 144-145 (*see also* Rectificers)
 single-phase
  availability in radiology departments, 142, 159
  generator, schematic representation, 142
  limitations, 142, 159
  waveform, schematic representation, 141, 142
 three-phase
  advantages of, 142, 159
  explanation of, 142
  out of phase, 142
  study question, 521-522
 waveform of
  features of, 141, 159
  schematic representative, 141
Aluminum
 use as interspace material, 122
  advantages, 122
 use for added filter, 232
Amipaque®, 460
Analog computer, 360, 392
Anatomically programmed radiography
 advantages of, 22
 description, 22
 touch key for, illustration, 20
Angiography

grid-controlled switching used for, 53, 65
 study question, 514
rating chart for
 illustration, 101
 use of, 103
use of grids in, 136
Angiotron®, 450, 451
 control field, photograph, 452
 diagramic layout, 451
 Digitron®, 452
 photograph, 450
 real-time image processing on-line, 451
 technique, 450
Angio-table, film changer, 329
Anode (*see also* Stationary-anode x-ray tube)
 composition
  focus, 72
  material used, 72, 73, 104
  target, 72
 copper used for, 72, 104
  study question, 515
 definition, 71
 factors in efficiency of x-ray production, 73
 faults, causes and effects, table, 102
 formula used, 73
 heat production, 73
 line focus principle, 72
  schematic representation, 72
 materials used to construct, 72, 73, 104
  requirements for, 73
  use of tungsten, 73, 104
 properties of tungsten, 73, 104
 rotating anode tube (*see* Rotating anode disc)
 saturation current, 71
 space-charge, 71
 stationary-anode tube, 74
  limitations, 104-105
 target angle, 72
  schematic representation, 72
 tungsten filament, 70-71
  electrons from 71
  study question, 515

563

M

Y

Z